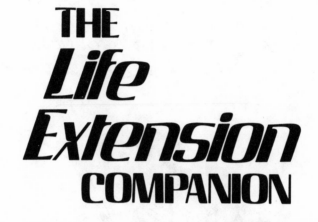

THE Life Extension COMPANION

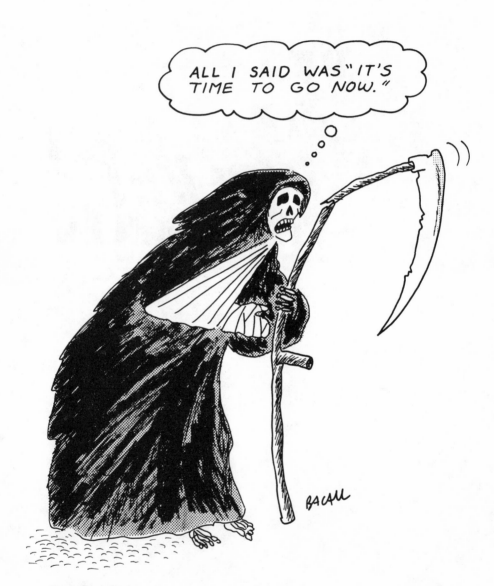

Idea by Sandy Shaw
© A. Bacall 1983

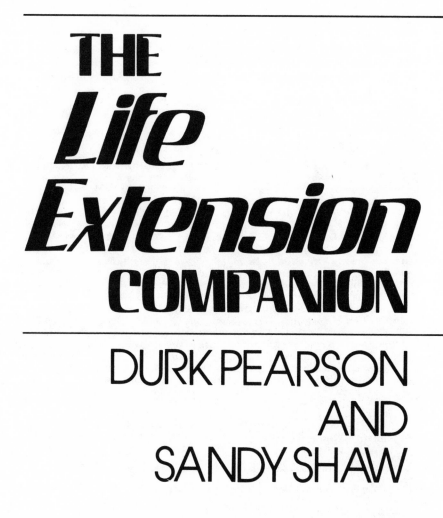

THE Life Extension COMPANION

DURK PEARSON
AND
SANDY SHAW

 WARNER BOOKS

A Warner Communications Company

The authors gratefully acknowledge William Morrow & Company, Inc. for permission to reprint the author's foreword in *The Life Extension Revolution*, a Morrow Quill Edition, Copyright © 1983 by Saul Kent.

All royalties for this book are payable directly to the Laboratory for the Advancement of Bio-Medical Research, a non-profit research foundation for Life Extension.

The following articles were previously copyrighted as follows:

Executive Stress: How to Protect Yourself from It, © 1981 by Durk Pearson and Sandy Shaw. *Biochemistry for Success,* © 1982 by Sandy Shaw. *How to Stay Well, or Helping Your Immune System,* © 1981 by Sandy Shaw and Durk Pearson. *A New Pharmaceutical Marketplace,* © 1983 by Durk Pearson and Sandy Shaw. *Better Hair and Better Health with Cysteine,* © 1981 by Durk Pearson and Sandy Shaw. *Improving Your Skin's Health and Appearance with Nutrients,* © 1981 by Sandy Shaw and Durk Pearson. *New Views on Pollution,* © 1982 by Durk Pearson and Sandy Shaw. *Chelating Agents and Life Extension,* © 1981 by Durk Pearson and Sandy Shaw. *Getting Rid of Phobias for Good,* © 1981 by Sandy Shaw and Durk Pearson. *Jet Lag or How to Reset Your Biorhythms,* © 1981 by Sandy Shaw and Durk Pearson. *Sleep and Your Health,* © 1982 by Durk Pearson and Sandy Shaw. *DMSO: Its Uses and Mode of Action,* © 1981 by Durk Pearson and Sandy Shaw. *Sex Play and Sexual Rejuvenation,* © 1982 by Durk Pearson and Sandy Shaw. *The Herpes Epidemic: A Possible Solution,* © 1982 by Durk Pearson and Sandy Shaw. *Synthetic Versus Natural: Which is Better?,* © 1981 by Durk Pearson and Sandy Shaw. *Back to Butter, or The Truth About Polyunsaturated Fats,* © 1981 by Sandy Shaw and Durk Pearson. *The Facts About Food Preservatives,* © 1981 by Durk Pearson and Sandy Shaw. *Sources of Information About Aging and Maintaining Your Health,* © 1981 by Durk Pearson and Sandy Shaw.

Volume I

Warner Books, Inc., 666 Fifth Avenue, New York, New York, 10103

⚫ A Warner Communications Company

Printed in the United States of America
First printing: March 1984
10 9 8 7 6 5 4 3 2 1

Library of Congress Cataloging in Publication Data
Pearson, Durk, and Shaw, Sandy.
    The life extension companion.

"We intend this book as a supplement to our Life
extension"—Foreword.
    "Volume 1."
    Bibliography: p.
    Includes index.
    1. Health.   2. Longevity.   I. Shaw, Sandy.   II. Pearson,
Durk. Life extension.   III. Title.
RA776.5.P344 1984   613   83-42692
ISBN 0-446-51277-X

Book design: H. Roberts Design

This Book is Dedicated To:

Jack Wheeler, the professional adventurer and explorer who introduced us to Merv;

and

Merv Griffin, whose TV show lead to our contract for *Life Extension*, among many other surprising opportunities, and who introduced us to many of our readers;

and

Seymour I. Feig, Esq., our media and communications counsel, an outstanding negotiator, Professor of Entertainment Law, New York Law School, and several times Chief Panelist of the American Arbitration Association, without whom there would have been neither a *Life Extension* nor a *Life Extension Companion*.

Special Thanks To:

You, the reader, who care enough about life extension to help both yourself and our research by purchasing, studying, and carefully using our books.

THE LIFE EXTENSION COMPANION

Contents

Introduction, Jeffrey A. Fisher, M.D., F.C.A.P.   xi
Foreword   xv

HEALTH MAINTENANCE FOR MIND
AND BODY   1

Executive Stress: How to Protect Yourself from It   3
Biochemistry for Success   32
How to Stay Well, or
    Helping Your Immune System   45
A New Pharmaceutical Marketplace   62
Selenium, an Anti-Cancer, Anti-Aging Nutrient   70
Better Hair and Better Health with Cysteine   75
Improving Your Skin's Health
    and Appearance with Nutrients   84
New Views on Pollution   91
Chelating Agents and Life Extension   96
Getting Rid of Phobias for Good   101
Jet Lag, or How to Reset Your Biorhythms   108

Sleep and Your Health   117
DMSO: Its Uses and Mode of Action   126
Hydergine®, an Effective Treatment for Sickle Cell Anemia,
    Predicted by Free Radical Pathology Theory   133

SEX   137

Sex Play and Sexual Rejuvenation   139
The Herpes Epidemic: A Possible Solution   150
Sex Hormones: Some Uses and Their Risks   158

FADS AND FALLACIES   163

FDA Notice: Prescribing Approved Drugs
    for Unapproved Uses   165
The Fallacy of Perfect Safety   168
Synthetic Versus Natural: Which Is Better?   174
Natural Versus Synthetic Vitamin E:
    A Reply to Henkel Corporation   179
Back to Butter, or The Truth
    About Polyunsaturated Fats   194
The Facts About Food Preservatives   201
Hydergine® Is Not a Vasoconstrictor   209

MORE LIFE EXTENSION INFORMATION   211

How to Use Case Histories and
    Anecdotal Evidence   213

SAVES - Study of Aging Volunteer Experimental Subjects
DATA - Doctors' Registry for the Treatment
    of the Aging   218

Sources of Information About Aging
    and Maintaining Your Health   230

You Can Use the National Library of Medicine:
    MEDLARS and MEDLINE -
    Computer Searches by Mail   242

        Example of a Search Request:
            Growth Hormone Secretion   248

        Example of a Search Printout:
            Growth Hormone Secretion   251

SOME ORIGINAL SCIENTIFIC LITERATURE   251

"Atherosclerosis: Possible Ill-Effects of the Use of Highly
    Unsaturated Fats to Lower Serum-Cholesterol Levels," by
    Dr. Denham Harman (from *The Lancet*, 30 Nov. 1957, pp.
    1116-1117)   259

"Dietary Carcinogens," by Philip H. Abelson (from *Science*,
    vol. 221, p. 1249, 23 September 1983)   263

"Dietary Carcinogens and Anticarcinogens," by Bruce N.
    Ames (from *Science*, vol. 221, pp. 1256–1264, 23
    September 1983)   265

"Free Radical Theory of Aging: Effect of Dietary Fat on
    Central Nervous System Function," by Denham Harman,
    M.D., Ph.D, Shelton Hendricks, Ph.D, Dennis E. Eddy,
    Ph.D, and Jon Seibold, M.A. (from *The Journal of the
    American Geriatrics Society*, vol. 24 (7), pp. 301-307,
    1976)   292

APPENDIX

A Few More Life Extension Suppliers   299

GLOSSARY

A Layman's Guide to Word Usage   311

INDEXES

Index of Indexes   337

Comprehensive Computer-Generated Index to *The Life Extension Companion*   343

Comprehensive Computer-Generated Index to *Life Extension, A Practical Scientific Approach*   367

Safety Index to *The Life Extension Companion*   421

Safety Index to *Life Extension, a Practical Scientific Approach*   424

Introduction

Preventive medicine and its analogs (nutrition, gerontology) have become important to the lives of millions of Americans. The social and political events which shaped the self-help consciousness of the 1960's and 70's have been chronicled in numerous volumes and discussed in university classrooms throughout the country. The influence this philosophy (or conglomeration of philosophies) has had upon the attitudes toward health care is evident. Some of the consequences have been positive, others negative.

The changes that arose were as much a backlash against traditional medical care as anything else. As people became distrustful of institutions and of authorities, a deterioration of the standard physician–patient relationship occurred. No longer are patients content to accept the doctor's word as a proclamation from Mt. Olympus. Physicians began to be questioned about side-effects of drugs and even as to why a drug was being prescribed in the first place. The idea that at the first sign of a minor illness one should telephone his physician for advice began to fade and was replaced with the notion that, fundamentally, each of us is responsible for our own health. Physicians began to be looked upon more as educators than as drug-dispensers.

Another positive aspect of alternative health care has been the emphasis on the contribution of the mind to the state of one's health. The excellent book by Carl Simonton, M.D., (*Getting Well Again*) is a concrete example. Somewhere in between placebo effect and the pharmacology of the brain's neurotransmitters is a nebulous area of mind control over bodily functions. Admittedly, these are difficult (if not impossible) to document via double-blind crossover studies, but positive results have been reported time and again. Even though these have been in the form of testimonial evidence, in the eyes of the keen observer (as pointed out in a recent *New England Journal of Medicine* by Louis Lasagna, M.D., a former head of F.D.A.), these observations can make a positive contribution.

As is common with backlash occurrences, however, the pendulum swung too far. Not only was there a general distrust of diagnoses rendered without documentation and of drugs dispensed without explanation, but there arose an anti-technological, anti-scientific bias. Merely by the fact that a substance was produced in a laboratory in stainless-steel reaction vessels made it inherently dangerous. Natural became holy, synthetic anathema. White laboratory coats and stethoscopes were replaced by sandals and shiatsu. Publications espousing the "natural way" abounded. Health care practitioners, with strange degrees (many of them mail-order) grew up as rapidly as mung bean sprouts in cheesecloth-covered jars.

Obviously this is not to indict all forms and concepts of alternative health care. The positive effects have already been mentioned. But quackery proliferated, with many fringe practitioners who, knowingly or unknowingly, took advantage of an unsuspecting public. This is somewhat ironic because it is part of what the rebellion against traditional medicine was attempting to correct.

The *Life Extension Companion*, like its more inclusive predecessor (*Life Extension, A Practical Scientific Approach*), takes a giant step towards correcting the prevalent anti-technological bias. This infusion of science is necessary if the positive aspects of preventive health care are to survive.

The authors have struck the proper balance between the maintenance of the individual's control over his own life and the application of scientific data to do so. On the one hand it is reiterated that, although a particular lifestyle may be espoused, it is not necessarily the only approach. They certainly recognize one's right to seek any form of health care even if non-scientifically-documented techniques are employed. On the other hand, they do caution against this and advise us to be discerning when choosing a particular approach.

A large portion of this book is devoted to dispelling predominant notions in preventive health care that appear to have little basis in scientific fact. We are told that it is no longer advisable to consume large amounts of polyunsaturated fats, as the American Heart Association preached for years. This increased consumption of readily oxidizable lipids is a likely explanation for the increased incidence of certain types of cancer epidemiologically associated with a reduced serum cholesterol. This is certainly consistent with Denham Harman's free radical theory of aging. Dr. Harman has recommended reduced consumption of polyunsaturated fats for many years. Other questions that are examined are the natural versus synthetic controversy and the dangers of purchasing vitamin E in oil containing gelatin capsules.

Both of these subjects are in part attended to in an eloquent reply to a letter from the Henkel Corporation, the country's largest supplier of natural vitamin E. These topics are scrutinized analytically and the conclusions are difficult to dispute. In view of Dr. Harry Demopoulos' findings that all four brands of vitamin E in gelatin capsules that he tested contained potentially hazardous levels of peroxidized lipids, we would do well to heed this advice and begin to consume our vitamin E in powder or tablet form.

This book represents a pragmatic approach in the use of biochemistry to cope with today's stressful lifestyle and at the same time helping to retard the aging process. It is stated throughout the book that these techniques, while *apparently* non-toxic, do amount to making oneself a guinea pig of sorts and that proper laboratory monitoring and clinical consultation by a physician well-versed in these techniques is essential. This should be *taken seriously*! *No one* should ingest large amounts of antioxidant nutrients (or any other related substances) without having baseline laboratory studies and periodic monitoring. We are embarking upon an era where nutritional pharmacology is becoming a recognized discipline. Taking megadoses of nutrients, be they vitamins or accessory food factors is *not* natural. (This is not dependent on whether the substances are manufactured synthetically or occur naturally.) This is not an implication that nutritional supplements should come under government control, but is offered as a caution against indiscriminate non-scientific application of those techniques.

If one follows the appropriate warnings and embarks upon a prudent course, the material is here to significantly reduce one's risk of developing the diseases that accompany aging (heart disease, cancer, diabetes, arthritis) and for improving the quality of one's life now. One realizes in reading this book that science and technology are not necessarily impersonal but, if correctly applied, can be life-enhancing.

Jeffrey A. Fisher, M.D., F.C.A.P.
Extensis Preventive Medical Center
Roslyn, New York

Foreword

Ever since the publication of our 858 page book *Life Extension, A Practical Scientific Approach* in June 1982, readers have been asking where they could find the articles and columns we have written that have appeared in several small circulation publications during the past two years. This anthology brings together some of these hard-to-find articles (including some extensively rewritten for this book), together with much new, never-before-published material. Since many of the chapters in this book were originally written as articles to stand alone, there is a degree of overlap of background material between some of them. We have carefully pruned this background explanatory material so that the emphasis is on particularly important and helpful information.

This book is *NOT* a simplified version of *Life Extension*, a book which contains FAR more information than is contained in this volume. We intend this book as a supplement to our *Life Extension* and many specific references will be made to it. This book may also interest many people in life extension (and possibly *Life Extension*!) who might otherwise have been intimidated by the size of that work. By referring to *Life Extension* during the reading of this anthology, the reader can greatly enhance his or her understanding of this book.

A unique feature of this volume is a comprehensive index to *Life Extension*, allowing readers to find their particular topics of interest with great ease and convenience. Although the Warner Books-prepared index to *Life Extension* was one of the best and longest to ever appear in a popular book, it was far from a comprehensive one and, as a result, it is sometimes hard to find what you are looking for. You can't get any benefit from information that you can't find, so we have corrected this by generating the complete index contained in this book.

To solve the index problem, we purchased software for one of our trusty sidekicks, our Intersystems Encore hard disc cache memory computer system, which reads the book (as recorded on computer disc) and relentlessly, comprehensively, and automatically indexes all occurrences of all technical terms, diseases, medical conditions, nutrients, drugs, chemicals, contraindications, cautions, warnings, scientists' names, institutions, and everything else that is not an ordinary, everyday word. We have done this for both *The Life Extension Companion* and *Life Extension, A Practical Scientific Approach*.

Computers play another very important role in this book. As a result of many requests, we have published herein a worked-out example of a MEDLARS computerized literature search of the National Library of Medicine's data base, and have included part of the computer printout of the search results. This tool puts you in touch with most of the biomedical information published during the past 15 years and as it is generated by the scientific community in the top 3000 biomedical journals. Having access to this information CAN SAVE YOUR LIFE! According to the National Cancer Institute, survival rates using state-of-the-art multimode (eg., surgery + radiation + (sometimes) immunotherapy) cancer therapy are often about twice the survival rates found with the most common therapeutic approaches (often a decade behind the most recent scientific research). By using MEDLARS, you can find out what combination of therapies gives you the best chance of survival. For $30 or less, you can help yourself and your physician by obtaining this information. To make it easy for you to use this incredibly powerful tool to improve your health and extend your life, we have included a sample MEDLARS search form with instructions on how to fill it out.

Possible applications for MEDLARS searches by readers are many. Are you interested in the long-term outcome of cardiac bypass operations? Perhaps you want to know if the balloon and catheter method of squashing atherosclerotic plaques is reasonably safe and effective. Do you need to know more about your rare disease? Just fill out a MEDLARS form as directed (your physician can help formulate your search statement), send it in to a MEDLARS center, enclose a small check, and ZAP, you and your doctor will have access to custom-designed information about your health, the sort of information that has heretofore been available only to research scientists!

The book's appendix, "A Few More Life Extension Suppliers," will help you to obtain more life extension compounds, and will introduce more supplier competition, to the reader's benefit.

The cartoons contained in *Life Extension* were particularly welcomed and enjoyed by readers, who often commented that they were helpful in understanding the material. Consequently, we have included another large collection in this volume. Most of these cartoons were especially commissioned for this book.

WARNING: Watch for sections marked **CAUTION** and **WARNING:** these are meant to be read carefully and taken seriously. In addition, remember that this book is designed to be used in conjunction with *Life Extension, A Practical Scientific Approach*. Before taking anything, you should check all the index entries for that substance in *Life Extension*, or, at the very least, all relevant **CAUTION**s and **WARNING**s in *Life Extension*.

We'd like you to know that 100% of the proceeds received from *The Life Extension Companion* have been assigned to an IRS-approved non-profit biomedical research foundation. When you purchase this book, you are contributing to biomedical research. In addition to our thanks, you may be able to deduct the royalty portion of the book price (10%) from your taxes as a charitable donation. We are not tax lawyers, however, so you had better ask your professional tax advisor to be sure. We are not donating the book money to a biomedical research foundation because we are philanthropists, but because scientific research is what we want to spend most of our time doing and that will use most of our funds. We are grateful that we will not have to spend 75% to 80% of our time chasing after government grant money, as several of our scientific colleagues tell us they do.

Live Long and Prosper,

Durk Pearson and Sandy Shaw
19 September, 1983

Health Maintenance for Mind and Body

Executive Stress: How to Protect Yourself from It

"The doctor of the future will give no medicine, but will interest his patient in the care of the human frame, diet, and in the cause and prevention of disease."

Thomas A. Edison

A SCENARIO FOR SUDDEN DEATH

You work and think long, hard productive hours. You live with uncertainty. You make difficult decisions every day, often under severe schedule pressures. Your professional stature, position, and compensation as an executive rises. Your advice is sought more and more often at the highest corporate levels. You are promoted again and again. You love all this hard work and you do it very well. Then one day, you wake up in an oxygen tent, with a catheter up your nose, an intravenous drip in your arm, and a ghastly pain in your chest. You have had your first heart attack. Must this be the inescapable price of diligent, productive, hard work and success? Not at all! This does not have to happen to you. Unlike other advice on this problem, our solution does not require that you take it easy, or avoid stress and overwork. **We will tell you**

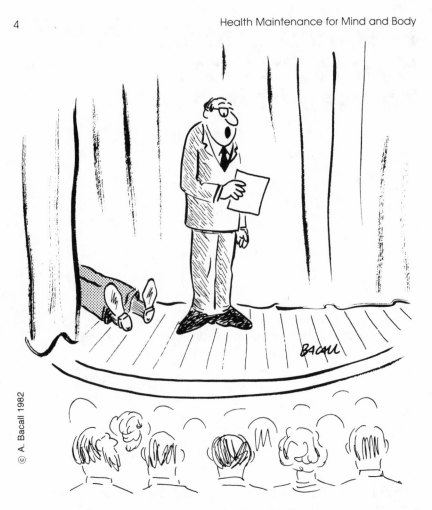

© A. Bacall 1982

"Is there a nutritional therapist in the audience?"

how to greatly increase your resistance to stress by the rational use of nutritional supplements and, optionally, certain prescription drugs. You can reduce the risks of stress *without* significantly altering your executive lifestyle.

WHAT IS "STRESS"?

Stress is "the sum of all non-specific biological phenomena elicited by adverse external influences, including damage and defense ..." according to *Dorland's Illustrated Medical Dictionary*. Although this definition specifies "adverse" external influences, similar stress physiological states also occur in response to beneficial external influences. In other words, being promoted can be as physiologically and psychologically stressful as not being promoted, even though we may feel quite differently about these two outcomes.

Our stress responses evolved over a long period of time. In fact, we share many common stress adaptation mechanisms with the reptiles. Often the physiological states that are produced by stressful conditions are harmful rather than helpful to our bodies because the conditions under which these mechanisms evolved may not necessarily be appropriate to present-day conditions. For example, the "fight or

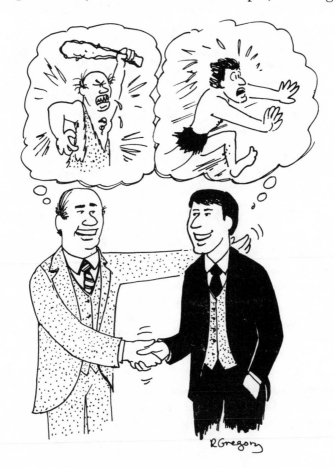

flight" state that is a common result of stress causes a massive release of adrenaline in our bodies and noradrenaline (also called norepinephrine or NE) in our brains. Corticosteroids, in response to the high levels of adrenaline, are released by our adrenal cortex to help maintain cell membrane integrity in case of injury. As a result of the speeded-up metabolism of the "fight or flight" state (appropriate if one actually has to fight or flee), people often eventually become depleted of norepinephrine (NE). This can cause depression and can also result in degraded performance of the immune system, which requires adequate NE for proper function. Corticosteroids suppress the immune system, and high circulating corticosteroid levels in the bloodstream, as a response to high levels of stress, could further impair immune function severely. This can be lethal, since your immune system is responsible for destroying invading bacteria, viruses, cancer cells, and even atherosclerotic plaques.

Different types of stress have somewhat different effects on physiological and biochemical functions. A hard-working and ambitious executive is exposed to many different stresses. With the right nutrition and, in some cases, prescription drugs, it is possible to provide very substantial protection against the damaging effects of these stresses.

DEPRESSION, EXHAUSTION, AND OVERWORK

When people become depressed, often called nervous exhaustion or severe overwork, they generally have low levels of NE in their brains (as inferred from the low levels of NE metabolites in the cerebrospinal fluid of depressed patients). Low levels of NE are hazardous to the health because the immune system requires the proper level of NE stimulation. The two nutrient amino acids the brain uses to make NE are tyrosine and phenylalanine. They can be purchased in some health food and drugstores. In human studies, both of these have been effective in bringing people out of their depressions in a few days at reasonable doses. In one study, phenylalanine worked for about 80% of depressed patients who took 100 to 500 milligrams a day for two weeks. The severe stress caused by the loss of a wife increased the chances of death to the surviving spouse by about 40% in the six months following the loss in a British study. The chances of contracting cancer are also markedly increased by the physiological responses to a loss of this magnitude. The use of the amino acids tyrosine or phenylalanine may help in coping with such a situation. Although the amino acids cannot change the nature of reality, the severity of the personal loss, they may help the survivors to recover from their grief more quickly and with less severe immune system depression. (See *Life Extension, A Practical Scientific Approach*, pages 181-188.)

CAUTION: People who have high blood pressure should take these amino acids ONLY under the supervision of their physician, as a few sensitive persons might have an increase in blood pressure while using them. Tyrosine often has a normalizing effect on blood pressure, decreasing it in hypertension and increasing it in hypotension. **WARNING:** These amino acids must *not* be used in conjunction with MAO inhibitors (a class of prescription antidepressants which is rarely used anymore). Consult your physician.

The brain has to use vitamins B-6 and C to turn the tyrosine or phenylalanine into NE, so it is a good idea to take supplements of B-6 and C with these amino acids.

THE IMMUNE SYSTEM, GUARDIAN OF YOUR HEALTH

In injuries or other stresses, the thymus gland can be severely depleted. The thymus is the master gland of the immune system, instructing special thymus-derived white blood cells called T-cells when and what to attack. Some of the T-cells in turn give orders to the antibody-manufacturing B-cells, made by the bone marrow. Following puberty, the thymus shrinks considerably in man. After an injury or other severe stress, the thymus further involutes (atrophies). This involution may be reduced or prevented by taking moderate

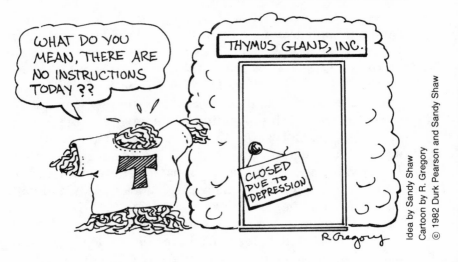

doses of vitamin A and chelated zinc supplements. A reasonable adult dose depends upon your intake of other fat-soluble antioxidants (such as vitamin E) because the vitamin A lasts longer in the bloodstream before it is destroyed by oxidation if you have taken other fat-soluble antioxidants. We usually take 10,000 to 20,000 units of A and 50 milligrams of chelated zinc per day. **CAUTION:** Too much vitamin A can be very hazardous. Overdosage symptoms, which may occur at doses above 20,000 i.u. of vitamin A per day, include sparse, coarse hair; loss of hair on the eyebrows; dry, rough skin; and cracked lips (particularly at the corners). Other nutrients which have been shown to stimulate immune function are vitamins C and E, the nutrient amino acids cysteine, arginine, ornithine, and L-Dopa (a prescription amino acid drug), and the mineral selenium. (Also, see *Life Extension, A Practical Scientific Approach*, pages 81-90.)

SUGGESTED IMMUNE SYSTEM STIMULANT NUTRIENTS

(All except the fat soluble vitamins A and E are best taken in three divided doses with meals; the A and E can be taken once per day. The arginine or ornithine will be more effective if taken on an empty stomach, such as an hour before meals. These are total daily doses.)

vitamin A	10,000 I.U.
vitamin B-1	100 milligrams
vitamin B-6	100 milligrams

WARNING: Do not use B-6 supplements if you have Parkinson's disease and are being treated with L-Dopa. Vitamin B-6 can counteract the brain effects of the L-Dopa and can result in increased side effects.

vitamin C	3-10 grams
vitamin E	1000 I.U.
beta carotene	25,000 I.U.
cysteine (not cystine)	1 gram

CAUTION: Do not take supplemental cysteine unless you take at least 3 times as much vitamin C supplement as your total cysteine consumption. In figuring your cysteine consumption, remember that the number of eggs you eat is relevant; each egg contains about ¼ gram of cysteine. While cysteine is quite water soluble, its oxidized form, cystine, is rather insoluble in water. If large amounts of cysteine are taken without the other water soluble antioxidants such as C, and without adequate quantities of fluids, cystine stone formation could conceivably occur in the kidneys and urinary bladder, especially if there is a urinary tract infection.

arginine (or half as much of ornithine)	2-3 grams
selenium (preferably as sodium selenite)	200 micrograms
chelated zinc	50 milligrams

JET LAG AND BIORHYTHMS

Many executives must travel frequently as part of their profession. Jet lag is a serious form of stress because many of our hormonal outputs exhibit circadian (24 hour) biological rhythms and are dependent on day-night cyclic cues for their regulation. During the roughly one day of acclimation per hour of time zone change for your biorhythms to adapt to a new day-night cycle, our immune response may be seriously impaired. In fact, frequent travel across time zones has been correlated with higher rates of cancer. (There may also be other factors involved, such as exposure to high levels of jet fuel combustion products and cigarette smoke during frequent flying. The nutritional supplements recommended here may provide protection from these hazards.) It is possible to avoid many of the difficulties of jet lag by re-setting

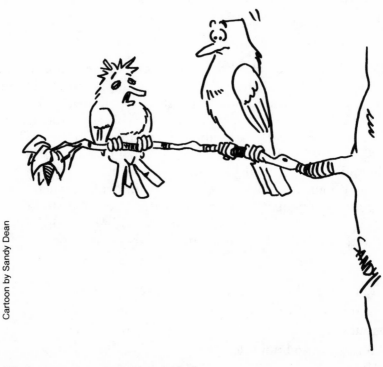

Cartoon by Sandy Dean

"It's the same story every spring—jet lag"

your own biological clocks with the right nutrients. See "Jet Lag or How to Reset Your Biorhythms" later in this book.

PHOBIAS

Another stress that may plague many executives is a fear of flying or public speaking. These are very common phobias that may bother you. It is now possible to get over phobias entirely, permanently, and without much will power or fear and without expensive and time-consuming psychotherapy by using a common prescription high blood pressure medication. This method of overcoming phobias has become quite popular in Europe and in Australia. Rules forbidding pharmaceutical manufacturers from informing physicians and the public about non-FDA-approved uses for approved drugs have prevented many phobic Americans from taking advantage of this scientifically well-established practice. This method is described fully in "Getting Rid of Phobias for Good" later in this book.

ALCOHOL AND SMOKING

Why do so many overworked, heavily stressed people smoke and drink? Alcohol and smoking often cause severe physiological stress. In fact, these two stressors kill over 500,000 Americans per year. Their behavior is not the pointless self-destruction that is so often attributed to them by opponents of smoking and drinking. Alcohol and the nicotine in tobacco act as stimulus barriers. A stimulus barrier might be described as a neurochemical version of sunglasses or earplugs. Your brain's stimulus barriers, whether natural (for example, acetylcholine, made from choline) or artificial (such as alcohol or nicotine) help your brain to filter out distracting stimuli, allowing your mind to focus. The supersalesman with five ringing phones on his desk and a big cigar in his mouth, drinking a martini with his left hand while holding the phone with his right, is relying on the nicotine and alcohol and also his lunch to help him cope with distracting stimuli. (See *Life Extension, A Practical Scientific Approach*, page 250, for data on a nutrient, choline, that acts as a stimulus barrier.)

Most of us have to put up with stresses of alcohol and

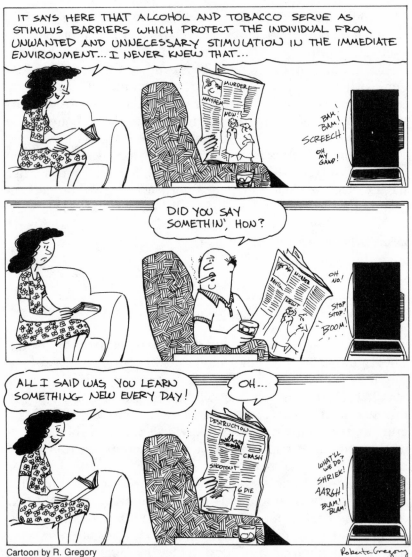

Cartoon by R. Gregory
© 1982 Durk Pearson and Sandy Shaw

smoking. Even if we don't smoke, we can be damaged by being exposed to the smoke from the cigarettes of people who do smoke. In one study in Japan, non-smoking women who lived with a husband who smoked were 50 to 100% more likely to get lung cancer than non-smoking women who lived with a husband who didn't smoke. The sidestream smoke, which comes directly from the burning end of the cigarette, contains roughly 1000 times as much carcinogenic material as the smoke drawn through the cigarette by the smoker. The exposure to your or other people's smoke damages your lungs, increases the risk of lung cancer, destroys antioxidant vitamins such as A, C, E, B-1, and B-6, and acts as a severe physiological stressor. Whether we smoke voluntarily or involuntarily, there are nutrients we can take which will aid us in coping with these chemical stresses and reduce our risk of lung, throat, mouth, and other cancers associated with smoking and drinking. The nutrient combination of vitamin B-1, vitamin C, and the amino acid cysteine is very protective against acetaldehyde, a toxic chemical found in cigarette smoke. A group of rats were given a dose of acetaldehyde that killed 90% of them. Another group of rats were given the same dose of acetaldehyde, but also given B-1, C, and cysteine, and had NO deaths. A reasonable dose of these nutrients for a healthy adult might be 1 gram of B-1, 1 gram of cysteine, and 3 grams of C per day, divided into three doses and taken after meals. These and other antioxidant nutrients such as selenium have dramatically reduced the cigarette smoke-induced mutations and cancerous transformation of human lung cells grown in tissue cultures.

CAUTION: Do not take supplemental cysteine unless you take at least 3 times as much vitamin C supplement as your total cysteine consumption. In figuring your cysteine consumption, remember that the number of eggs you eat is relevant; each egg contains about $\frac{1}{4}$ gram of cysteine. While cysteine is quite water soluble, its oxidized form, cystine, is rather insoluble in water. If large amounts of cysteine are taken without the other water soluble antioxidants such as C, and without adequate quantities of fluids, cystine stone formation could conceivably occur in the kidneys and urinary

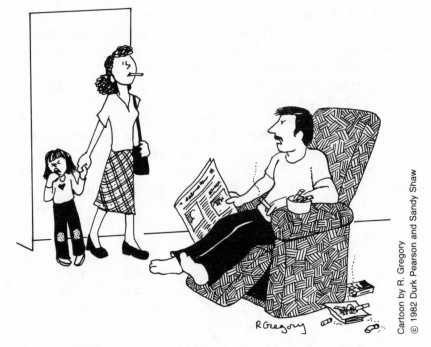

"What kind of crummy doctor would say a five-year-old has smoker's cough?"

Cartoon by R. Gregory
© 1982 Durk Pearson and Sandy Shaw

bladder, especially if there is a urinary tract infection. (For additional techniques for reducing the risks of smoking, see *Life Extension, A Practical Scientific Approach*, pages 239-258.)

Smoking, Lung Cancer, and Beta Carotene

Recently, beta carotene (the substance that makes carrots orange) was reported to provide very dramatic protection against lung cancer to smokers in a 19-year prospective epidemiological (the relationship of population, various conditions, and disease) study of about 2000 middle-aged men. In this study, smokers for up to 30 years who had the highest levels of dietary beta carotene had a risk of lung cancer no higher than that of non-smokers with an average or below average intake of beta carotene. The intake of beta carotene at the highest level was probably roughly 10,000 I.U. per day, expressed as vitamin A activity, or about 6 milligrams of beta carotene. We believe that 25,000 to 50,000 I.U. per day would be appropriate, taken as 15-30 milligrams of beta carotene, due to beta carotene's relatively poor absorption from the gut. Other antioxidants in the vegetables (the source of the beta carotene) may have contributed to this protection. And, of course, there is no guarantee that even a non-smoker will not get lung cancer.

Reducing Alcohol Damage and Hangovers

Alcohol intoxication can be hazardous, and not just because it increases the likelihood of an accident while driving.

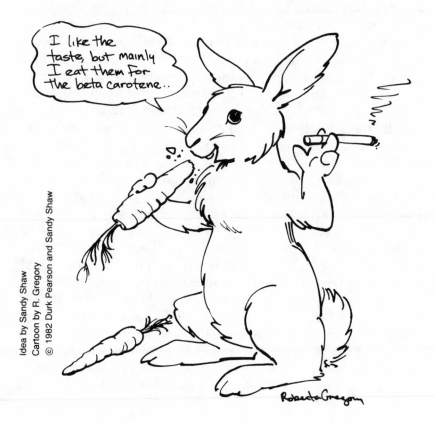

Idea by Sandy Shaw
Cartoon by R. Gregory
© 1982 Durk Pearson and Sandy Shaw

A Finnish study found even occasional intoxication increases the risk of stroke in young adults and even teenagers. Of young patients admitted to a hospital for a stroke, 43% had been drunk within 24 hours of their first symptoms. Neurosurgical researchers at New York University, led by Dr. H. B. Demopoulos, found that "drunk doses" of alcohol doubled the extent of experimental injuries to the brain and spinal cord of cats. At least some of this alcohol-caused damage may be preventable by taking the right nutrients.

You may have heard of the old wives' remedy for a hangover: you break an egg in a glass of orange juice, stir, and drink. Yech! It may not be too appetizing, but this drink really does work in providing help in recovering from a hangover. Your liver turns alcohol into acetaldehyde, and it is acetaldehyde, not alcohol itself, which leads to the damage in the brains and bodies of alcohol drinkers. The egg provides about ¼ gram of cysteine and the orange juice provides about 250 milligrams of vitamin C. Taking a dose of B-1, C, and cysteine (as in the paragraph above) is even more effective in preventing or getting over a hangover. Most of the alcohol damage is caused by free radicals, chemically reactive atoms or molecules with an unpaired electron, which are created by high energy x-ray radiation, during normal metabolism (for example, in the oxidation of food to carbon dioxide, water, and energy) and in the self-stimulated oxidation (called autoxidation) of many molecules, especially acetaldehyde. The acetaldehyde, made by the liver from alcohol, stimulates its own enzymatically uncontrolled autoxidation, which creates many free radicals. The symptoms of hangover resemble some of those of radiation sickness because both are caused by free radicals and both can be prevented or at least reduced by free radical scavengers like vitamins B-1, C, and the amino acid cysteine. Other effective free radical scavengers include E, A, B-5 (pantothenic acid or calcium pantothenate), B-6, PABA, selenium, and zinc. A scientist named Herbert Sprince and others gave rats a dose of acetaldehyde large enough to kill 90% of them. To a similar group of rats, he gave the same dose of acetaldehyde and the nutrients B-1, C, and cysteine. None of the rats given these three nutrients died.

STAMINA AND STRENGTH

Long grueling hours of work are an often unavoidable vocational hazard of the executive. Such stress can cause the body to perform less well than it would in the absence of the stress. It reduces the amount of work that muscles can do. It was found in a study by Ralli and Dumm (1953) that vitamin B-5, given as calcium pantothenate to rats, greatly increased the amount of time they could swim under the stress of being put into water at 18 degrees C (about 64 degrees F) and having to swim to exhaustion. The rats were divided into three groups, depending on how much pantothenate they received. The pantothenate deficient group swam $16 +/- 3$ minutes, the adequate pantothenate group swam $29 +/- 4$ minutes, and the high pantothenate group swam $62 +/- 12$ minutes. The authors of this study noted that these results reminded them of earlier work by Shock and Sebrell (1944) who were able to double the amount of work done by frog leg muscles by simply adding calcium pantothenate to the perfusing fluids which bathed the muscles.

The reason that vitamin B-5 works so well is that it is a required co-factor (acetyl coenzyme A) in an enzyme system that is necessary for the manufacture of the universal energy carrier molecule ATP. This molecule, ATP, carries chemical energy obtained by the oxidation of foods we eat. The principal chemical pathway for the production of ATP is called the Krebs Cycle (also called the Tricarboxylic Acid Cycle or the Citric Acid Cycle).

VITAMIN C AND HEALING

Vitamin C is required for the synthesis of collagen, the most common protein found in our bodies. Collagen is the connective tissue that holds our cells together. The requirement for vitamin C in healing has been recognized for decades by conventional medical texts; however, it is rarely found in hospitals, where it should logically be used extensively. For example, in one study the healing rate of broken bones in guinea pigs was speeded by giving larger vitamin C supplements than were required to prevent scurvy. Vitamin C should be included in intravenous drip solutions supplied to recovering surgery patients, too. Ask for it if you are going to the hospital. Such IV solutions are commercially available but may have to be ordered in advance.

PROTECTION AGAINST UBIQUITOUS FREE RADICALS

There are many other indications of the importance of vitamin C to the maintenance of health. A long-term study conducted on middle aged men in San Mateo showed that higher serum levels of vitamin C were the single best predictor of 5 year survival, surpassing even smoking and drinking (which severely deplete vitamin C) in predictive significance. For example, the brain and spinal cord have specially constructed blood capillaries that constitute the blood-brain barrier, that is very picky about what it allows to pass through. It contains special vitamin C pumps so that it can increase the concentration of vitamin C within the fluid bathing the brain and spinal cord to *ten times* that in the rest of the body. The individual nerve cells in the brain and spinal cord also contain special vitamin C pumps so that they increase the concentration of vitamin C inside these cells to a *hundred times* the concentration of vitamin C in the rest of the body. This vitamin C is very important in protecting nerve cells from free radical damage, to which they are very susceptible because of their high content of polyunsaturated lipids (fats and oils). Polyunsaturated lipids contain carbon-to-carbon double bonds, which are easy to autoxidize, with the resulting creation of a chain reaction of free radicals which can then attack RNA or DNA (causing mutations that can impair cell function or even result in cancer), proteins (possibly altering molecular shape, which can impair function), and lipids, creating more free radicals, and inactivating important membrane-dependent enzymes. For example, prostacyclin synthetase, the enzyme that makes the anti-clotting hormone prostacyclin (also called PGI_2), is very easily inhibited by free radicals and the organic peroxide autoxidation products that they form. Without PGI_2, the insides of blood vessels become as sticky as fly-paper and the blood sludges as it passes by.

Furthermore, researchers have found that leukocytes (a type of white blood cell), during a heart attack, carry vitamin C to the damaged region of the heart, even to the point of severely depleting the rest of the body. This vitamin C is very important in helping limit the damage done to the heart muscle and its pacemaker nerve by the large number of free radicals generated when a part of a coronary artery is either blocked by a clot or ruptures, resulting in hypoxia (inadequate quantities of oxygen available to cells). Poor blood flow, with hypoxia, has been shown to cause free radical damage in the brain, heart, and intestines.

For more about free radicals, see *Life Extension, A Practical Scientific Approach,* pages 100-119, 322-330, 363-369, 402-407, and 408-418.

SHOCK

When we are stressed in a situation involving physical damage, whether it is a heart attack, an accident, or surgery, we may experience a massive release of histamine in our bodies. The histamine release has a protective function, since histamine is a necessary factor for cell division, but in excessive quantities it can do a lot of damage, even causing death by shock. One mechanism of histamine damage is increasing the permeability of capillaries—in other words, these small blood vessels become more leaky. The copper and iron contained in the blood that leaks into the tissues are potent stimulants (catalysts) of free radical production. It has recently been discovered that one of the functions of vitamin C is to detoxify this excess histamine. The amount of vitamin C needed for this detoxification is four or five times the amount of C usually adequate in animals such as guinea pigs.

In one experiment, weights of differing amounts were

dropped onto the legs of anesthetized guinea pigs to produce a frequently lethal wound shock. There was a definite relationship between the amount of the crushing energy absorbed by the limb and the tissue damage and mortality that resulted. When vitamin C (as ascorbic acid) was given in concentrations over 100 milligrams per kilogram of body weight by injection shortly after the crushing injury was received, all the treated animals survived, even when all untreated animals died from identical wounds. Untreated animals received normal doses of vitamin C in their food (adequate to prevent scurvy) but did not receive the extra supplement of C given the treated animals.

SUDDEN DEATH

It is possible for animals or people to be stressed to death. In some cases, people's beliefs that they were going to die resulted in their death. This may be a result of the depletion of brain NE, as discussed earlier in this chapter.

One type of emotional (acute NE overstimulation) stress that caused sudden death has been studied in dogs. It was possible to psychologically stress dogs to death (ventricular fibrillation heart failure), but if the vagus nerve (which is a nervous pathway from the brain to the heart) was cut, the animals could no longer be stressed to death by psychologically induced heart attack. Some people who die suddenly and seemingly without cause may have died in this way. The vagus nerve, when overstimulated, can cause the heart to go into unsynchronized spasms called fibrillation, which do not pump blood. If rhythmic heart action is not quickly restored, death results. The prescription drugs Timolol®, Anturane® and propranolol can provide very effective protection against this type of sudden death by preventing the vagus nerve from being overstimulated. Indeed, in a clinical study in Canada, Anturane® reduced the death rate from a second or subsequent heart attack by 74% when given during the first six months after an initial heart attack. Even though the FDA approves Anturane® only for the treatment of gout (Durk used it for a few years for this condition), about 90% of the new Anturane® prescriptions in the U.S. are now being written for heart patients.

HIGH BLOOD PRESSURE: CONTROL BY MEDICATION AND BIOFEEDBACK

High blood pressure is a major killer. If you have high blood pressure, you should be under the care of a physician. He or she is likely to prescribe drugs to control your high blood pressure. The most common medication is the beta blocker propranolol (also mentioned above for phobias), which blocks the beta receptors sensitive to adrenaline (called adrenergic receptors) on certain cells. More severe cases of high blood pressure receive drugs that stimulate a separate class of these adrenergic receptors, the alpha receptors, such as clonidine or Loniten®. These beta adrenergic receptor blockers and alpha agonists (alpha adrenergic receptor stimulants) have saved over 250,000 lives in the U.S. over the last decade. Other common medications are diuretics, which increase water and sodium excretion to help control high blood pressure, particularly in those who are sensitive to salt and other dietary sodium. **If your physician gives you a prescription for high blood pressure medication, take it as if your life depends on it. It does!** Get several small pill boxes and make sure that you have them in your desk, in each suit, in your car (under the seat is much cooler than the glove compartment; some drugs are temperature sensitive) and in your travel kit. Also, remember to follow your doctor's prescription of a very low salt diet, and take in extra potassium by eating bananas or oranges. Many diuretics deplete the body of potassium.

Biofeedback is also useful in controlling high blood pressure. Sears, Ward's, JS & A Sales (mail order) and even some drugstores now sell home blood pressure monitoring equipment. The old-fashioned device uses a stethoscope to monitor the arterial blood flow sounds as the arm pressure cuff is deflated. This requires reasonably good hearing and a little special training from a doctor or nurse. The new generation of equipment contains a microphone in the cuff and a micro-processor to interpret the blood flow sounds and to compute and display your blood pressure. Although these modern bio-medical electronic devices are more expensive ($100 to $200), they are much easier to use. Timex is about to introduce a microprocessor-controlled digital blood pressure gauge for sale (about $60) through drugstores.

Regular self measurement of your own blood pressure may actually lower your blood pressure. In a study of high blood pressure patients, 43% were able to reduce their blood pressure (systolic and/or diastolic) by 10 mm Hg or more by twice-a-day self measurement for a month.

The inexpensive microprocessor containing a pocket-sized pulse rate meter can also be used for biofeedback. An infra-red source and sensor clip over your fingertip, and the device digitally reads out your pulse rate. With about 15 minutes of practice, you will find that you can slow your pulse rate (and usually lower your blood pressure) by a substantial amount. After this, a few one minute biofeedback sessions per day can help to keep your pulse rate and blood pressure down. You can also use these instruments to quantitatively measure various stressors in your life. How does a phone call to a bureaucrat compare to daily commuting, for example?

Several other types of biofeedback can also lower blood pressure, including alpha wave EEG (electroencephalograph, or brain waves), GSR (galvanic skin response), and EMG (elec-tromyography, a measure of muscular tension).

PERSONAL APPEARANCE

Executives have to look good because their appearance is often the vital first impression that they make on a new acquaintance. Because a suntan gives a person a good appear-ance, many businessmen spend time in the sun to get one. The sun, however, ages skin prematurely because of the ultra-violet light energy that penetrates the skin and damages the DNA of many skin cells, leading to improper cell function, or even cancer or cell death. Indeed, sunshine is the most frequent cause of human skin cancer, which is by far the most common type of human cancer! Worse yet, the weekend golfer or sun seeker is far more likely to get skin cancer than somebody who spends most of his time outdoors, such as a farmer. Why? Probably because the constant sun exposure stimulates the production of protective enzymes within the skin, whereas this does not occur when exposure is intermittent. A better way to get the good-looking skin color of a tan is to use a new prescription product called Orobronze® that is available in Canada. The active ingredient is a red carotenoid (a plant pigment related to the yellow beta carotene in carrots) called canthaxanthin. This material does not cause skin damage and aging like the sun's ultraviolet, in fact, it provides a degree of protection against it. Indeed, carotenoids in general are powerful cancer preventive nutrients. Over a period of a few weeks, you can get a beautiful bronze tan skin color simply by taking a few tablets a day. A recent Canadian study found some minor, microscopic eye changes, which do not affect vision, in canthaxanthin users; these changes appear to be insignificant. This carotenoid is FDA approved as a food

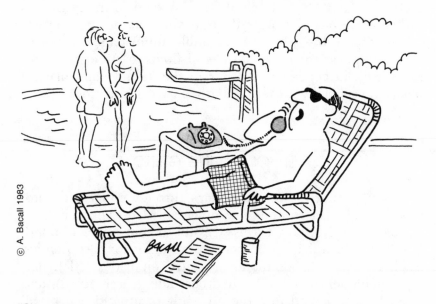

© A. Bacall 1983

"Oh, nothing much; just catching some rays and forming some undesirable cross-linking bonds. What's happening with you?"

coloring agent, but is not yet approved for tanning. Nevertheless, there are several mail order vendors offering this material in the U.S. However, we suggest that you consult with your physician first.

Smoking and drinking are major causes of premature skin aging, including wrinkles and loss of elasticity and the ability to retain moisture. The acetaldehyde and other readily autoxidizable aldehydes from alcohol and smoke actually embalm your skin, like the formaldehyde used to preserve cadavers. These compounds are crosslinkers; they make uncontrolled and undesired chemical bonds between your collagen (connective tissue) molecules, which is the basis for these effects. The antioxidant nutrients B-1, C, and cysteine are very effective at preventing this type of damage. Another antioxidant nutrient, vitamin B-5, often markedly improves skin appearance after a few weeks of use at a dose of 1 gram per day.

CAUTION: Do not take supplemental cysteine unless you take at least 3 times as much vitamin C supplement as your total cysteine consumption. In figuring your cysteine consumption, remember that the number of eggs you eat is relevant; each egg contains about ¼ gram of cysteine. While cysteine is quite water soluble, its oxidized form, cystine, is rather insoluble in water. If large amounts of cysteine are taken without the other water soluble antioxidants such as C, and without adequate quantities of fluids, cystine stone formation could conceivably occur in the kidneys and urinary bladder, especially if there is a urinary tract infection.

THE COMMUTING GRIND

Commuting to and from work through congested automobile traffic is a thoroughly unpleasant stress you may have to face daily. Not only is this stressful to your peace of mind, but it is stressful to your body, too. Many toxic substances (such as ozone, carbon monoxide, nitrogen oxides, aldehydes, lead, polynuclear aromatic hydrocarbons (carcinogens), and others) are released into the atmosphere around you by all those automobiles. And you have to breathe it, even if your car is air-conditioned. Fortunately, many nutrients offer protection against these poisons. Some of the most serious health hazards are caused by free radicals that are created by the chemical reactions of aldehydes, nitrogen oxides, and ozone. Nutrients that may provide protection include vitamins A, E, C, B-1, B-5, B-6, PABA, the amino acid cysteine, the minerals zinc and selenium. Vitamin C can help keep heavy metals like lead dissolved in our bloodstreams where they can be eliminated via the urine, rather than being deposited in our brains and bones. Beta carotene may protect you from lung cancer caused by the combustion tars, the polynuclear aromatic hydrocarbons.

You may also find driving in traffic to be aggravating. This psychophysiological response is stressful in itself. If you do become more aggressive under these conditions, you may find the amino acid tryptophan of help. It is used in the brain to make an inhibitory neurotransmitter called serotonin. Neurotransmitters are chemicals used by nerve cells to communicate with each other. Inhibitory neurotransmitters and neuromodulators (such as glycine, inositol, or serotonin) reduce nerve cell response to stimulation, whereas excitatory neurotransmitters (like norepinephrine or glutamate) increase nerve cell response to stimulation. Excessively aggressive men have been found to have low levels of the serotonin breakdown product 5-HIAA in their urine. Treatment with tryptophan can bring these levels up and reduce aggression. The tryptophan won't make the traffic any more pleasant, but it might reduce your unpleasant response to it. Remember, it is your psychophysiological response to the traffic congestion that causes your ulcers or heart problems. A reasonable dose for an adult is about 1 to 2 grams. It may make you somewhat sleepy if you are not used to it, so keep this in mind if you are going to be driving.

WARNING: We know of one case (a Chinese woman in her mid thirties) where, on three separate occasions, a 500 milligram dose of tryptophan caused excitation and insomnia rather than the expected sedation. Since we do not know the biochemistry of this rare excitatory effect, *prudence demands* *that one NOT use tryptophan supplements if one finds them excitatory rather than sedative.* The nutrient amino acid glycine (available in many health food and drugstores) also has soothing effects in some people in a dose of 3 to 10 grams. The nutrient carbohydrate inositol has Valium®-like anti-anxiety effects at doses of 1 to 5 grams; in fact, inositol is a natural activator of the brain's benzodiazepine (Valium® and Librium®) receptors, as is the B vitamin niacinamide. A reasonable dose of niacinamide is 250 milligrams to 3 grams. In our experience, the vitamin complex niacinamide ascorbate has anti-anxiety effects in the dose range of 500 milligrams to 5 grams.

SUMMARY

Stress is inherent in the life of an executive. This does not mean that you, as an executive, are doomed to stress-induced illness and death. You can protect yourself from the health hazards of stress to a substantial degree by fortifying your natural physiological protective mechanisms with the proper nutrients. You must accept responsibility for rationally managing the way your body and mind cope with executive stress.

SUGGESTED NUTRIENTS FOR STRESSED EXECUTIVES

total daily amount, to be taken with meals, divided into three daily doses

A	10,000 to 20,000 I.U.
B-1	1 gram
B-2	100 milligrams
B-3	300 milligrams
B-5	1 gram
B-6	250 milligrams

WARNING: Do not use B-6 supplements if you have Parkinson's disease and are being treated with L-Dopa. Vitamin

B-6 can counteract the brain effects of the L-Dopa, and can result in increased side effects.

cysteine (not cystine)   1 gram

CAUTION: Do not take supplemental cysteine unless you take at least 3 times as much vitamin C supplement as your total cysteine consumption. In figuring your cysteine consumption, remember that the number of eggs you eat is relevant; each egg contains about ¼ gram of cysteine. While cysteine is quite water soluble, its oxidized form, cystine, is rather insoluble in water. If large amounts of cysteine are taken without the other water soluble antioxidants such as C, and without adequate quantities of fluids, cystine stone formation could conceivably occur in the kidneys and urinary bladder, especially if there is a urinary tract infection.

C	3 grams
selenium	200 micrograms
E	1000 I.U.
chelated zinc	50 milligrams
PABA	300 milligrams

WARNING: PABA will counteract sulfa type A. Do not use concurrently with sulfa drugs.

beta carotene   25,000 I.U.

Optional:

tryptophan   1–3 grams, in the evening or
                                     when irritated

WARNING: We know of one case (a Chinese woman in her mid thirties) where, on three separate occasions, a 500 milligram dose of tryptophan caused excitation and insomnia rather than the expected sedation. Since we do not know the biochemistry of this rare excitatory effect, ***prudence demands***

that one NOT use tryptophan supplements if one finds them
excitatory rather than sedative.

glycine	3-10 grams when irritated
niacinamide	250 milligrams to 3 grams, when irritated, or
niacinamide ascorbate	500 milligrams to 5 grams when irritated
inositol	1-5 grams when irritated
phenylalanine, or tyrosine	50 milligrams to 1 gram in the morning; dose must be individualized.

WARNING: Do NOT use phenylalanine or tyrosine with MAO inhibitors.

CAUTION: Persons with high blood pressure must use these two amino acid supplements only with the advice of their doctor, with tyrosine probably preferable. Monitoring of blood pressure is essential. We recommend that all persons with high blood pressure purchase and learn to use a home blood pressure measuring device.

REFERENCES

Pearson and Shaw, *Life Extension, A Practical Scientific Approach*, Warner Books, June 1982; 858 pages with hundreds of references to the primary scientific literature.

Laughlin, Fisher, and Sherrard, "Blood Pressure Reductions During Self Recording of Home Blood Pressure," *Amer. Heart J.* 98(5): 629-634, Nov. 1979

Chope and Breslow, "Nutritional Status of the Aging," *Amer. J. Publ. Health* 46: 61-67, 1955

Drake et al, "A Seven-Year Following of the San Mateo Nutrition Study Population," presented before the Western Branch of the American Public Health Association, Long Beach, Calif., May 31, 1957

Benditt, "The Origin of Atherosclerosis," *Sci. Amer.*, Feb. 1977 (available as *Scientific American* offprint #1351 from W. H. Freeman and Co., 660 Market St., San Francisco, CA 94104)

Ralli and Dumm, "Relation of Pantothenic Acid to Adrenal Cortical Function," *Vit. Horm.* 11: 133-158, 1953

Ungar, "Effect of Ascorbic Acid on the Survival of Traumatized Animals," *Nature* 1: 637-38, 1942

Keller et al, "Suppression of Immunity by Stress: Effect of a Graded Series of Stressors on Lymphocyte Stimulation in the Rat," *Science* 213: 1397-1400, 1981

Lattime and Strausser, "Arteriosclerosis: Is Stress-Induced Immune Suppression a Risk Factor?" *Science* 198(4314): 302-303, 1977

Riley, "Psychoneuroendocrine Influences on Immunocompetence and Neoplasia," *Science* 212: 1100-1109, 1981.

Pao and Mickle, "Problem Nutrients in the United States," *Food Technology*: 58-79, Sept. 1981.

"Nonsmokers affected by tobacco smoke," *Science News*, 5 April 1980, p. 221.

Repace and Lowrey, "Indoor Air Pollution, Tobacco Smoke, and Public Health," *Science* 208: 464-472, 1980.

Sprince, Parker, Smith, Gonzales, "Protective Action of Ascorbic Acid and Sulfur Compounds against Acetaldehyde Toxicity: Implications in Alcoholism and Smoking," *Agents and Actions* 5(2): 164-173, 1975

Hume et al, "Leukocyte Ascorbic Acid Levels After Acute Myocardial Infarction," *Brit. Heart J.* 34: 238-243, 1972

Spallholz et al, "Immunologic Responses of Mice Fed Diets Supplemented with Selenite Selenium," *Proc. Soc. Exp. Med. Biol.* 143: 685-689, 1973

Anderson et al, "The Effects of Increasing Weekly Doses of Ascorbate on Certain Cellular and Humoral Immune Functions in Normal Volunteers," *Am. J. Clin. Nutr.* 33: 71-76, Jan. 1980.

Nockels, "Protective Effects of Supplemental Vitamin E Against Infection," paper presented at 62nd annual scientific meeting (Apr. 9 to 14, 1978) of the Federation of American Societies for Experimental Biology

Barbul et al, "Arginine: A Thymotropic and Wound-Healing Promoting Agent," *Surgical Forum* 28: 101-103, 1977

"Dietary Tryptophan and Aggressive Behavior in Rats," *Nutr. Rev.* 39(7): 284-285, 1981

Shekelle et al, "Dietary Vitamin A and Risk of Cancer in the Western Electric Study," *The Lancet*, 28 Nov. 1981, pp. 1185-1190 [beta carotene and the risk of lung cancer]

Wurtman, "Nutrients That Modify Brain Function," *Sci. Amer.*, April 1982

Finnish study of the relation of alcohol and stroke in young persons appeared in the July/Aug. *Stroke*, as reported in "Alcohol and Stroke" in the 1982 Update-Best of Hotline, *The Medical Hotline*

Hess et al, "Involvement of Free Radicals in the Pathophysiology of Ischemic Heart Disease," *Canad. J. Physiol. & Pharmacol.* 60: 1382-1397, 1982.

Flamm et al, "Ethanol Potentiation of Central Nervous System Trauma," *J. Neurosurg.* 46: 328-335, 1977.

Demopoulos et al, "The Free Radical Pathology and the Microcirculation in the Major Central Nervous System Disorders," *Acta Physiol. Scand.* Suppl. 492: 91-119, 1980.

McCord and Roy, "The Pathophysiology of Superoxide: Roles in Inflammation and Ischemia," *Canad. J. Physiol. & Pharmacol.* 60:1346-1352, 1982.

Biochemistry for Success

INTRODUCTION

Your intellectual and emotional limits probably pose a far greater barrier to your success than other factors do and they are far more easily improved than you may realize. Scientists have discovered enough in the past two decades so that it is now possible to enhance your intelligence and modify your emotional states with nutrients and, optionally, prescription drugs. If you weren't born with quite the right biochemistry to be a great leader, you may be able to make yourself a better leader by biochemical means.

Altering *your* biochemistry does not in any way improve the rationality of those with whom you must deal. But you have a choice. You can improve your own chances or not. You do not have the choice of altering the behavior of others. In the not too distant future, the genetic factors and the corresponding biochemistry underlying some persistent irrational mental biases (such as sexism) will be much better understood, leading to greater opportunity for individual change.

In this article, we describe techniques that have been used to enhance human and animal intelligence, increase assertiveness, overcome depressions and phobias, and control anxiety through an understanding of some of the biochemistry involved and the appropriate use of certain nutrients and, optionally, prescription drugs. It is important to keep in mind that NOTHING IS PERFECTLY SAFE; the precautions and data about side-effects are meant to be taken seriously. Even common nutrients have side-effects when taken in excessive doses. For these purposes, doses must often be individualized.

ASSERTIVENESS AND DEPRESSION

No matter how talented you are, your success may be limited by your aggressiveness in pursuing your goals. An important brain chemical (technically called a neurotransmitter, a substance that nerve cells use to communicate with each other) involved in aggressive behavior is norepinephrine. It is also called noradrenaline, the brain's version of adrenaline. Norepinephrine (NE) is important in areas of the brain involved in primitive drives and emotions (such as dominance, acquisition, and sex), memory, and in other functions as well. The brain uses the nutrient amino acids tyrosine and phenylalanine to manufacture NE. Assertiveness may be increased by taking these amino acids, but the dose is a very individual matter and may range from 50 milligrams to 1 or 2 grams per day. If you decide to try these after understanding the precautions, you should begin use at a low dose (50 milligrams) and slowly increase the dose over a few weeks. These amino acids compete with other amino acids to be carried into the brain, across the blood-brain barrier, a highly selective barrier composed of specially constructed capillaries in the brain and spinal cord. This is why taking them on an empty stomach is most effective. They work best when used either just before bedtime or just upon arising in the morning. Too much phenylalanine or tyrosine can cause excess aggressiveness or a "wired" feeling. If this occurs, reduce your dose or discontinue use.

CAUTION: In a few susceptible individuals, phenylalanine in high doses (probably higher than those mentioned here) may cause the blood pressure to rise. People with high blood pressure should use these amino acids only with the supervision of their physician and with frequent monitoring of blood pressure. Tyrosine seems to have a normalizing effect on blood pressure, increasing it in hypotension and decreasing it in hypertension.

WARNING: Do not use phenylalanine and tyrosine if you are taking an MAO inhibitor antidepressant drug, since the combination could result in potentially dangerous, extremely high blood pressure. If you have a heart rhythm irregularity or malignant melanoma, you should *NOT* use these substances.

Phenylalanine and tyrosine are very effective in depression, too. In one study of people suffering from various types of depression (endogenous, schizophrenic, the depressive phase of manic-depressive illness, amphetamine abuse, and others), 80% of them were entirely relieved of their depres-

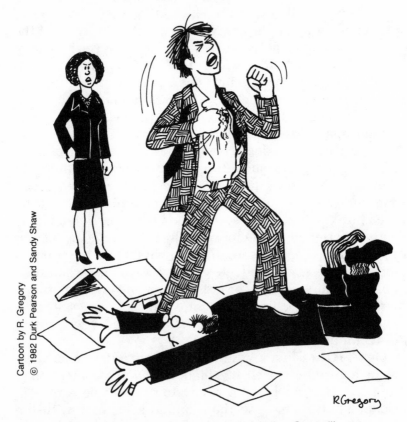

Cartoon by R. Gregory
© 1982 Durk Pearson and Sandy Shaw

"Maybe you'd better cut down a little on the phenylalanine, George!"

sions within two weeks by taking 100 to 500 milligrams of phenylalanine per day. Tyrosine is effective at similar doses. Amphetamine and cocaine abuse are very common causes of depressions that are responsive to tyrosine and phenylalanine. That is because both these drugs cause the brain to release its NE and then block NE recycling, resulting in a high concentration in the gaps (synapses) between nerve cells that is responsible for the drugs' excitatory effects; however, they do not cause the brain to make any more NE. Eventually after heavy use, the brain is depleted of NE, and depression, poor memory, and lack of energy and motivation result. Vitamins B-6 and C are required for the brain's manufacture of NE. (For more information on depression, see *Life Extension, A Practical Scientific Approach*, pages 181-188.)

One final thought: you can easily adjust your aggressiveness to that of a dominant male, but you will not instantly acquire the experience to use this high power drive productively. Be careful.

PHOBIAS

Four years ago, it was difficult for Sandy to ask a clerk at a hardware store the price of nails. Public speaking was out of the question, despite her extensive scientific knowledge. Yet, Sandy appeared on dozens of TV shows, including the "Merv Griffin Show," during our recent book promotion tour (*Life Extension: A Practical Scientific Approach*) with co-author Durk Pearson. These public appearances were possible for Sandy because of new understanding of what causes phobias and the discovery of a class of widely used drugs that can block them, so that you can quickly unlearn your phobias. See "Getting Rid of Phobias for Good" in this book for a complete discussion of the problem and a solution for many people.

ANGER

Your unwanted anger may be controllable through the use of the nutrient amino acid tryptophan. The brain uses tryptophan to make serotonin, a calming neurotransmitter which is responsible for inducing the sleep state. A dose of 1 to 2 grams at bedtime or when excessive anger or aggression appear can often provide a desirable soothing effect. The tryptophan does not change the nature of reality or your perception of it, but it can alter your angry response to it. Vitamins B-6 and C are required by the brain to make serotonin from the tryptophan, so be sure to take supplements of these as well. Excess tryptophan may make you sleepy, make your nose run, or cause a headache.

Angry Depression

One type of depression which is responsive to tryptophan features excess aggressiveness and violence, including sometimes violent attempts at suicide. A group of Navy men displaying these symptoms were found to have low levels of 5-HIAA, a breakdown product of serotonin, in their urine, an indication of inadequate levels of serotonin. Treatment with tryptophan was very effective in reversing this type of depression.

Tryptophan is effective in modulating the increased aggressiveness resulting from phenylalanine or tyrosine use. It can give you greater control over the aggressive state so that you can use it constructively.

WARNING: We know of one case (a Chinese woman in her mid thirties) where, on three separate occasions, a 500 milligram dose of tryptophan caused excitation and insomnia rather than the expected sedation. Since we do not know the biochemistry of this rare excitatory effect, *prudence demands that one NOT use tryptophan supplements if one finds them excitatory rather than sedative.*

Inositol and Glycine Help Control Anger

Two other nutrients that can be helpful in controlling anger include inositol (a sugar) and glycine (an amino acid). Glycine is an inhibitory neurotransmitter (that is, it reduces the activity of nerve cells, exerting a calming effect) for

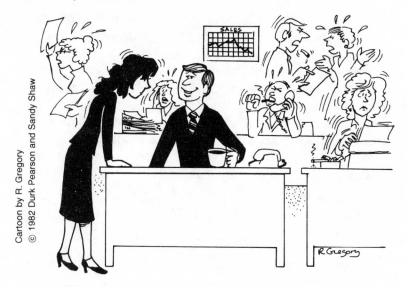

"What's my secret for staying calm? I sweeten my coffee with inositol and tryptophan!"

primitive areas of the brain. Inositol increases the effectiveness of natural anti-anxiety receptors in the brain (more on that below). A dose of 3 to 10 grams of glycine and 1 to 5 grams of inositol would be reasonable; you will have to determine the most effective doses for yourself through experimentation.

ANXIETY

Recently, scientists discovered that Valium® and Librium® produce their anti-anxiety effects by binding to receptors on brain cells now called the benzodiazepine receptors. Since these receptors exist naturally in the brain, it was immediately realized that there had to be natural substances in the brain which fit into them. Some substances that affect the benzodiazepine receptors have been identified and these can be useful in controlling anxiety. Their use has allowed some people to reduce the amounts of Valium® and Librium® or alcohol that they use. Niacinamide is a nutrient that is believed to bind to the benzodiazepine receptors. The sugar inositol enhances this binding, increasing the anti-anxiety effects. Alcohol exerts its anti-anxiety effects at least in part because of its effects on these receptors. Unfortunately, in long-term excess use of alcohol, the benzodiazepine receptors are damaged, so that there is a great increase in anxiety. A daily dose of 250 milligrams to 3 grams of niacinamide and 1 to 5 grams of inositol are reasonable for a healthy adult.

Anxiety may be a more common problem for women than it is for men, judging by the far larger number of prescriptions for Valium® and Librium® written for women.

INTELLIGENCE

There are over a dozen substances now known to enhance human intelligence, including some nutrients (available at most health food and drugstores) and prescription drugs. Intelligence is a broad term and covers many different aspects of mental function, including memory, abstract reasoning, serial learning (as in learning lists of words), ability to focus, and so on. The intelligence enhancing chemicals (we call them smart pills) do not improve every aspect of intelligence, but only parts of it. Some of the effects are subtle and not always subjectively detectable and may take a period of learning for effective use.

The reason for the recent progress in enhancing human intelligence is because we now have some understanding of how intelligence works, that is, the biochemistry that underlies it. Our understanding is still crude, but since information in this field is doubling roughly every five years, we can expect further improvements in the relatively near future. (For more information, see *Life Extension, A Practical Scientific Approach*, especially pages 167-180.)

Choline and Vitamin B-5

Choline is a B vitamin nutrient that can be bought at most health food and drugstores. In a study of MIT students, a dose of 3 grams of choline a day resulted in an improved memory and a greater ability to learn a list of words. The brain requires vitamin B-5 (pantothenic acid or calcium pantothenate) to convert the choline into acetylcholine, a neurotransmitter. Acetylcholine is involved in memory, long-term planning, filtering sensory stimuli that enter the brain, primitive drives and emotions, and focus and concentration, among other functions. In people over about 50, the use of choline frequently causes an increase in libido. It is often helpful in improving verbal fluency. A dose of 3 grams of choline and a gram of vitamin B-5 per day is reasonable. Begin at a low dose and work your way slowly up. Excess choline can result in headaches or muscular tension. Some people note a fishy body odor, as a result of gut bacteria turning choline into trimethylamine. Although we have not observed this, it may be a problem for some people. If this occurs, you can try increasing dietary fiber or eating yogurt, either of which will alter the gut bacteria and may solve the problem.

Vasopressin

Diapid® is a prescription drug that enhances intelligence. It is a synthetic version of a natural hormone, vasopressin, released by your brain's pituitary gland. In one study of men in their fifties and sixties, 16 I.U. (about 8 gentle snorts of the vasopressin nasal spray) per day resulted in better memories, an enhancement of intelligence in tests requiring focus and concentration, and a faster reaction time. At this dose level, there were no side effects. Vasopressin has also been used successfully to help amnesia victims recover their memories. One effect of vasopressin that was not mentioned in any of the scientific papers is its intensification and prolongation of orgasm! Cocaine causes the pituitary to release vasopressin and this is responsible for part of cocaine's reputation as an enhancer of sexual activities. Unfortunately, cocaine does not cause the brain to make more vasopressin, so after using cocaine heavily for a couple of weeks or so (depending on the individual), the pituitary runs out of vasopressin, helping to cause a poor memory and difficulty in reaching orgasm. Excessive doses of vasopressin can cause temporary intestinal cramping. **CAUTION:** Vasopressin should not be used by angina patients because it may precipitate an angina attack in these people. Do *not* snort the vasopressin as part of a deep breath, as some people have experienced spasm of the larynx. The idea is to snort it into the upper part of your nasal cavities (from which it is transported to your brain), *not* into your larynx and lungs.

Vasopressin is interesting for other reasons. It is associated with brain theta wave activity, a correlate of creative thinking. And vasopressin improves the ability to visualize. On the *average*, women have better verbal abilities than men but do less well on tasks requiring visual-spatial or complex spatial relations. This is probably why there are so few female architects, topologists, or grand prix race car drivers. Diapid®

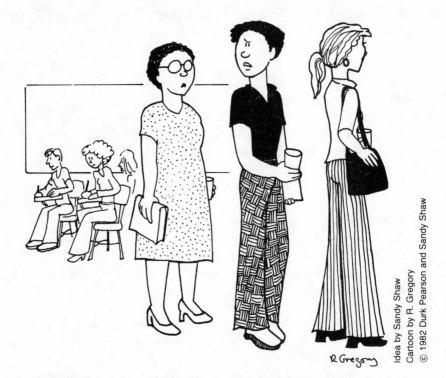

Idea by Sandy Shaw
Cartoon by R. Gregory
© 1982 Durk Pearson and Sandy Shaw

"I don't mind the exam—but I hate these urine tests afterwards, checking for the presence of 'smart drugs'!"

is one way to overcome this natural inequality. One reason that some children have an eidetic ("photographic") memory (which tends to disappear as they become older) is that they have higher levels of vasopressin. Vasopressin release precedes REM (rapid eye movement sleep, where dreaming takes place). It is also released during orgasm.

Hydergine®

Another smart pill of particular interest is the prescription drug Hydergine®. Hydergine® has biochemical effects similar to that of caffeine, but much more selective than caffeine, so that it provides a lift but usually not the letdown or jitters that often accompany caffeine use. In doses of 12 milligrams a day for two weeks, normal human subjects showed an improvement in their memories and intelligence, including their ability to do abstract reasoning. Long term use of Hydergine® can provide improvements to people with mild to moderate amounts of brain damage, including senility, damage from strokes, damage resulting from hypoxia (too little oxygen) at birth, and other conditions. Hydergine® stimulates the growth of connections between nerve cells called neurites which are necessary for such functions as learning. It appears to work via a similar mechanism to the natural NGF (nerve growth factor), which, as we grow older, is less abundant in the brain.

Hydergine® Has an Enviable Safety Record

Hydergine® is a particularly safe drug. Nobody is known to have died from an overdose or even to have done permanent damage to themselves, even though a few people have attempted suicide with it. It has been used for over 25 years and is the 5th most prescribed drug in the free world (outside of the United States). Hydergine® protects the liver from many harmful chemicals, including alcohol, and slows aging in the brain resulting from free radical aging mechanisms. Initial use may cause a mild degree of nausea, but this is not a

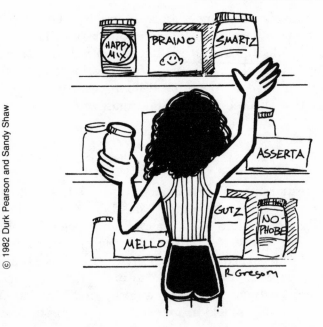

Cartoon by R. Gregory
© 1982 Durk Pearson and Sandy Shaw

toxic effect and will usually disappear after a few days of use and can usually be avoided by starting at 1 milligram per day and slowly increasing the dose. Although 3 milligrams a day is recommended by the FDA, 9 to 12 milligrams a day are more typically used in Europe. We would not expect to see dramatic improvements in mental function at the low 3 milligram dose. Conditions under which an individual should not use Hydergine® include individual sensitivity to it and, possibly, acute psychosis. Hydergine® also dramatically increases the effects of caffeine when they are used together, so watch your caffeine consumption, particularly when increasing your dose of Hydergine®. Overdoses can lead to temporary headache, nausea, insomnia, or excessive excitation.

We wish you much success. Live Long and Prosper!

REFERENCES

Pearson and Shaw, *Life Extension, A Practical Scientific Approach*, Warner Books, June 1982

Kielholz, *A Therapeutic Approach to the Psyche via the Beta Adrenergic System* [phobias and beta blockers], University Park Press, 1977

Sitaram et al, "Choline: Selective Enhancement of Serial Learning and Encoding of Low Imagery Words in Man," *Life Sci.* 22: 1555-60, 1978

Wurtman, "Nutrients That Modify Brain Function," *Sci. Amer.*, April 1982

Legros et al, "Influence of Vasopressin on Memory and Learning," *Lancet*, 7 Jan. 1978, p. 41

Berde and Schild, eds., *Ergot Alkaloids and Related Compounds*, Springer-Verlag, 1978 [Hydergine® data]

Gelenberg et al, "Tyrosine for the Treatment of Depression," *Am. J. Psychiat.* 137(5): 622-23, 1980

"Dietary Tryptophan and Aggressive Behavior in Rats," *Nutr. Rev.* 39(7): 284-85, 1981

Korda, *Power!* Ballantine Books, 1975

"Workshop on Advances in Experimental Pharmacology of Hydergine," *Gerontology* 24 (1978), Suppl. 1:1-154

Moehler et al, [benzodiazepine receptors and their endogenous ligands], *Nature* (London) 278: 563-565, 1979

Braestrup, Nielsen, "Searching for endogenous benzodiazepine receptor ligands," *Trends in Pharmacological Sciences*, 424-427, Nov. 1980

Snyder, *Biological Aspects of Mental Disorder*, Oxford University Press, 1980

Hindmarch et al, "The Effects of an Ergot Alkaloid Derivative (Hydergine) on Aspects of Psychomotor Performance,

Arousal, and Cognitive Processing Ability," *J. Clin. Pharmacol.* 19(11-12):726-732, 1979

Weingartner, Gold, Ballenger, Smallberg, Summers, Rubinow, Post, Goodwin, "Effects of Vasopressin on Human Memory Functions," *Science* 211: 601, 1981

How To Stay Well, or Helping Your Immune System

Potentially deadly bacteria and viruses are all over and within our bodies, ready to take advantage of any chink in our defensive armor. Why, then, are we not all dead? Because our immune system, which protects us from these enemies, as well as from cancer cells and atherosclerotic plaques, is busy all the time. Diseases like the flu, colds, arthritis, and cancer occur when our defenses fail. Recent research has discovered much about how our immune system keeps us well and how to help it to do a better job, whether we are healthy or already sick.

Your immune system is made up of white blood cells (of which there are several types), the thymus gland (behind your breastbone), the spleen, bone marrow, lymph glands, and a variety of large molecules such as antibodies, interferon, and complement. There are two main types of white blood cells: the T-cells identify enemies, then kill them so scavenger cells can eat them; the B-cells make antibodies, generally under instructions from the T-cells. The thymus gland serves as the master programmer of the T-cells, educating them to kill only certain specified enemies and only when they are told to do so. The thymus is supported by growth hormone, supplied by the pituitary gland in the brain. Without adequate quantities of growth hormone, the thymus shrinks and becomes less effective in defending the body.

Immunity begins in childhood with exposure to various organisms, either through contracting the diseases or via immunization against those diseases. Some parents believe that it is no longer necessary to immunize their children against childhood diseases. But what they don't realize is that if the child does not develop immunity, he or she may contract a childhood disease as an adult, when it may have much more serious consequences. For example, when a baby gets polio, the disease is usually like a bad cold, the infant recovers and then has immunity for life. But when an older child or adult gets polio, the risk of paralysis is much higher. The education that a child's immune system receives early in life is very important to his or her later health.

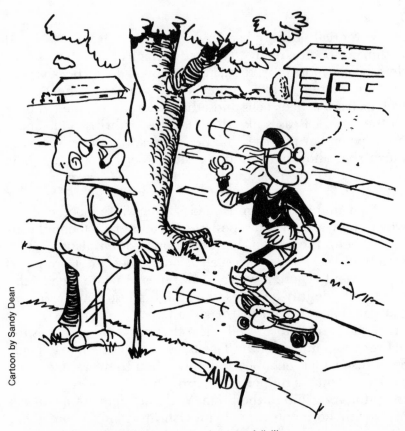

Cartoon by Sandy Dean

"Confound it, Mary Elizabeth! You're not aging gracefully!"

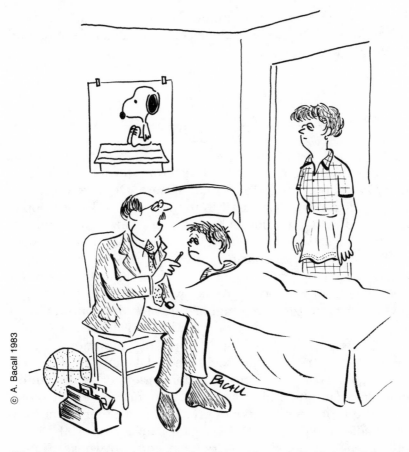

"The bad news is that he has an infection. The good news is that he's educating his immune system."

CANCER

The immune system is also responsible for detecting and killing cancer cells in our body. Cancer begins when the DNA programs regulating cellular growth are damaged. Nobel Prize winning tumor biologist P. B. Medawar has said that everyone probably develops cancer cells thousands or perhaps even millions of times in his life. But most of the time, our immune system destroys the cancer before we ourselves can detect it. When our immune system is not working up to par, however, those few cancer cells may escape notice and develop into a tumor.

DEPRESSION

What impairs the ability of our immune system to do its job? One important factor is mental state. Depressed individuals tend to have depressed immune systems. Depression is associated with depletion in brain stores of the neurotransmitter (chemical which nerve cells use to communicate with each other) norepinephrine, NE. NE causes the pituitary gland to release growth hormone. It is also an important neurochemical for mood. We know that people suffering a severe personal loss have higher rates for the contraction of cancer for a period of several months following the loss. It is possible to replete the brain's stores of norepinephrine by taking the nutrient amino acid phenylalanine. In a clinical study, 70 to 80% of patients with depressions of several different types (amphetamine abuse, schizophrenic, endogenous, depressive phase of manic-depressive, and others) were entirely alleviated of their depressions by taking 100 to 500 milligrams of phenylalanine per day for two weeks. Similar doses of the nutrient amino acid tyrosine also work well and are probably better suited to individuals with high blood pressure, since tyrosine often reduces blood pressure in hypertension.

(**CAUTION:** People with high blood pressure should use tyrosine and phenylalanine cautiously and *only* under a physician's care since blood pressure elevations may occur in sensitive individuals.)

WARNING: Tyrosine and phenylalanine must *not* be used with MAO inhibitor drugs (a seldom prescribed class of antidepressants), since extremely hazardous hypertension could result. Individuals with irregular heart rhythms or malignant melanoma should *not* use these substances, either.

GROWTH HORMONE

As people age (in the absence of intervention) the pituitary gland releases less growth hormone, resulting in a decline in the function of the thymus gland and contributing to the older person's far greater risk of contracting infectious diseases, cancer, and cardiovascular disease.

Growth hormone is also involved in tissue repair, such as the healing of injuries, and in burning up body fat and increasing lean muscle mass. (See pages 222-225, 226-238, and 284-295 in *Life Extension, A Practical Scientific Approach.*)

FREE RADICALS

Another important factor which reduces the effectiveness of our immune system is free radicals, chemically reactive and destructive entities with an unpaired electron created in our bodies as part of normal metabolism, by the breakdown in our bodies of peroxidized (rancid) fat, by white blood cells as weapons for killing enemies, and by radiation. (Radiation sickness is a pure free radical disease, although, normally, radiation contributes only a very small part of the total free radicals to which we are exposed.) Although we have special protective enzymes (such as superoxide dismutase, glutathione peroxidase, and catalase) and protective antioxidant nutrients (including vitamins A, C, B-1, B-5, B-6, E, the amino acid cysteine, the triple amino acid glutathione, and the minerals zinc and selenium), protection is not perfect and, as time passes, damage tends to build up throughout the body. Free radicals are implicated as causative agents in aging, cancer, heart disease, arthritis, and many other abnormal conditions.

When oils and fats in the body, especially polyunsaturated fats, are exposed to oxygen (or chemical oxidizers such as the air pollutants nitrogen oxides and ozone), they become peroxidized (rancid). These rancid fats directly inhibit immune function and also break down, releasing lots of free radicals, which further impairs the performance of our immune system. Peroxidized (rancid) fats are mutagenic (can damage DNA) and carcinogenic (can cause cancer). Many anti-cancer compounds have anti-free radical properties. After rabbits were fed a small quantity of rancid polyunsaturated vegetable oil, the activity of the macrophages (a type of white blood cell) in the lungs was measured. The macrophages were greatly inhibited—they didn't move about actively seeking out and killing enemies as they should have—because of the presence of the organic peroxides and the free radicals released in the breakdown of these organic peroxides in the rancid oil. Peroxidized lipids (oils and fats) are also thrombogenic (cause abnormal blood clots) and atherogenic (cause atherosclerosis). Your immune system (if healthy) destroys these clots and atherosclerotic lesions. These are some reasons why overweight people are so much more susceptible to diseases of all types, including heart disease and cancer, than normal weight individuals: they are full of peroxidized fat. People of normal weight who eat significant quantities of polyunsaturated oils without also taking large supplements of antioxidant nutrients, such as those mentioned above, also run a serious risk of immune system depression.

STIMULATING YOUR IMMUNE SYSTEM

What can we do to stimulate the function of our immune system? We may do a great deal with some simple nutrients, available without a prescription, which have been shown in animal experiments to improve immune system surveillance. Certain prescription drugs are also of value. These materials include:

1. Vitamin A—A can prevent the decrease in thymus weight and numbers of thymic lymphocytes (a thymus derived type of white blood cell) that occurs in injuries. It can increase the

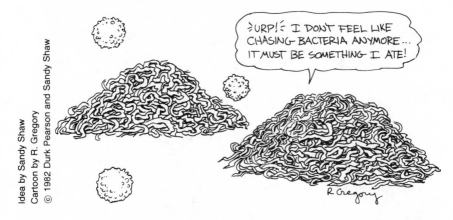

size of the thymus, even doubling it. Vitamin A has also been shown to inhibit the development of cancers in epithelial tissues (including the linings of lungs and gastrointestinal system). 15,000 I.U. per day is a reasonable adult dose of vitamin A. Zinc is required for mobilization of vitamin A stores from the liver. A supplement of 50 milligrams a day of chelated zinc is a reasonable dose for a healthy adult. **CAUTION:** In excess quantities, vitamin A can cause liver damage. Symptoms of vitamin A overdosage include cracks in the corners of the lips, irritability, headaches, loss of appetite, itching, and hair loss. If these symptoms appear, reduce or temporarily discontinue your dose of vitamin A; usually these signs and symptoms disappear within a week or two.

2. Vitamin C—C increases the activity of certain white blood cells which patrol the body looking for bacteria, viruses, cancer cells, and atherosclerotic plaque cells. It also increases the quantity of interferon made in lymphocytes and fibroblasts (connective tissue cells). Vitamin C is lost rapidly via the urine, so it should be taken four times daily. (A convenient schedule is to take it after breakfast, lunch, and dinner, and then at bedtime.)

3. Vitamin E—In several species of animals (chicken, lamb, turkey, and rat), vitamin E supplementation at a level of 200 to 2000 I.U. of E per kilogram of food resulted in improved

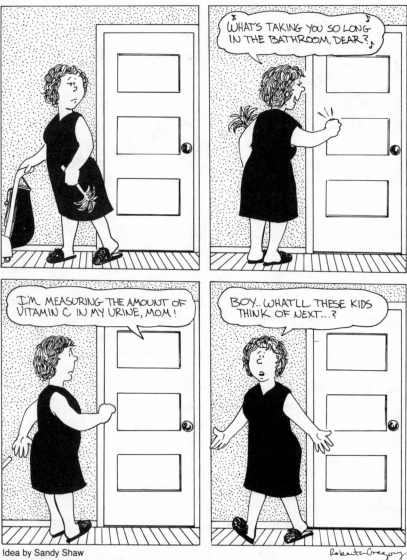

Idea by Sandy Shaw
Cartoon by R. Gregory
© 1982 Durk Pearson and Sandy Shaw

immune system responses, 10 times greater for B-cells and 3 to 5 times greater for T-cells. 200 to 2000 I.U. of vitamin E per day is a reasonable daily dose for healthy adults. Bruce and his associates found mutagenic substances in the feces of normal humans. These substances may be causative agents for colon cancer. When Bruce fed vitamins C and E to volunteers, they found a reduction in mutagens to 25% that of the control (no vitamin supplements) group. In a recent study, 600 milligrams a day of vitamin E (about 800 I.U.) reversed and completely eliminated the development of fibrocystic breast disease in 22 out of 26 women with the condition. About 20% of women in the U.S. get fibrocystic breast disease and then seem to have a higher risk of developing breast cancer.

4. Arginine and ornithine, nutrient amino acids—In mice inoculated with MSV (Moloney Sarcoma Virus, a potent cancer causing agent), arginine and ornithine were able to block formation of tumors. Arginine and ornithine increased the thymus weight in both the MSV and non-MSV injected mice. These two amino acids cause the brain's pituitary gland to release growth hormone, important in the maintenance of the immune system. 3 to 10 grams of arginine (or half as much ornithine as arginine) at bedtime is a reasonable adult daily dose.

CAUTION: If you have a herpes infection: While arginine and ornithine are immune system stimulants, they are also required for viral replication. They may increase the severity of the symptoms. We do not know whether their use during a herpes infection would be beneficial or detrimental. See "The Herpes Epidemic: A Possible Solution" in this book for a way to deal with herpes.

5. L-cysteine, a sulfur-containing amino acid—Cysteine is an immune system stimulant. It is not as powerful as the chemically related thiol, mercaptoethanol, which has been able to restore the immune system function of aged mice (the equivalent of 80 years old for a human) to that of young adult mice; however, we do not have long-term use data for mercaptoethanol and, consequently, more research is needed before people use it on a regular basis.

CAUTION: Do not take supplemental cysteine unless you take at least 3 times as much vitamin C supplement as your total cysteine consumption. In figuring your cysteine consumption, remember that the number of eggs you eat is relevant; each egg contains about ¼ gram of cysteine. While cysteine is quite water soluble, its oxidized form, cystine, is rather insoluble in water. If large amounts of cysteine are taken without the other water soluble antioxidants such as C, and without adequate quantities of fluids, cystine stone formation could conceivably occur in the kidneys and urinary bladder, especially if there is a urinary tract infection. 1 or 2 grams per day of cysteine taken with 3 to 6 grams or more of vitamin C in divided doses are reasonable daily doses for a healthy adult.

6. Zinc, a mineral (taken in chelated form)—Zinc deficiency can cause severe thymus gland shrinkage; this can be reversed with zinc. 50 milligrams of chelated zinc is a reasonable daily dose for adults. Zinc is required to mobilize vitamin A from its storage sites in the liver.

7. Selenium, a mineral—Selenium is an important antioxidant in the body. It is estimated by some researchers studying selenium that if people were to take 200 micrograms per day that the incidence of cancer and cardiovascular disease could be cut by 70% and the incidence of cataracts reduced by 80%. In a 1965 epidemiological study, higher levels of selenium in soil and crops correlated with lower human cancer death rates in the U.S. and Canada. Selenium is an essential part of the antioxidant enzyme glutathione peroxidase, which is important in preventing damage to the immune system and other systems by organic peroxides, like those formed by the abnormal non-enzymatically controlled oxidation (via a free radical route) of body fats and oils. In a number of experiments, selenium has demonstrated powerful anti-carcinogen (inhibits development of cancer) and anti-mutagen (prevents damage to DNA) properties. Sodium selenite is an effective, relatively safe, and the least expensive form.

8. Other growth hormone releasers include serotonin (a neurotransmitter the brain makes from the amino acid tryptophan), Parlodel® (a prescription drug), L-Dopa (a prescription drug amino acid), and vasopressin (a pituitary hormone available in a synthetic form as Diapid®, a prescription drug). In people younger than about 30, vigorous exercise also releases growth hormone. Sleep and moderate fasting are two other stimuli that release growth hormone.

9. Parlodel® was given to a strain of mice which has a very high rate of spontaneous breast cancer. At the doses used, the spontaneous breast cancer rate was reduced to zero. It also reduced the cancer rate of mice given a combustion tar carcinogen (PAH) from 100% to 0%. Hydergine®, a chemically related compound (prescription drug), was also effective in suppressing spontaneous breast cancer in experimental animals. Hydergine® is a powerful antioxidant, possibly the most powerful yet measured.

10. BHT and BHA, antioxidant food additives, inhibited the development of cancer under conditions where there was contact between a carcinogen and a target organ (such as cancer of the stomach in mice fed the PAH carcinogens benzoalphapyrene or dimethylbenzanthracene, found in combustion tar) and also where the target organ was located far from the site of administration of the carcinogen, such as mammary tumors in rats given oral dimethylbenzanthracene. The American Cancer Society has recently made a grant of $900,000 to two scientists at Johns Hopkins Medical School Hospital to study the effectiveness of BHA for both prevention and treatment of cancer in animals and humans.

BHT destroys herpes viruses at doses that do no detectable damage to mammalian cells. Herpes viruses are associated with higher risks of cancers in animals and even in some human cancers, such as nasopharyngeal, uterine, colon, Burkitt's lymphoma, and liver. Scottish deerhounds, a breed of dogs, usually die after only 4-6 years of a type of sarcoma, a muscle tumor. Given BHT, their lifespans were increased to 8-10 years and they did not die of sarcomas, but of the usual causes of death among non-cancer-prone dogs.

BHT, vitamins C and E, and selenium inhibited chromosome breakage by the PAH carcinogen dimethylbenzanthracene.

FAT CONSUMPTION, SMOKING, ALCOHOL, AND RISK OF CANCER

There are specific factors that increase the risks of cancer. A number of studies in experimental animals have shown that an increase in fat consumption, especially of polyunsaturated fats, increases the risk of developing cancer. It is important to take adequate quantities of antioxidants along with any polyunsaturated fats ingested in the diet. Smoking, of course, greatly increases the risks of lung, mouth, and throat cancer. Sidestream smoke, the smoke coming off the burning tip of a cigarette, contains even more carcinogens than the smoke inhaled by the smoker, which is filtered through a tobacco mat. A recent Japanese study showed that women living with a smoking husband had a significantly increased risk of lung cancer compared to women living with a non-smoking husband. Antioxidants, especially beta carotene, have been shown to provide substantial protection against lung cancer. The proper air cleaners (both the HEPA filter type and the electronic precipitator type) can remove smoke and tars from the air.

People that both smoke and drink heavily have much higher cancer risks than people who either smoke or drink. The risks are multiplied, not just added. Alcohol is converted in the liver to acetaldehyde and then to acetate, in the process of detoxification. Acetaldehyde, chemically related to the embalming and tanning agent formaldehyde, is a potent mutagen and carcinogen. In the process of its formation and in its self-catalyzed spontaneous oxidation, acetaldehyde releases free radicals and can chemically convert combustion tars to their carcinogenic epoxides. Antioxidants provide significant protection against these free radicals. Sprince and others gave a group of rats a dose of acetaldehyde large enough to kill 90% of them. To a similar group of rats, he

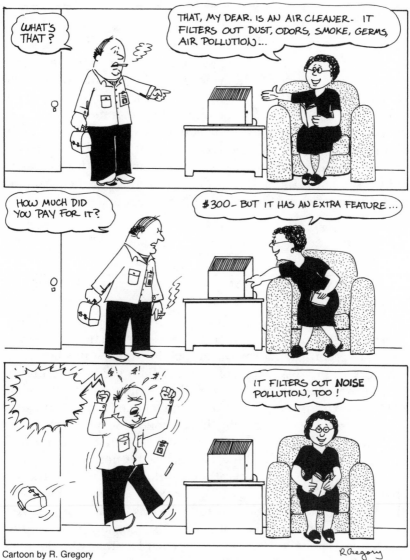

Cartoon by R. Gregory
© 1982 Durk Pearson and Sandy Shaw

gave the same dose of acetaldehyde and also a combination of antioxidants: vitamins B-1 and C and the amino acid cysteine. None of the rats given the antioxidants died. This combination also makes a good hangover remedy. (For more on smoking and drinking, see *Life Extension, A Practical Scientific Approach,* pages 239-258 and 267-283.)

SKIN CANCER

Ultraviolet light (UV) in sunlight is responsible for most cases of skin cancer, which accounts for about 90% of all human cancers. Although generally curable when detected early, skin cancer can be deadly. Many commercially available sunblock remedies now contain esters of PABA (a B vitamin) that provides excellent skin protection by absorbing the ultraviolet light before it has a chance to damage skin cells, especially their DNA. The carotenoids beta carotene and canthaxanthin also provide UV protection.

SMOKING, LUNG CANCER, AND BETA CAROTENE

In a 19 year epidemiological study (comparing populations living under different conditions for particular disease states, e.g., comparing the difference in cancer rates between smokers and non-smokers) of about 2000 men, beta carotene, a carotenoid (which gives carrots their yellow color), provided very powerful protection against lung cancer to both smokers and non-smokers. Men who had smoked 30 years or more who were in the highest carotenoid ingestion quartile had about the same risk of lung cancer as the non-smokers who were below average in carotenoid intake. (However, the lethal cardiovascular effects of smoking were not reduced by the beta carotene.) The carotene in this study was derived from dietary sources. The beta carotene consumption rate in the highest quartile averaged somewhat less than 10,000 units a day. We take 75,000 to 150,000 units a day of beta carotene as a supplement. Although this substance can be converted to vitamin A in the body, there is no danger of hypervitaminosis A (excess vitamin A) because the conversion is under feedback control. The only side effect is yellowing of the skin at high doses. Skin yellowing will not occur at 25,000 I.U. per day.

REFERENCES

Pearson and Shaw, *Life Extension, A Practical Scientific Approach*, Warner, 1982

Anderson et al, "The Effects of Increasing Weekly Doses of Ascorbate on Certain Cellular and Humoral Immune Functions in Normal Volunteers," *Am. J. Clin. Nutr.* 33: 71-76, Jan. 1980

Barbul et al, "Arginine: A Thymotropic and Wound-Healing Promoting Agent," *Surgical Forum* 28: 101-103, 1977

Bjelke, "Dietary Vitamin A and Human Lung Cancer," *Int. J. Cancer* 15: 561-565, 1975

Brown and Reichlin, "Psychologic and Neural Regulation of Growth Hormone Secretion," *Psychosom. Med.* 34 (1): 45-61, 1972

Burnet, *Immunology, Aging, and Cancer*, Freeman, 1976

Campbell, Reade, Radden, "Effect of Cysteine on the Survival of Mice with Transplanted Malignant Thymoma," *Nature* 251: 158-159, 1974

Goetzl et al, "Enhancement of Random Migration and Chemotactic Response of Human Leukocytes by Ascorbic Acid," *J. Clin. Invest.* 53: 813-818, 1974

Spallholz et al, "Immunologic Responses of Mice Fed Diets Supplemented with Selenite Selenium," *Proc. Soc. Exp. Med. Biol.* 143: 685-689, 1973

Pauling, Linus, *Vitamin C, the Common Cold, and the Flu*, Freeman, 1976

Nockels, "Protective Effects of Supplemental Vitamin E Against Infection," paper presented at the 62nd Annual Scientific Meeting (April 9-7 14, 1978) of the Federation of American Societies for Experimental Biology (FASEB)

Khandwala and Gee, "Linoleic Acid Hydroperoxide: Impaired Bacterial Uptake by Alveolar Macrophages, a Mechanism of Oxidant Lung Injury," *Science* 182: 1364-1365, 1973

Marx, Jean L., "Thymic Hormones: Inducers of T Cell Maturation," *Science* 187: 1183, 1975

Borison et al, "Metabolism of an Amino Acid with Antidepressant Properties," *Res. Commun. in Chem. Pathol. and Pharmacol.* 21 (2): 363-366, August 1978

Shekelle et al, "Dietary Vitamin A and Risk of Cancer in the Western Electric Study," *The Lancet*: 1185-1190, 1981

Shamberger, "Is Peroxidation Important in the Cancer Process?" Chapter 33 in *Autoxidation in Food and Biological Systems*, edited by Simic and Karel, Plenum Press, 1980

Shamberger, "Antioxidants in Cereals and in Food Preservatives and Declining Gastric Cancer Mortality," *Cleveland Clinic Quarterly* 39(3): 119-124, 1972

Snipes et al, "BHT Inactivates Lipid-containing Viruses," *Science* 188: 64-66, 1975

Franklyn, "BHT in Sarcoma-prone Dogs," *The Lancet*, p. 1296, 12 June 1976

Sprince, Parker, Smith, Gonzales, "Protectants Against Acetaldehyde Toxicity: Sulfhydryl Compounds and Ascorbic Acid," *Fed. Proc.* 33(3), Pt. 1, March 1974

Sundaram et al, "Alpha-tocopherol and Serum Lipoproteins," *Lipids* 16(4): 223-227, Apr. 1981 [remission of fibrocystic breast disease with alpha tocopherol]

Greeder and Milner, "Factors Influencing the Inhibitory Effect of Selenium on Mice Inoculated with Ehrlich Ascites Tumor Cells," *Science* 209:825-827, 1980

Pecile and Muller, eds., *Growth and Growth Hormone*, Excerpta Medica, 1972

Green, "Cigarette Smoke: Protection of Alveolar Macrophages by Glutathione and Cysteine," *Science* 162: 810-811, 1968

Koreh, Seligman, Demopoulos, "The Effect of Dihydroergotoxine on Lipid Peroxidation in vitro," *Lipids* 17(10): 724-726, 1982

Sasaki, Kurokawa, Tero-Kubota, "Ascorbate Radical and Ascorbic Acid Level in Human Serum and Age," *J. Gerontol* 38(1):26-30, 1983 [The ratio of dehydroascorbic acid to ascorbic acid in serum has never been found higher than 1.0 in human subjects.]

Riley, "Psychoneuroendocrine Influences on Immunocompetence and Neoplasia," *Science* 212: 1100-1109, 1981.

A New Pharmaceutical Marketplace

There are three usual sources of drugs (defined as any substance that alters the body's biological function): (1) prescription, (2) over-the-counter (e.g., aspirin), and (3) under the counter (e.g., cannabis). In recent years, we have seen the development of a growing alternative to these traditional sources of drugs in the health food trade, in which vitamins and other nutrients plus other drugs are offered without seeking FDA approval. Any vitamins sold at levels higher than can be obtained in a good diet may qualify technically as drugs, because the quantities required to catalyze certain metabolic reactions are quite small. Above these amounts, vitamins act as drugs. The same is true of other nutrients offered in health food stores; the doses may be high enough to permit unusual functions that ordinarily, because of limited dietary supply, are not possible. For example, cysteine is a relatively scarce dietary amino acid. The best dietary source is eggs (each egg contains about a quarter gram). This amino acid is useful in a number of ways. It is required in many proteins, such as insulin. Cysteine also acts as a potent antioxidant in the body. It also constitutes about 8% of human hair. Since cysteine is in such limited quantity in typical human diets, it is used by the body for the most important functions first. Hair is probably the very last to get its share. However, if a person supplements his or her diet with cysteine, it is possible for hair to have an abundance of cysteine. A person's head of hair may even be doubled in density. (See "Better Hair and Better Health with Cysteine" in this book. Also, see *Life Extension, A Practical Scientific Approach*, especially page 217 and pages 758-759 in the case histories section.)

The Proxmire Act of the early 1970's spared the vendors of vitamins and other nutrients the requirement that they have FDA approval before making them available to consumers. Thus, drugs which are also nutrients are not necessarily subject to tight FDA restrictions which result in an average truly new drug taking 8–12 years and about $50 million to achieve approval and reach the marketplace.

There are other substances offered in health food stores, however, which constitute yet another category of drug-non-nutrient chemicals which never received FDA approval, but which seem to be offered with impunity nevertheless. A good example is DMSO. DMSO is not a nutrient (although it does occur naturally in beets). It was offered in health food and drugstores long before it received limited approval as a pharmaceutical. (RIMSO-50® is listed in the 1982 *Physician's Desk Reference* and is FDA approved only for "symptomatic relief of interstitial cystitis.") It continues to be offered without a prescription at health food stores. Although the FDA has declared it illegal to continue to sell DMSO for drug use without a prescription, it is still being offered all over the United States. The 18 & 25 December 1982 *Science News* says that an estimated 5 to 10% of the U.S. population is using non-prescription DMSO solutions to treat muscle strains, arthritis, and the like.

The FDA has made no serious attempt to control DMSO sales. In fact, it could not do so because it would never be able to shut down the small fly-by-night firms offering the material by mail order. And the cost of any attempt to sweep DMSO out of stores would be astronomical. Canthaxanthin, which is a natural carotenoid nutrient, is only approved in this country as a food coloring agent, but it is sold, mostly by mail order, as a sun tanning pill. Although the FDA alleges this is illegal, it has not successfully halted these sales. Yet another example is BHT, a synthetic antioxidant approved as a food additive, but being sold all over the U.S. for use against herpes infections

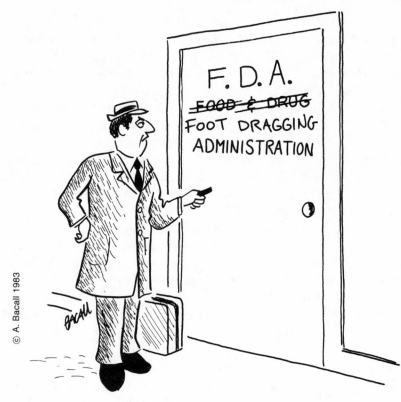

© A. Bacall 1983

(see "The Herpes Epidemic: A Possible Solution"). The marketing strategies of two would-be vendors of "sober up" products are discussed in "Sobriety Aid Marketers Seeking Cure for FDA" on page 35 of the 20 December 1982 issue of *Advertising Age.* One is proceeding with an application for FDA drug approval, while the other is redesigning their label and advertising to position it as a health food store nutrient supplement. Guess which product will be the first to reach the market?

As long as no claims are made on the label, it is possible to market these unapproved drugs. Books, other media, and health food store personnel make the claims which motivate consumers to go buy these substances. The FDA's powers are limited. We recently saw DMSO that had been packaged in an underarm roll-on style bottle. The marketers told us that the FDA required that they remove from the label the designation that the DMSO was 99.996% pure and that it had been purchased from a French pharmaceutical company, but they couldn't make them change the dispensing bottle! What did the FDA accomplish by these actions? The FDA simply made it easier for vendors of potentially hazardous industrial solvent grade DMSO to compete against the high purity product which could no longer be identified as such. The FDA claims that they are "protecting the consumer" by doing this.

What about future offerings? A prime substance to be sold in this fashion is a CCK nasal spray for weight control. CCK is cholecystokinin, a natural hypothalamic and polypep-

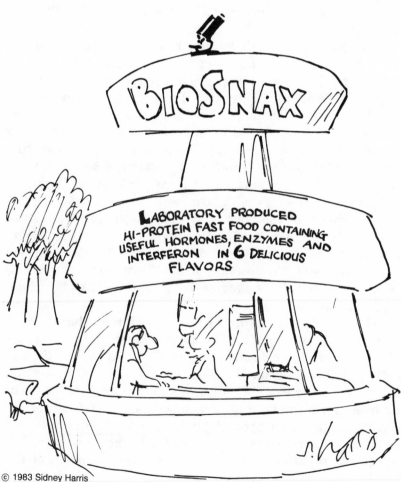

BioSNAX

LABORATORY PRODUCED HI-PROTEIN FAST FOOD CONTAINING USEFUL HORMONES, ENZYMES AND INTERFERON IN 6 DELICIOUS FLAVORS

tide (amino acids connected together in a particular pattern) gut hormone that is released after a meal to signal satiation. A rat given enough CCK will never eat, even with food piled up around it, and will eventually starve to death. On the other hand, preventing the release of CCK in a rat will result in the rat eating and eating until its gut explodes and it dies. Although it is known that CCK works as the satiation signal in humans as well, more animal experiments and double blind, placebo controlled human clinical trials must be conducted to determine proper dose levels and safety factors for weight control. For people who are not eating enough, such as anorexia nervosa victims during the starvation phase, monoclonal antibodies against CCK might be an effective treatment.

We see, therefore, that a fourth source of drugs is rapidly emerging: new health food store offerings packaged without therapeutic label claims or package inserts, the labels merely stating the contents. This new development is not an unmixed blessing. Many new health food store products are worthless and a few could even be hazardous (e.g., capsules containing easily peroxidized polyunsaturated oils). Nevertheless, the FDA's approach to drug regulation is so bad that, in many respects, no regulation at all is preferable. Thanks to the FDA and the excessively stringent Kefauver drug approval amendments of 1962, we now find ourselves in the bizarre situation of new drugs being developed, manufactured, prescribed, and sold entirely outside of the health profession. We do *not* welcome the absence of health professionals in this new market. But this is a logical result of the FDA's "consumer protection."

One important feature of the prescription pharmaceutical market is the use of FDA approved drugs for purposes different from their approved uses. (See also the "Fallacies" section of this book for the FDA's new policy statement on this subject.) For example, propranolol is approved for treating heart arrhythmias and high blood pressure. It is not approved for the treatment of phobias, for which it has been shown in numerous human clinical trials (most conducted in Europe) to be effective. Diapid®, a synthetic version of the

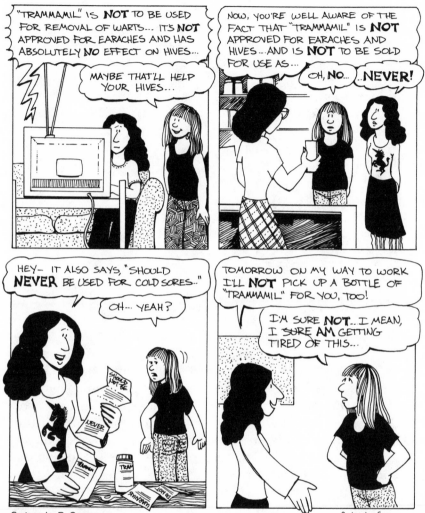

Cartoon by R. Gregory
© 1982 Durk Pearson and Sandy Shaw

natural hormone vasopressin, is approved to treat diabetes insipidus, not for the improvement of human memory and learning. Hydergine® is approved only for the treatment of Alzheimer's disease and of selected symptoms in the elderly, not to prevent sickle cell anemia attacks or to improve human intelligence. Once a drug has been approved for a particular purpose, costing on the average about $50 million and taking

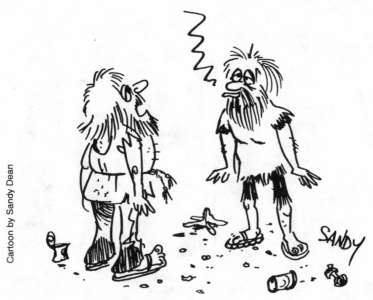

Cartoon by Sandy Dean

"I *know* laetrile is illegal, but it *still* won't get ya high, no matter how you use it"

about 8 to 12 years, receiving approval for another purpose costs additional tens of millions of dollars and usually takes several years more. A strategy we have seen some pharmaceutical manufacturers taking is to get a new drug approved for any purpose that is likely to receive approval, even if the market for that use is small, knowing that information about other, non-approved uses, will eventually reach physician publications. Physicians may legally prescribe an FDA approved drug for any purpose (with the exception of "controlled substances" such as narcotics), whether the FDA has approved that particular use or not.

The Physician's Desk Reference, a very useful book, contains information only on the FDA approved uses for the pharmaceuticals described therein. Basically, the book is a collection of FDA approved (censored) pharmaceutical package inserts. Other publications are emerging that provide information on non-approved uses. We expect these sources to become even more widely circulated among physicians and their patients, who should work together in the use of such sources.

REFERENCES

Pearson and Shaw, *Life Extension, A Practical Scientific Approach*, Warner Books, 1982

Landau, Richard, editor, *Regulating New Drugs*, Univ. of Chicago Center for Policy Study, 1973 [See particularly pp. 113-211 by Peltzman]

"Sobriety Aid Marketers Seeking Cure for FDA," *Advertising Age*, 20 December 1982, pg. 35

Much good data on unapproved uses for approved drugs may be found in:

Trends in Pharmacological Sciences, Elsevier/North Holland, Inc., 52 Vanderbilt Ave., New York, NY 10164, $42.50/12 issues; aimed toward the research scientist and clinical research oriented physician

Medical Hotline, 119 W. 57th St., New York, NY 10019, $24/year, telephone orders to (212)977-9585; aimed toward physicians and intelligent laymen (who should work together in the use of this information) with an emphasis on new unapproved uses for approved drugs

Selenium, An Anti-Cancer, Anti-Aging Nutrient

Selenium, a trace mineral, has recently become the focus of a number of research studies. Results of studies already completed indicate that selenium, taken in the proper doses, may greatly reduce the susceptibility of animals and humans to the development of cancer and cardiovascular disease. In fact, it is thought by some scientists doing ground breaking work in this area that the risk for these conditions as well as for cataracts could be reduced by 70% or so by regular supplements of selenium of about 200 micrograms a day. This tiny amount of selenium costs only a fraction of a cent.

Epidemiological studies are surveys of particular populations to observe the patterns of disease occurrence and how they relate to other factors, such as nutrition. In epidemiological studies involving several large cities in the United States and Canada, scientists found that the incidence of cancer was inversely proportional to the amount of selenium in the drinking water. That is, larger amounts of selenium were associated with smaller incidences of cancer. Other variables might also be at work, and more extensively controlled studies need to be carried out with humans. In feeding studies, experimental animals receiving supplements of selenium along with carcinogens such as polynuclear aromatic hydrocarbons (the product of the burning of fuels, tobacco, etc.) developed fewer cancers than controls (animals receiving a normal diet with no selenium supplement which were exposed to the same carcinogens).

Selenium is an antioxidant. That is, it can react with oxidants such as free radicals, chemically reactive entities with an unpaired electron, to prevent their reaction with sensitive cellular components (such as DNA, RNA, enzymes, cell membranes, and fats), which would be damaged in such reactions. Selenium is required as part of the antioxidant enzyme glutathione peroxidase, an important substance in cellular free radical control mechanisms. Each molecule of glutathione peroxidase requires four atoms of selenium. This enzyme helps prevent the formation and accumulation of toxic, mutagenic (mutation causing), carcinogenic (cancer-causing) substances, such as peroxidized (rancid) fat. Organic peroxides have been shown to promote the development of

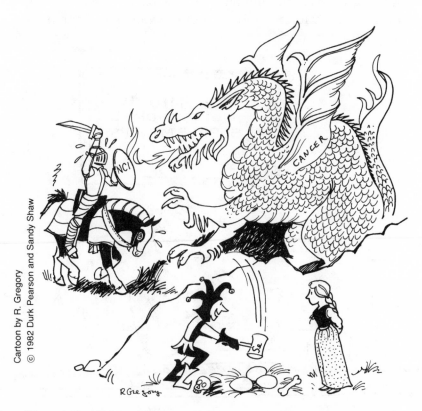

Cartoon by R. Gregory
© 1982 Durk Pearson and Sandy Shaw

"*Preventative Medicine:* It just seems to make a lot more sense."

cancer, damage DNA, inhibit the immune system (which is responsible for destroying cancers, atherosclerotic plaques, bacteria, and viruses), and promote the formation of abnormal blood clots and atherosclerotic plaques.

A relatively nontoxic form of selenium that may be used is the inorganic form, sodium selenite. Two common organic forms of selenium, selenomethionine and selenocystine, are potentially more toxic because the body cannot readily separate selenomethionine and selenocystine from your normal sulfur-containing amino acids and may make a mistake by incorporating the selenium-containing amino acids into a protein where it is not supposed to be. Such proteins may not function properly because of the differing electronic distributions of selenocystine and cysteine, for example. These substitutions do not occur with moderate doses of inorganic sodium selenite, as long as the animal does not have a severe sulfur amino acid (methionine and cysteine) deficiency. Your body

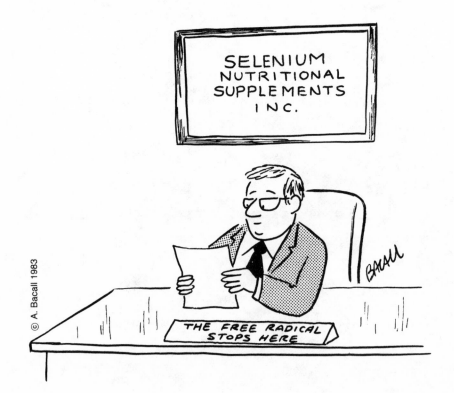

cannot directly use selenium-containing amino acids in glutathione peroxidase; they must first be broken down into inorganic selenium. Hence, we take the inorganic sodium selenite directly. The FDA recognizes 50 to 200 micrograms of selenium as a safe daily dose. Higher doses should only be taken with the advice of a physician. A common early symptom of selenium overdose is garlic breath, urine, and sweat.

REFERENCES

Pearson and Shaw, *Life Extension, A Practical Scientific Approach*, Warner, 1982

Schrauzer, "Selenium and Cancer: A Review," *Bioinorg. Chem.* 5:275-281, 1976

Latshaw and Biggert, "Incorporation of Selenium into Egg Proteins After Feeding Selenomethionine or Sodium Selenite," *Poultry Science* 60: 1309-1313, 1981

Greeder and Milner, "Factors Influencing the Inhibitory Effect of Selenium on Mice Inoculated with Ehrlich Ascites Tumor Cells," *Science* 209: 825-826, 1980

Sunde and Hoekstra, "Structure, Synthesis and Function of Glutathione Peroxidase," *Nutr Rev* 38(8): 265-273, 1980

Spallholz et al, "Immunologic Responses of Mice Fed Diets Supplemented with Selenite Selenium," *Proc. Soc. Exp. Med. Biol.* 143: 685-689, 1973

Shamberger, "Relationship of Selenium to Cancer. I. Inhibitory Effect of Selenium on Carcinogenesis," *J. Nat'l. Cancer Institute* 44(4): 931-936, April 1970

McBrien and Slater, eds., *Free Radicals, Lipid Peroxidation and Cancer*, Academic Press, 1982

Smith, *Autoxidation*, Plenum Press, 1981

O. H. Muth, in *Selenium in Biomedicine*, O. H. Muth et al, Eds. (Avi, Westport, Conn., 1967), pp. 2-6 [Muth states that at least half of states in the U.S. have deficient selenium availability such that selenium-responsive deficiency diseases may be detected in farm animals. In general, farm animals are provided better nutrition than are humans.]

Better Hair and Better Health with Cysteine

This chapter is about a remarkable amino acid nutrient that can extend animal life span, increase the growth rate of human hair, decrease significantly the health risks of smoking and drinking, stimulate the body's disease-fighting immune system, and block reactive hypoglycemia. Cysteine, a sulfur-containing amino acid, can do all these things and more. Scientists have discovered a good deal about *how* cysteine produces these results, too. Below we tell you about some of these effects and their molecular causes.

Cysteine is relatively uncommon in our food supply. The best dietary source is eggs, which contain about 250 milligrams of cysteine per egg. We have each been taking a supplement of 2 grams per day of this amino acid for the past ten years. We use it in the form of pure crystals of cysteine hydrochloride monohydrate that we buy directly from a manufacturer. It is now available as an individual supplement in some health food or drugstores. Interestingly, cysteine is usually obtained by extracting it from hair, of which it comprises 8%.

Cysteine gives hair its structural form and shape because of the chemistry of its sulfur-to-hydrogen (sulfhydryl) bond. When the sulfur in the sulfhydryl group bonds to another such sulfur, the process is called cross-linking and creates a sulfur-sulfur (disulfide) bond. (Such sulfur-sulfur bonds are also

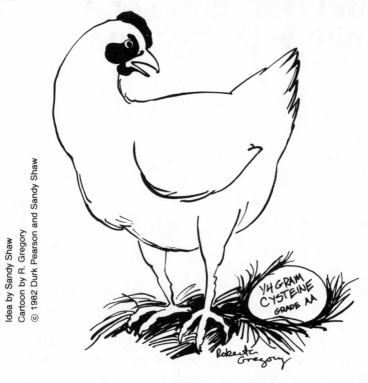

Idea by Sandy Shaw
Cartoon by R. Gregory
© 1982 Durk Pearson and Sandy Shaw

created in the process of vulcanization which turns soft latex gum into a hard rubber comb.) Cross-linking of hair is desirable. However, abnormal uncontrolled cross-linking is an important mechanism of aging, as we explain later.

The amino acid cysteine is a particularly limiting factor in hair growth because it is in relatively short supply even in a person eating a good diet. The best dietary source for cysteine is eggs; an egg contains about ¼ gram of cysteine. We use cysteine crystals purchased from a Japanese manufacturer of amino acids. Many people with thin or slow growing hair have reported readily noticeable improvements with a 1 to 2 gram per day cysteine supplement. In some cases, the amount of hair has been doubled. (See *Life Extension, A Practical Scientific Approach*, case histories in Appendix L, pp. 757-759.) Male pattern baldness is caused by a developmental aging clock, not by cysteine deficiency. The progression of male pattern baldness can be readily stopped, and in most cases significant hair regrowth can be achieved by using the proper techniques. (Complete how-to-do-it information is given in *Life Extension, A Practical Scientific Approach*, pp. 212-221.)

Another thing you can do to promote longer, thicker hair is to prevent free radical damage to hair follicles. Free radicals are highly chemically reactive molecules (or atoms) with an unpaired electron. These are formed during normal metabolism and as a result of various pathological processes, including as a byproduct of non-enzymatic fat autoxidation (self-catalyzed oxidation of fats, resulting in what is commonly

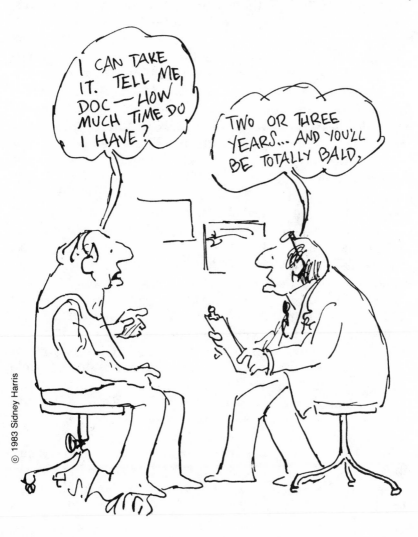

© 1983 Sidney Harris

called rancid fats). The scalp contains a considerable quantity of fatty materials which may become oxidized due to exposure to oxygen in the air. Dandruff is an example of a condition resulting from free radical damage. The organic peroxides formed as a result of the oxidation of the scalp's lipids (fats and oils) are irritants. The skin cells in contact with these irritant organic peroxides are stimulated into excess cell division, resulting in the proliferation of excess skin cells, which fall off as dandruff when pushed out by other skin cells growing underneath. Free radicals can also "turn off" or destroy hair follicles or their pigment-producing melanocytes. Free radicals are mutagens (cause mutations) and carcinogens (cancer causing). Use of shampoos containing antioxidants (substances which block uncontrolled oxidation reactions) such as zinc (zinc pyrithione, Head and Shoulders® shampoo) or selenium compounds (selenium sulfide, Selsun Blue® shampoo) provide some protection against free radical damage to hair follicles and may result in a thicker, more luxuriant hair growth. Use of oral supplements of sodium selenite (200 micrograms per day), chelated zinc (50 milligrams per day), and vitamin E (1000 I.U. per day) often provides dramatic relief from dandruff, itchy scalp, and rancid hair odors. Cysteine is a potent antioxidant which, in addition to acting as a structural part of hair, can also help protect hair follicles from free radical damage.

CAUTION: When you do take cysteine for hair or any of the other purposes we discuss here, it is important to make sure that you do not take supplemental cysteine unless you take at least 3 times as much vitamin C supplement as your total cysteine consumption. In figuring your cysteine consumption, remember that the number of eggs you eat is relevant; each egg contains about ¼ gram of cysteine. While cysteine is quite water soluble, its oxidized form, cystine, is rather insoluble in water. If large amounts of cysteine are taken without the other water soluble antioxidants such as C, and without adequate quantities of fluids, cystine stone formation could conceivably occur in the kidneys and urinary bladder, especially if there is a urinary tract infection.

Antioxidants like cysteine and the vitamins A, C, E, B-1, B-5, B-6, and the minerals zinc and selenium can do a good

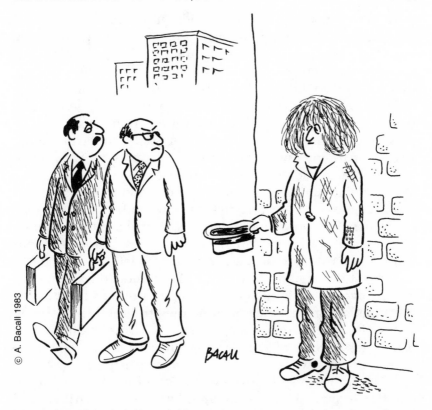

© A. Bacall 1983

"Just look at all that hair. He probably spends every cent on cysteine, zinc, sodium selenite, and vitamin C."

many things to improve our health. Research has shown that they can provide protection against the most important of the damage mechanisms that cause aging, cancer and cardiovascular disease. These antioxidants and others block some of the damage of free radicals, implicated as causative factors in aging, cancer, cardiovascular disease, and other pathological conditions. Radiation (except for neutrons) sickness is caused entirely by free radical damage. But most of the free radicals in our bodies do not come from exposure to radiation. Free radicals are created by our bodies as natural parts of many biochemical pathways, as mentioned earlier. Our bodies contain several potent antioxidant enzymes (e.g., superoxide dismutase, glutathione peroxidase, and catalase) and antioxidant nutrients such as cysteine to provide protection against these free radicals. Unfortunately, such protection isn't perfect and, over the years, our bodies are damaged. For example, your body's manufacture of prostacyclin, a natural anti-clot hormone found in healthy arteries, can be prevented by free radicals and free radical generated organic peroxides. In one study, cysteine increased the survival rate of mice and guinea pigs (but not female rats). In another study, the average life span of male mice was increased significantly by 25% when given large supplements (1%) to their diet.

Cysteine can also inhibit the cross-linking reactions described above. These enzymatically uncontrolled reactions, which can be caused by free radicals, contribute to hardening of the arteries and to skin wrinkling. These same reactions cause the hardening of plastic containers left out in the sun and the stiffening and brittleness of automobile rubber parts as they age. Undesirable cross-linking of proteins can destroy the function of enzymes or alter the structural property of supportive connective tissue (collagen). Cross-linking of nucleic acids (DNA and RNA) can result in improper cell function, which may cause cell death or even cancer.

The immune system is a collection of entities which patrol the body, looking for enemies like bacteria, viruses, and cancer cells, which are then killed and eaten. The system includes the thymus gland (behind the breastbone), several types of white blood cells, and your own chemical disease-fighters like antibodies, interferon, and complement. As people age, the ability of their immune systems to stave off these enemies declines. Part of the reason for this is that free radicals inhibit the activity of parts of the immune system, such as macrophages (a type of white blood cell). Several antioxidants, including cysteine, are able to stimulate aspects of immune system performance. In animal studies, cysteine has shown the ability to increase survival of animals given transplanted tumors. Cysteine also provides powerful protection against radiation damage.

Cysteine helps prevent damage in smokers and drinkers, too. The damage caused by smoking and drinking is largely due to the creation of free radicals. Alcohol is metabolized by the liver into acetaldehyde. This acetaldehyde is what causes the harm we blame on alcohol, including hangovers. Acetaldehyde is easily autoxidized (it stimulates its own free radical chain reaction oxidation), in the process of which free radicals are created. That horrible hangover in the morning has symptoms similar to radiation sickness because they are caused by the same type of damaging agent: free radicals. Tobacco smoke contains acetaldehyde and other aldehydes which produce free radicals that can cause cross-linking and other damage. Emphysema is caused at least in part by such cross-linking of lung tissues. Dr. Herbert Sprince and others found that the combination of vitamins B-1, C, and cysteine was a very potent one for protection against acetaldehyde. He gave one group of rats a dose of acetaldehyde large enough to kill 90% of the animals; he gave another group of rats the same dose of acetaldehyde and B-1, C, and cysteine. None of the rats receiving the nutrient combination died. Cysteine alone prevented the death of 80% of rats in a similar group receiving the same dose of acetaldehyde.

Cysteine is a strong reducing agent (it can prevent oxidation of some other substances). In fact, it has been found that too much cysteine in a cell culture medium can inactivate the hormone insulin contained in the medium. The insulin molecule contains three disulfide bonds, at least one of which can be reduced by cysteine. When this happens, the insulin molecule can no longer maintain the proper shape to function normally to stimulate the metabolism of sugar. In hypoglycemia attacks there is too much insulin and too little sugar in the blood stream. Cysteine can inactivate insulin, thereby allowing the sugar level to begin to rise again. We and others have used the combination of B-1, C, and cysteine to successfully abort severe attacks of hypoglycemia. A reasonable dose for a healthy adult is 5 grams of C, 1 gram of B-1, and 1 gram of cysteine.

CAUTION: Although cysteine is a nutrient, its use on a long-term basis should be considered *experimental*. Start with a low dose (250 milligrams per day) and work your way up. Always use at least three times as much vitamin C as cysteine. Be sure to consult with your physician and have regular clinical tests of basic body functions, especially liver and kidney.

WARNING: Diabetics should not use cysteine supplements due to its anti-insulin effects, except under the guidance of their physician.

Cysteine or cystine? Many nutritional supplements contain cystine rather than cysteine. Does cystine work as well as cysteine? Frankly, we don't know for sure. We do know that the bioavailability of large doses of cystine may be a problem; although cysteine is freely soluble in water, cystine is relatively insoluble, only 112 milligrams dissolving in a liter of water at 25 degrees C. We also know that cystine (but not cysteine) can form dangerous kidney and bladder stones. We know that your body must chemically reduce cystine to cysteine before you can use it. Finally, all of our experimental experience has been with cysteine rather than cystine, and the reports that we have found in the scientific life extension literature have also dealt with cysteine. Personally, we would not use cystine with our present state of knowledge, but we do use cysteine.

REFERENCES

Pearson and Shaw, *Life Extension, A Practical Scientific Approach*, Warner, 1982

Sprince, H., Parker, C., Smith, G., "L-Ascorbic Acid in Alcoholism and Smoking: Protection Against Acetaldehyde Toxicity As an Experimental Model," *Int. J. Vit. Nutr. Res.* 47 (Suppl 1G): 185-212, 1977

Hayashi, Larner, Sato, "Hormonal Growth Control of Cells in Culture," *In Vitro* 14 (1): 23-30, 1978

Oeriu, Vochitu, "The Effect of the Administration of Compounds Which Contain Sulfhydryl Groups on the Survival Rates of Mice, Rats, and Guinea Pigs," *J. Gerontol.* 20: 417-419, 1965

Harman, "Free Radical Theory of Aging: Effect of Free Radical Reaction Inhibitors on the Mortality Rate of Male LAF$_1$ Mice," *J. Geront.* 23 (4): 476-482, 1968

Harman, "Role of Free Radicals in Mutation, Cancer, Aging, and the Maintenance of Life," *Radiation Res.* 16: 753-764, 1962

Campbell, Reade, Radden, "Effect of Cysteine on the Survival of Mice with Transplanted Malignant Thymoma," *Nature* 251: 158, 1974

Sprince, Parker, Smith, Gonzales, "Protective Action of Ascorbic Acid and Sulfur Compounds against Acetaldehyde Toxicity: Implications in Alcoholism and Smoking," *Agents and Actions* 5 (2): 164-173, 1975

Bacq and Alexander, "Importance for Radio-protection of the Reaction of Cells to Sulfhydryl and Disulphide Compounds," *Nature* 203: 162-164, 1964

Bjorksten, Johan, "The Crosslinkage Theory of Aging as a Predictive Indicator," *Rejuvenation* VIII (3): 59-66, 1980

Bjorksten, Johan, "The Crosslinkage Theory of Aging," *J. Amer. Geriatrics Soc* 16: 408-427, 1968

Verzar, "The Aging of Collagen," *Scientific American*, pp. 2-8, April 1963

Green, "Cigarette Smoke: Protection of Alveolar Macrophages by Glutathione and Cysteine," *Science* 162: 810-811, 1968

Improving Your Skin's Health and Appearance with Nutrients

The skin is the largest and most visible of your body's organs, subject to all the aging mechanisms of other organs and, in addition, exposed to and damaged by the sun's ultraviolet light. Your skin's health and good looks depend on a complex interaction between various biochemical systems. We report here two major mechanisms of skin aging and some actions that can be taken to correct them.

Young skin tends to be smooth, soft, and supple, whereas old skin tends to be rough, hard, and inelastic. These changes are caused by two major factors: (1) Cross-linking: this is the same process as tanning, in which skin is converted into leather by forming chemical bonds that link macromolecules such as collagen, a protein, together. Although some cross-linking is normal and necessary, sometimes it occurs in an uncontrolled manner, forming undesirable cross-linking chemical bonds. In arteries, cross-linking contributes to hardening of the arteries. Skin cross-linking is caused largely by ultraviolet light and free radicals. (2) A loss of the skin's ability to bind and hold water; the missing moisturizing ingredient is water, not oil. You can demonstrate this for yourself by suspending an old piece of hard shoe leather in a glass of oil, and another piece in a glass of water. After allowing the pieces of leather to soak overnight, examine them. The water-soaked strip will be soft, whereas the oil-soaked strip will still be hard.

Old skin holds less water for two reasons: cross-linked prot ___ such as collagen in skin have fewer water binding sites (as in old, hardened Jell-O®, which "weeps"), and older skin has less of the specific natural water binding moisturizer compounds.

The skin contains natural moisturizers, the most important being NaPCA (the sodium salt of pyrollidone carboxylic acid). By the time a person reaches old age, his or her skin contains only about half the amount that a healthy young person's skin has. NaPCA is a remarkable substance. If a quantity of dry powdered NaPCA is placed in a bowl in the middle of the Sahara desert, it soon becomes a puddle because it absorbs moisture from the dry desert air. NaPCA can sometimes be found in premium grade cosmetics, but it is not easy to find even though it has FDA approval for this purpose. Apparently, the cosmetics industry has not discovered this substance yet (possibly due to poor marketing by its manufacturer). See the supplier section of this book for sources of NaPCA. For best results, it should be used in a cosmetic formulation in which it constitutes about 10% and in which there are cosolvent carriers and surfactants to get the NaPCA into the skin; in 50% aqueous solution, NaPCA is sticky and non-penetrating and, therefore, unsuitable for comfortable use on skin. Use of NaPCA in a properly compounded cosmetic gives skin a moist, youthful "glow." Note that this is *not* a cosmetic coverup; it is a physiological correction of an age-related deficiency state. We ourselves develop cosmetic formulations on a contract R & D basis, and this is helping to support our research. We currently have a NaPCA skin lotion formula available on a non-exclusive basis.

Skin contains more unsaturated fats than any other organ in the human body, after only the brain and spinal cord. Unsaturated fats are highly susceptible to damage by uncontrolled nonenzymatic oxidation reactions, which makes the skin subject to cross-linking damage. Fats which have been damaged in this process are called rancid (the layperson's description), autoxidized (self-catalyzed oxidation), or peroxidized (organic peroxides contain highly reactive -O-O- groups). Peroxidized (rancid) fats are cross-linkers, mutagens (can damage DNA) and carcinogens (cancer-causing substances). The damage is done largely via the formation, dur-

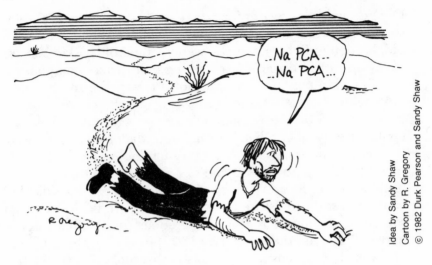

ing the breakdown of the peroxidized fats, of highly reactive entities called free radicals. Free radicals are implicated as causative agents in aging, cardiovascular disease, cancer, arthritis, the damage from strokes, skin wrinkling, and in many other pathological conditions.

The skin and the rest of the body contain special protective enzymes (e.g., superoxide dismutase, catalase, glutathione peroxidase) and antioxidants (nutrients such as vitamins A, E, C, B-1, B-5, B-6, beta carotene, the amino acid cysteine, glutathione, and the minerals zinc and selenium) which are major defenses against free radical damage. The quantities of antioxidants which you can obtain in a natural diet are very limited. Antioxidant supplements can provide even greater protection to the unsaturated fats in your skin, brain, and other tissues.

Vitamin A, in addition to being an important antioxidant, increases your skin's supplies of receptors for the natural growth and healing hormone, EGF (epidermal growth factor). Even by the standards of the FDA's minimal Recommended Dietary Allowances, about 40% of the U.S. population is vitamin A deficient. Vitamin A is very important for the regulation of the growth and repair of epithelial tissue (rapidly dividing cells lining skin, lung, mouth, nose, and gut).

Deficiency of vitamin A increases susceptibility of these tissues to carcinogenesis (development of cancer) and to cancer promoters. Indeed, in the case of certain carcinogens, vitamin A can actually reverse the earliest stages in the process by which normal skin cells are transformed to cancerous cells. Serum levels of the antioxidant nutrients are depressed in smokers and drinkers; both the latter groups exhibit a greatly elevated incidence of epithelial cancer.

CAUTION: Excess intake of vitamin A can be hazardous. Early symptoms of hypervitaminosis A are: sparse, coarse hair; loss of hair on the eyebrows; dry, rough skin; headache; irritability; and cracked lips (especially at the corners). If

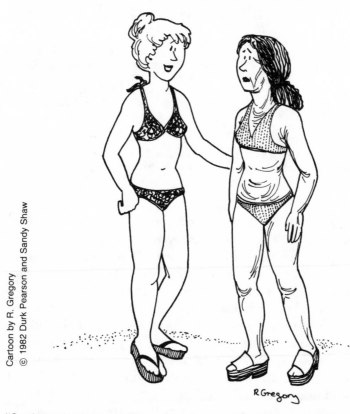

Cartoon by R. Gregory
© 1982 Durk Pearson and Sandy Shaw

R Gregory

"Canthaxanthin may not be the *most* natural way to get a tan . . . but then, wrinkles are a little *too* natural for me!"

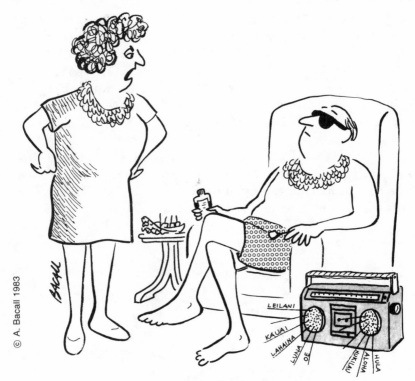

"Well, eating pineapples, wearing a lei, listening to Don Ho tapes, and using canthaxanthin is not a substitute Hawaiian vacation in my book."

these symptoms occur, reduce or temporarily eliminate your dose of vitamin A. The use of other antioxidants along with vitamin A increases the time for vitamin A to be destroyed in the body by oxidation, so people taking antioxidant supplements may need less vitamin A. Zinc is required by the liver to mobilize its stores of vitamin A; a dose of 50 milligrams of chelated zinc a day is reasonable to take along with vitamin A.

Vitamin B-5 (calcium pantothenate or pantothenic acid), vitamin B-1 (thiamine), and vitamin H (biotin) are central to the synthesis of essential skin lipids (fats and oils). A number of people we know who take relatively large doses of these vitamins frequently tell us that they have received compliments about the appearance of their skin within a few weeks of beginning the use of these supplements. Reasonable adult daily total doses (taken in four divided doses during the day) are 1 milligram of biotin, 1 gram of B-5, and 1 gram of B-1.

Exposure to the sun's UV (ultraviolet) light causes most wrinkling and other visible signs of skin aging in people who neither smoke nor drink. Smoking and drinking cause extensive free radical-induced cross-linking of skin and other tissues. The antioxidant nutrients also provide protection against damage due to UV. Beta carotene, the carotenoid which gives carrots their yellow color, is used by people who have erythropoietic protoporphyria (a condition of hypersensitivity to sunlight) to provide UV protection; it has been reported that some such people, who could not go into the sun at all before using beta carotene, can even develop a suntan! Similar results have been reported in human victims of xeroderma pigmentosa, a genetic defect in UV damage repair. The only problem with beta carotene is that it can color your skin yellow or orange. Another carotenoid, canthaxanthin, is available in Canada (Orobronze®, Rohrer) as a way of getting a suntan without going into the sun because canthaxanthin colors the skin a beautiful golden-bronze color over a period of a few weeks; it also provides UV protection to the skin.

The skin provides a unique window into the brain because of the similarities between nerve and skin cells, which are derived during fetal development from the same cell type. The brain, which contains a great deal of highly unsaturated fats, also requires plenty of antioxidants to maintain function and slow aging there. Smoking- and drinking-caused skin damage is a reflection of similar damage in the brain caused by the same underlying free radical mechanisms.

REFERENCES

Pearson and Shaw, *Life Extension, A Practical Scientific Approach*, Warner, 1982

"The Salts of PCA and Their Moisturizing Effects," Technical Bulletin, Ajinomoto Company (with 8 references)

Jetten, "Retinoids Specifically Enhance the Number of Epidermal Growth Factor Receptors," *Nature* 284: 626-631, 17 April 1980

Tanzer, "Cross-linking of Collagen," *Science* 180: 561-566, 1973 Elden, ed., *Biophysical Properties of the Skin,* Wiley Interscience, 1971

Verzar, "The Aging of Collagen," *Sci. Amer.*, April 1963

Laden and Spitzer, "Identification of a Natural Moisturizing Agent in Skin," *J. Soc. Cosmet. Chemists* 18: 351, 1967

New Views on Pollution

One fascinating thing about science is that you are sometimes confronted with surprises, data which don't fit earlier thinking or which even appear to contradict what you think you already know. Then you have to decide whether your old model needs modification, or possibly even abandonment.

Consider, for example, these recent findings about radiation and pollution:

1. The average life spans of rats were increased when they were continually exposed to levels of radiation about three times normal background. (At higher levels, average life spans are decreased.)

2. There was no detectable increase in genetic defects or cancer levels in multi-generation studies of rats exposed to radiation at levels about three times normal background.

3. In one region of China (as recently reported in *Science*), the population lives at a level of natural background radiation three times that of populations in surrounding areas. No significant difference in cancer rates or birth defects has been found in this large-scale human epidemiological study.

4. Which city do you think has the highest cancer rate? Birmingham, Alabama; Pittsburgh, Pennsylvania; Newark, New Jersey; Los Angeles, California; or San Francisco, California? Curiously, the city with the lowest level of air pollution by far—San Francisco—has the highest cancer incidence, ad-

justed for population age distribution. Newark, New Jersey, which twenty miles downwind still smells like an oil refinery, has the same incidence of cancer as the United States as a whole.

These are data which do not fit the popular media theories of radiation and pollution effects, namely, that every level of radiation is unsafe and causes cancer and that we have to control all air pollution because it causes cancer. But these seemingly confusing results do fit into an emerging understanding of some of the biochemical events in the interaction between living organisms and radiation and other pollutants.

Damage from ionizing radiation such as x-rays is an example of a free radical disease. Radiation kills by creating free radicals, molecules or atoms with an unpaired electron, which are extremely chemically reactive and dangerous. These free radicals are mutagens (cause mutations) and carcinogens (cause cancer) when they damage DNA. They attack fats in the body, causing them to become peroxidized (rancid) fats which, besides being mutagens, carcinogens, atherogens (atherosclerosis-causing), thrombogens (clot promoting), and immune suppressants, can break down to form more free radicals, causing a free radical chain reaction of further damage. But external radiation is not usually an important source of free radical damage to organisms. Free radical reactions are a necessary part of normal metabolism. For example, the manufacture of ATP (the universal energy storage molecule) requires free radical reactions. Thus, free radicals are constantly created in the body and, as suggested by Dr. Denham Harman (the originator of the free radical theory of aging), can be considered internal radiation. In fact, all air breathing organisms on this planet have elaborate defense and control systems for free radicals.

But free radical control systems are not perfect and damage occurs throughout life. Free radicals are now considered by scientists studying them to be major causative factors in aging, cardiovascular disease, cancer, arthritis, immune system incompetence, and other less serious conditions including bruises and even dandruff. Our sophisticated free radical control system includes special antioxidant enzymes such as

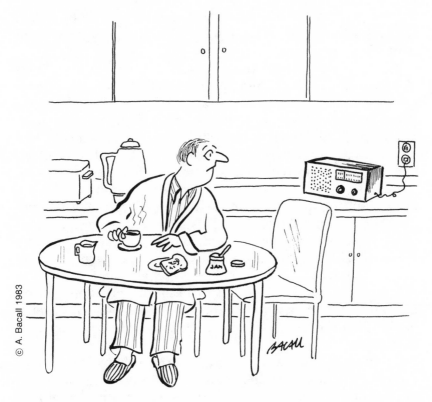

"Air quality is unacceptable today . . . without antioxidants."

superoxide dismutase (SOD), glutathione peroxidase, catalase, compounds such as reduced glutathione, and antioxidant nutrients, such as vitamins A, C, E, B-1, B-5, B-6, PABA, the amino acid cysteine, and the minerals zinc and selenium.

One important feature of the antioxidant enzymes is that they are substrate inducible. That means that when there are more free radicals in your body, these enzymes are manufactured in greater quantities. Thus, when radiation levels are increased (up to the limit of inducibility), more protective enzymes are produced. The maximum life span of individuals of several mammalian species is directly proportional to their concentration of SOD divided by the level of metabolic free radical generating activity. The research findings mentioned above probably reflect a life span increasing effect of that increase in the levels of protective enzymes. In other words, zero radiation may not be optimal from the point of view of longevity.

The principal eye irritants in Los Angeles type photochemical smog are organic peroxides called PAN, peroxyacetylnitrile and peroxyacetylnitrate. Again, the increase in pollutants increases production of protective enzymes. You've probably noticed that when you are first exposed to a heavy smog, your eyes burn and your lungs feel uncomfortable. But after you've been in heavy smog for a few days or so, the smog no longer produces these physical symptoms. This is *not* a result of your "getting used" to the smog or becoming insensitive to the discomfort. This is caused by an increased production of glutathione peroxidase (detectable in one's tears) which destroys the PAN. Other protective enzymes may be involved as well. Ozone, a principal damaging chemical found in air pollution, also causes the creation of free radicals as its primary method of damaging lungs. This probably leads to the increased production of protective enzymes in the lungs.

In addition, it was reported very recently in *Science* that ozone in the concentration range of severe smog (0.3 to 0.8 ppm) is more toxic in tissue culture to cancer cells than it is to normal cells. Could it be helping to protect some people against the development of lung cancer? This remarkable finding brings up the question of whether, aside from aesthetic considerations, it is truly advisable to eliminate all air pollution!

In our opinion, studies of pollution should consider the relative biological effects of (1) potentially "desirable" pollutants which have relatively low damage potential, but are inducers of protective enzymes, (2) pollutants which have a relatively high damage potential but which induce protective enzymes, and (3) particularly dangerous damaging pollutants which are relatively ineffective at inducing protective enzymes. All pollutants are *not* equally undesirable.

REFERENCES

Demopoulos and Gutman, "Cancer in New Jersey and Other Complex Urban/Industrial Areas," *J. Environ. Pathol. Toxicol.* 3(4): 219-235, March 1980

Demopoulos, Pietronigro, Flamm, Seligman, "The Possible Role of Free Radical Reactions in Carcinogenesis," *J. Environ. Pathol. Toxicol.* 3(4): 273-303, March 1980

Tolmasoff, Ono, Cutler, "Superoxide Dismutase: Correlation with Life-span and Specific Metabolic Rate in Primate Species," *Proc. Nat'l Acad. Sci. USA* 77(5):2777-2781, May 1980

Luckey, *Hormesis with Ionizing Radiation*, CRC Press, Inc., 1982 [beneficial effects of low levels of ionizing radiation on biological systems]

Chelating Agents and Life Extension

What does a black and blue bruise on your leg have to do with the greenness of a package of frozen brussels sprouts? And what do either of these have to do with life extension? Plenty!

When you open up that package of frozen vegetables, such as brussels sprouts, you are immediately struck by the almost unnaturally green color. But that color is not painted on. It is real. The reason the sprouts have not turned a drab brownish green color, as they do naturally, is that they have been given a special bath with an EDTA solution before packaging. EDTA is a commonly used food additive, a chelating agent which removes heavy metals (such as copper and iron) from the surface of green vegetables like brussels sprouts. "Chelate" comes from the Greek word for "claw"; chelating agents chemically capture and bind many metal ions. Copper and iron in the leaves catalyze (stimulate) the production of free radicals during the oxidation of many of the plant's constituents as it ages after harvesting. These free radicals are what normally make the sprouts and other green vegetable matter wilt (by damaging the cell walls) and turn brown after death. In fact, the lovely colors leaves turn in the fall come about partly as a result of free radical reactions. First, the green chlorophyll in the leaves is destroyed by free radicals. The leaves are then beautifully colored by the carotenoids (such as yellow-orange beta carotene in carrots) they contain. Finally, the carotenoids themselves are destroyed by free radicals, and the leaves turn brown.

Free radicals are highly chemically reactive entities with an unpaired electron, which are created in the bodies of animals and plants, while they are alive and even after they die. Because these free radicals are required for many necessary biochemical reactions, both plant and animal organisms have developed an array of protective enzymes (including superoxide dismutase, glutathione peroxidase, and catalase) and antioxidant nutrients (including vitamins A, B-1, B-5, B-6, C, E, the amino acid cysteine, reduced glutathione, and the minerals zinc and selenium) to protect themselves against free radical damage. When these radicals get out of control, they can do serious damage to cellular membranes, fats, enzymes, DNA, and RNA to cause cell damage, death, or even cancer. Free radicals are a major mechanism of damage that causes our own aging.

But back to the brussels sprouts for a moment. What is the relation of the browning of the sprouts to your bruise? The same copper and iron that catalyze free radical production in the sprouts do the same to your tissues in crushing injuries, whenever blood (red blood cells contain lots of iron and copper) leaks into the tissues from broken capillaries. Those black, blue, and yellow colors in a bruise are created by the uncontrolled chemical attack of free radicals on substances in the tissue. Chelating agents, which can bind, inactivate, and remove these heavy metals from an injury, can greatly reduce the damage and speed healing.

Spinal cord injuries, far more serious than mere bruises, have been treated with some success with D-penicillamine, a powerful chelating agent. It is possible to reduce the degree of paraplegia that would ordinarily result from an experimental spinal cord injury in cats by prompt injection of D-penicillamine. By chelating the heavy metals in the injured area, the D-penicillamine inhibits the development of a free radical chain reaction which can literally destroy the spinal cord tissue by converting the highly polyunsaturated lipids (fats and oils) there into organic peroxides, which generates more free radicals in a chain reaction. Without chelation of the iron and copper leaking from the hemolyzing (breaking down) red blood cells which have escaped from broken capillaries, free radical activity in the crushed area increases by more than 100,000 times within four hours! D-penicillamine has also been used in the successful treatment of some cases of severe rheumatoid arthritis. **CAUTION:** D-penicillamine chelation therapy should be done ONLY by a physician experienced in this type of therapy. **WARNING:** L-penicillamine, a different substance, is very dangerous and can be lethal.

Chelation has been tried successfully for extending the life span of experimental animals. Sincock and his co-workers treated microscopic organisms (the rotifer *Mytilina brevispina*) by immersing them briefly in solutions of one of the chelating agents sodium citrate, sodium tartrate, EDTA, and EGTA. Their lives were extended by all the treatments, up to 75.9% with EGTA. The treated rotifers did not accumulate nearly as much calcium with age as the untreated rotifers did.

Chelating agents are now being used to treat people for a number of conditions. In heavy metals poisoning, such as lead intoxication, the combination of EDTA and vitamin C has been found particularly effective, especially in removing lead from the brain, where it does the most harm. Vitamin C alone helps prevent the buildup of heavy metals by helping to keep them in solution in the blood where they can be eliminated via the urine.

Some good results have been obtained with EDTA chelation therapy for atherosclerosis in cases where there are abnormally high plasma lipids. Plasma lipid levels were lowered to normal or near normal in some patients that had elevated levels. Plasma levels returned back to their original levels after EDTA therapy was stopped, but fell again when it was re-initiated. In atherosclerosis patients with normal plasma lipid levels, there was little or no plaque reduction with EDTA.

Recently, a chelated form of copper, copper salicylate, has been found effective in destroying superoxide free radicals, thereby preventing some of their damaging effects to synovial fluids and joint membranes in some types of arthritis (e.g., rheumatoid arthritis). The anti-inflammatory effects of aspirin work in a similar way by inhibiting the synthesis of inflammatory prostaglandins which are formed via a free radical route. These copper salicylates work much like the natural anti-superoxide radical enzyme superoxide dismutase (SOD) and are sometimes called artificial superoxide dismutases. Since the SOD-like copper salicylate chelate is not FDA approved yet, you can't purchase it at your drugstore. Fortunately, you can easily make it in the convenience and privacy of your own stomach. Any drugstore will sell you 350 milligram sodium salicylate tablets without a prescription. Any health food and many drugstores have chelated copper nutritional supplements. These usually contain 2.5 milligrams of copper bound by a relatively weak chelator such as glycine or gluconic acid. Some arthritis sufferers have obtained relief by taking one tablet of each four times a day; the copper salicylate chelate promptly forms in your stomach.

Our bodies contain a number of natural chelating agents, several special metal-binding proteins (most of which contain the sulfur amino acids cysteine or methionine), citric acid, gluconic acid, and the amino acids glycine and aspartic acid, for example, to help control the quantities and availabilities of trace heavy metals in our blood required for certain metabolic reactions. Sometimes these natural control systems break down, resulting in illness. For example, some schizophrenics have excessive levels of copper in their blood. They can sometimes be treated by chelation. However, since all trace metals are removed by chelation, it is necessary to add some of these back. Only an experienced physician should administer treatments using powerful unselective chelating agents such as EDTA, EGTA, and D-penicillamine. However, small amounts of copper salicylate and nutrient chelating agents such as glycine, and citric and gluconic acids can be orally self-administered. Cysteine itself strongly binds heavy metals such as lead and mercury. This affinity is so great that cysteine will actually take most heavy metals away from most synthetic chelating agents.

CAUTION: Do not take supplemental cysteine unless you take at least 3 times as much vitamin C supplement as your total cysteine consumption. In figuring your cysteine consumption, remember that the number of eggs you eat is relevant; each egg contains about $\frac{1}{4}$ gram of cysteine. While cysteine is quite water soluble, its oxidized form, cystine, is rather insoluble in water. If large amounts of cysteine are taken without the other water soluble antioxidants such as C, and without adequate quantities of fluids, cystine stone formation could conceivably occur in the kidneys and urinary bladder, especially if there is a urinary tract infection.

REFERENCES

Pearson and Shaw, *Life Extension, A Practical Scientific Approach*, Warner Books, June 1982

Hourani and Demopoulos, "Inhibition of S-91 Mouse Melanoma Metastases and Growth by D-penicillamine," *Lab Invest* 21: 434, 1969

Bjorksten, Johan, "Possibilities and Limitations of Chelation as a Means for Life Extension," paper presented at the Conference of the American Academy of Medical Preventics, Denver, Colo., 3 Nov. 1979

Sincock, "Life Extension in the Rotifer *Mytilina brevispina* Var Redunca by the Application of Chelating Agents," *J. Gerontol.* 30(3):289-293, 1975

Oxygen Free Radicals and Tissue Damage, CIBA Foundation Symposium 65, Excerpta Medica, 1979, p. 55 [copper salicylates, "artificial superoxide dismutases"]

Olwin and Koppel, "Reduction of Elevated Plasma Lipid Levels in Atherosclerosis Following EDTA Therapy," *Proc. Soc. Exper. Biol. Med.* 128(3-4): 1137-1140, 1968

Brown et al, "Antiinflammatory Effects of Some Copper Complexes," *J. Med. Chem.* 23: 729, 1980

Julian, *Chelation*, Wellness Press, 1981 [popular book; James J. Julian, M.D. is director of the Julian Holistic Medical Center, Julian Medical Bldg., Hollywood Blvd. at Cahuenga, #1654, Hollywood, CA 90028]

Getting Rid of Phobias
for Good

Phobias are all too common. Surveys indicate that over half the population will admit to having a phobia, which probably means that most people have them. In many cases, people can probably live with their phobias without suffering excessively. The phobias may be inconvenient and even embarrassing, but are not necessarily a serious psychological problem. However, for the businessman who wants to fly but has a flying phobia, or the professional who wants to lecture but has a public speaking phobia, the consequences of their phobias are debilitating, expensive, and can decrease self-esteem. Women are even more likely to have a phobia (and they often come in clusters). In addition, phobias are serious stresses that can depress the activity of the immune system, possibly increasing the phobia victim's chances of contracting diseases, including cancer.

The reasons why women are more susceptible to phobias are not yet known. We suspect that phobias may be one of evolution's ways to assure reproductive success by inhibiting many women and some men from engaging in exploratory, potentially risky activities. It is interesting to note that phobias often appear in the late teens or early twenties, at the beginning of the prime reproductive period. Whether a genetic mechanism of this sort is involved or not, there is an effective way to get over phobias for good.

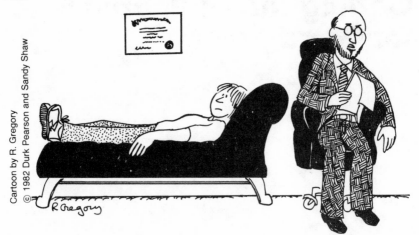

Cartoon by R. Gregory
© 1982 Durk Pearson and Sandy Shaw

"Contrary to what you told me, I see no indication whatsoever that you're suffering from claustrophobia, ailurophobia, acrophobia, or agoraphobia.... However, you *do* seem to have an acute case of phobiaphobia."

Although a therapy (gradual desensitization) is sometimes an effective way to get over a phobia, this method consumes a lot of time because the phobic fear has to be alleviated a tiny step at a time. Now there is a new way of very rapidly relieving the acute panic feelings associated with phobias as well as the unpleasant self-perception of being a coward. This approach uses no tranquilizers or sedatives, yet it enables one to quickly, relatively painlessly, and permanently unlearn a terrifying phobia. This new method of treatment, which has been used in many successful clinical studies, is based upon recent advances in understanding of the underlying psycho-biochemistry of phobias.

When a person enters a phobic situation, his body responds by releasing adrenaline, while his brain releases its own version of adrenaline, noradrenaline. As a result of this massive adrenaline-noradrenaline release, the body goes into a classic "fight or flight" state in which the blood is diverted into the muscles and, in the brain, diverted out of the higher cognitive centers in the cerebral cortex and into the primitive so-called reptile brain. This type of psychobiochemical response is a good evolutionary adaptation, well suited to a situation such as a saber tooth tiger suddenly leaping at you from behind a bush. But it just doesn't work well when this archaic mechanism is triggered when you are trying to make a speech or learn how to deal with your phobic fears. Your learning capacity is crippled when your thinking brain is shut down by your reptile brain. Phobias do not generally go away by themselves.

Adrenaline and noradrenaline are known to interact with cell receptors called the alpha and beta adrenergic receptors. Drugs which specifically block the beta receptors, so that adrenaline or noradrenaline cannot attach themselves to these receptors, have been used to enable people to get over their phobias with remarkable ease and speed. Three beta blockers are currently available in this country, although there are several available in some European countries. Propranolol is an FDA approved beta blocker for control of high blood pressure, a condition for which it is very effective. In fact, it is thought that the reduction in heart attack fatalities (especially of the sudden death variety) which has occurred during the past decade has resulted partially because of better control of high blood pressure using propranolol. Propranolol use for phobias may also lower your blood pressure, resulting in lightheadedness and possibly some dizziness, especially if you rise quickly from a sitting position.

CAUTION: Persons with asthma should *not* use propranolol for phobias, because propranolol blocks the beta receptors of bronchial smooth muscle, interfering with bronchodilating drugs. More selective beta blockers are available in England; asthmatics with phobias should explore the use of these drugs *only* with the advice and assistance of their physician.

CAUTION: Propranolol and other beta blockers should not be used by diabetics except under the advice and care of their physician.

In an English study using a somewhat more selective beta receptor blocker, a related European high blood pressure control medication called oxprenolol, violin players who had experienced pre-concert anxiety were judged by an independent panel of musical experts to have performed better using oxprenolol (because their fingers shook less!) and experienced much less anxiety. In another study, students suffering from chronic examination phobia who were treated with the beta blocker oxprenolol and then given an exam had much less anxiety with no decrement in their intellectual performance.

One of the authors (Sandy) has used propranolol to overcome a public speaking phobia of many years duration. Sandy was so afraid of addressing strangers a few years ago that, even with the psychological isolation provided by a telephone, she found it very difficult to make even the most routine business call. This severe phobia did not merely encompass telephone conversations where she was being evaluated by prospective consulting customers or professional peers; it extended to trivial matters, such as whether an electronics store stocked a certain part. In spite of her wide knowledge, public speaking was utterly out of the question. A businessman about to embark on a long phobia-filled flight can take a large dose of sedatives or tranquilizers each time. This is the most common means of dealing with phobias. But that businessman must pay the price of his relatively comfortable flight with impaired cognitive capacities at his destination, unless he has enough time to recover before his appointment. This approach is not viable when the phobic situation involves publicly addressing an audience of scientists; sedation would be intolerable. Instead, Sandy took 30 to 40 milligrams of propranolol about an hour before speaking and found that it prevented the bodily symptoms of anxiety (hands shaking, sweating, knots in stomach, etc.) and, of far greater significance, prevented her mind from "going blank." There was neither dulling of the intellect nor difficulty in the physical delivery of lectures. Outside of the phobic situation, she could subjectively sense no effect of the drug whatsoever. Best of all, Sandy found that after she had used propranolol to give two or three successful lectures, she no longer had to use the drug. It is now about two years since Sandy began using propranolol to get over her phobias; she is now relaxed, comfortable, and confident with public speaking—even when she is featured on a live network television show!

Sandy had two other phobias which promptly and permanently succumbed to propranolol. The first was a fear of flying whose symptoms had previously been temporarily mitigated through the use of meprobamate or Valium®. Each

© A. Bacall 1983

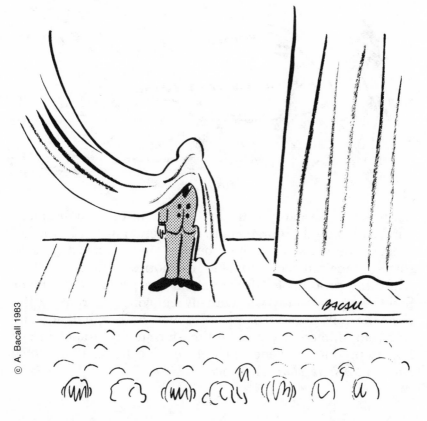

"This is my first attempt at public speaking and I seem to have misplaced my propranolol."

flight required the same tranquilization. A few flights taken with propranolol instead, and the phobia was eliminated, apparently forever. In fact, a few months ago, Sandy took a ride in an open cockpit aerobatic biplane which did a loop and a roll. She took 60 milligrams of propranolol about an hour before the flight. The physical sensations that would have caused terror before were ecstatic this time.

Sandy also had a severe roller coaster phobia. Attempting to ride the repeatedly upside-down, looping ride of the Knott's Berry Farm Corkscrew roller coaster was quite a substantial goal. Due to phobic projections of an expected terrifying experience and because a degree of sedation would

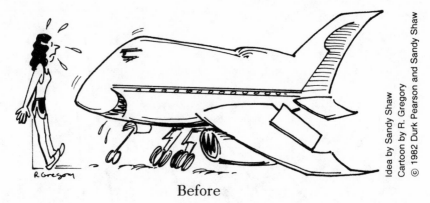

Before

not interfere seriously with the enjoyment of an amusement park, Sandy used propranolol in conjunction with a European anti-cholinergic drug called benactyzine. This latter substance impaired vivid phobic memories and projections, while the propranolol disconnected the primitive "fight or flight" system. Sandy was actually enjoying the ride by the time the roller coaster swooped down the first hill, and she was being filmed at the same time for an appearance in our Disney-produced science-adventure-educational film, *Black Holes, Monsters That Eat Space and Time!*

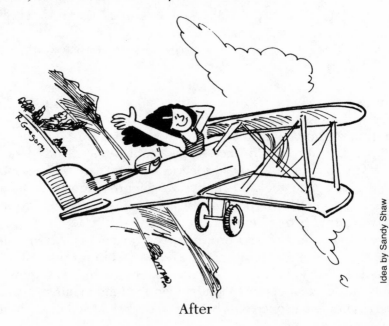

After

When your thinking brain is not shut down, you can learn how to benefit from your experiences. Propranolol does not eliminate the need for courage to enter a phobic situation, but it blocks the "fight or flight" syndrome which normally prevents the phobic individual from learning to overcome these fears. Your physician is exceptionally well informed if he has heard of this use of propranolol and other beta blockers (approved by the FDA only for the control of high blood pressure and certain cardiac arrhythmias). FDA regulations make it a criminal offense for a drug manufacturer to report to doctors on drug uses not specifically approved by the FDA no matter how scientifically justified, even if the drug has already been approved for some other purpose. The cost of FDA approval for additional drug uses is usually tens of millions of dollars, and the regulatory delay is generally several years. Since the patents on propranolol have expired, it is in no one's economic interest to pay this huge bill. Although safe (doses used a few times for phobias are typically about as much as those used a few times each and every day for hypertension) and remarkably effective, propranolol will probably never receive FDA approval for the treatment of phobias. **It is perfectly legal, however, for your physician to prescribe propranolol for any purpose whatsoever, including the treatment and cure of phobias.** You will probably have to provide copies of the scientific literature in the references section of this book before he or she is willing to explore this new use for an old drug. One of the references provides a number of original papers presented at a 1977 symposium. (See also the FDA notice in the "Fads and Fallacies" section of this book.)

REFERENCES

Kielholz, editor, *A Therapeutic Approach to the Psyche via the Beta-adrenergic System,* University Park Press, 1977

Pearson and Shaw, *Life Extension, A Practical Scientific Approach,* Warner Books, June 1982

Jet Lag, or How to Reset Your Biorhythms

Circadian (24-hour) biological rhythms play an important part in human functioning and health. Scientists have only a very sketchy understanding of mechanisms controlling changes taking place in biological rhythms as a result of travelling across time zones. But even at our present relatively crude levels of understanding, we know some causes of the most important phenomena and how to minimize some deleterious changes that can occur in long distance travelers. Acclimation to a new time zone doesn't happen instantly. In fact, most people require about one day at their destination for each one hour time zone change. Many large corporations forbid their executives to engage in the most critical of negotiations until this adaptation period is past. But what if you are flying between Los Angeles and New York and don't have three days to devote to the natural acclimation process?

Jet lag is a familiar phenomenon to many, if not most, frequent fliers. Waking up groggy and/or having a hard time getting to sleep, waking up frequently and finding it difficult to get back to sleep, and experiencing fatigue, depression, and inefficiency during the day are common. We have developed a way to prevent these symptoms in ourselves which is based upon a biochemical understanding of some of the day/night rhythms in the brain.

We know that sleep is induced by the release in the brain

of the neurotransmitter serotonin (neurotransmitters are chemicals used by nerve cells to communicate with each other). The serotonin release cycle appears to be disrupted by flying into different time zones. Therefore, when we decide that we want to sleep (a decision that may be better made by logic rather than gut feelings under conditions of jet lag!), we take about 2 grams of the amino acid nutrient tryptophan, which in most people is rapidly converted to serotonin in the brain. Since tryptophan has to compete with other aromatic amino acids to be transported into the brain through the finicky blood-brain barrier, best results occur in us when the tryptophan is taken alone and on an empty stomach immediately before going to bed. Exact dosage has to be individualized. We find it helpful to take, at the same time, a 100

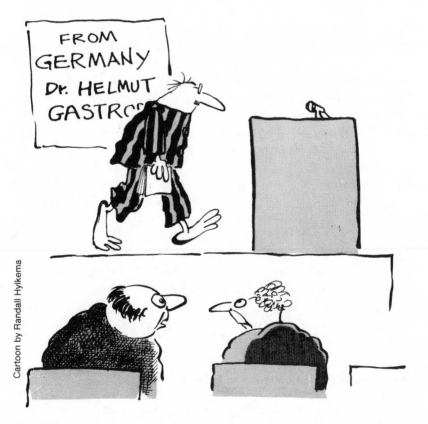

Cartoon by Randall Hylkema

"Talk about jet lag ..."

milligram supplement of vitamin B-6 and 1 gram of vitamin C, since both B-6 and C are required for the conversion of the tryptophan to serotonin.

WARNING: We know of one case (a Chinese woman in her mid thirties) where, on three separate occasions, a 500 milligram dose of tryptophan caused excitation and insomnia rather than the expected sedation. Since we do not know the biochemistry of this rare excitatory effect, *prudence demands that one NOT use tryptophan supplements if one finds them excitatory rather than sedative.*

The time-shifted traveler often suffers from interrupted or restless sleep. The neurotransmitter acetylcholine plays a major part in the control of responsiveness to external stimuli as well as regulating nerve signals sent to muscles. In normal sleep, adequate acetylcholine is released to turn down response to the environment and to inhibit restless movements. These symptoms can be modified or eliminated in the insomniac traveler by taking the nutrient choline (which is converted by the brain into acetylcholine) before bed. A dose of 3 grams is reasonable. Since Vitamin B-5 is required for the conversion of choline to acetylcholine, a supplement of 200 milligrams to 1 gram of B-5 (pantothenic acid or calcium pantothenate) with the choline can produce superior results.

Some frequent travelers take Valium® or Librium® as sedatives to make it easier to sleep. Scientists have discovered that the brain receptors which respond to Valium® and Librium® also respond to the nutrients niacinamide and inositol. A gram or two of niacinamide and 3 to 10 grams of inositol before bed can be very helpful in producing drowsiness and sleep.

To increase alertness, motivation, and energy the next day, we often take a quantity of the amino acid nutrients phenylalanine or tyrosine early that day (or just before bed the night before). Phenylalanine or tyrosine, after transport into the brain, are converted into the neurotransmitter norepinephrine (the brain's version of adrenaline). This conversion requires Vitamins C and B-6. Norepinephrine is important for memory and learning as well as for primitive drives and emotions, long term planning, and mood. Some popular stimulants, such as amphetamines and cocaine, cause the brain to release norepinephrine from its stores but, unfortunately, do not tell the brain to make more, eventually depleting the supply. Depletion of norepinephrine by excessive use of stimulants can result in severe depression. In one clinical study of people depressed as a result of a number of causes, including amphetamine abuse, endogenous, and schizophrenic depressions, etc., most were entirely relieved of their depressions by taking 100-500 milligrams of phenylalanine a day for two weeks. Doses have to be individualized. Tyrosine has similar antidepressant effects. Jet lag attenuation with tyrosine or phenylalanine is most important when flying from west to east. The dose required on the first night is generally larger than that required for chronic antidepressant use and is typically 250 milligrams to 1 gram taken at lights out, not an hour earlier.

CAUTION: Persons having high blood pressure should increase tyrosine or phenylalanine doses cautiously, while checking their blood pressure; some large doses can cause blood pressure elevation in a few susceptible individuals. Tyrosine usually seems to normalize blood pressure, decreasing it when it is too high and increasing it when it is too low. **WARNING:** Do not take tyrosine or phenylalanine with MAO inhibitors, a type of antidepressant prescription drugs that are rarely used nowadays, because hazardously high blood pressure could result. People who have irregular heart rhythms or malignant melanoma should *not* use these two amino acids.

Driving a car or operating hazardous equipment should be performed very carefully by the jet-lagged individual. Even our suggestions do not compensate perfectly. Reaction times are slower and judgement is likely to be impaired. The prescription drug Diapid® (Sandoz), a synthetic version of the natural pituitary hormone vasopressin, may help. Men in their 50's and 60's given 16 I.U. a day of Diapid® had improved memories and performed better intellectually in tasks requiring focus and concentration. The men also had faster reactions. Similar results have been obtained in other human clinical trials.

Relieving the unpleasant symptoms of jet lag is more than just a matter of comfort and convenience, though, be-

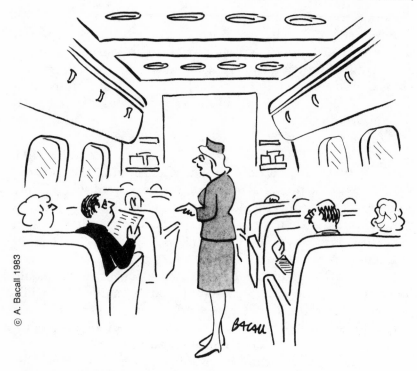

© A. Bacall 1983

"Please fasten your seatbelts . . . and remember to take some phenylalanine, and vitamins C and B-6, after we land."

cause we know that disrupted day/night neurotransmitter release patterns are hazardous to your health. When serotonin and norepinephrine release is disrupted, it affects the release of other important chemicals. Growth hormone is one of the most important. Without adequate growth hormone, the immune system does not function well. Since your immune system is your defense against viruses, bacteria, cancer, and atherosclerotic plaques, this is a serious matter. People who frequently travel long distances have been found to have higher rates of many illnesses including cardiovascular disease and cancer, both of which largely result from inadequate immune system surveillance. There are a great many ways to stimulate the performance of the immune system with nutrients you can buy in any health food store: see "How to Stay Well" in this book and pages 81-90 in *Life Extension, A*

Practical Scientific Approach. In the meantime, both seroto-nin and norepinephrine are important growth hormone re-leasers during sleep. Taking these nutrient supplements to prevent jet lag may help prevent both serious disease and the near-ubiquitous minor illnesses that dog the jet-lagged travel-er. Before embarking on your next trans-time-zone trip, stop by a vitamin shop or drugstore and purchase the nutrients mentioned above. We follow our own advice; we now wake up alert the first morning in New York City after a good night's sleep, having left Los Angeles the day before. Due to our personal late-to-bed late-to-rise sleeping habits, this in-volves a time shift of about five hours. Using the techniques described here, we both feel and perform better on the first morning than we did previously after three days of adapta-tion.

There are other suggested methods of overcoming jet lag. One program based largely on the experiments per-formed by Dr. Charles F. Ehret, Senior Scientist at the Ar-gonne National Laboratory, is reported to be highly successful

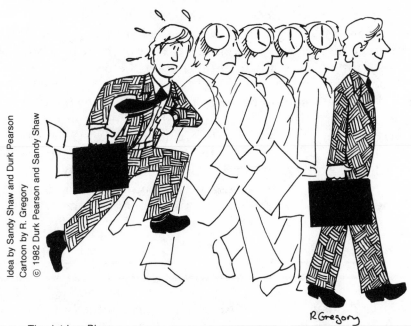

Idea by Sandy Shaw and Durk Pearson
Cartoon by R. Gregory
© 1982 Durk Pearson and Sandy Shaw

R Gregory

The Jet Lag Blues

in minimizing jet lag symptoms, although we have not yet tried it. The techniques are described fully in the book *Overcoming Jet Lag*, co-authored by Dr. Ehret, an expert in chronobiology (the timing of biological rhythms) and Lynne Waller Scanlon.

Dr. Ehret's program uses certain foods to accomplish a similar result to our suggested use of tryptophan and phenylalanine. For example, high carbohydrate dinners are suggested at specific times to aid sleep. The reason this works is that a high carbohydrate meal, as shown by Fernstrom and Wurtman, increases the passage of tryptophan into the brain, where it can be made into serotonin and put you to sleep. The high protein breakfasts and lunches suggested at other times supply phenylalanine and tyrosine.

Three closely related compounds—caffeine, theophylline (in tea), and theobromine (in chocolate)—are known to reset circadian (daily) biological rhythms. They can either set the daily cycle back to an earlier part of the phase (phase delay) or set the cycle forward to a later part of the phase (phase advance), depending on when they are taken. Dr. Ehret has performed experiments to determine when to use these substances to help reset circadian rhythms in order to avoid the effects of jet lag and provides very detailed, lengthy, specific recommendations. He also reports that experiments show that restricting caloric intake of rats the day before a circadian phase change and then feeding breakfast at the equivalent of the destination point made it easier for the rats to adapt to the phase change. He provides a suggested schedule of feasting one day and fasting (restricting caloric intake) the next day on the four days preceding the jet flight. Unfortunately, the authors (or the publisher) provide no bibliography or literature citations. Nevertheless, we are sufficiently familiar with the chronobiology literature to recommend this book.

REFERENCES

Pearson and Shaw, *Life Extension, A Practical Scientific Approach*, Warner Books, June 1982

Moehler, Polc, Cumin, Pieri, Kettler, [benzodiazepine receptors and their endogenous ligands], *Nature* (London) 278: 563-565, 1979

Braestrup, Nielsen, "Searching for Endogenous Benzodiazepine Receptor Ligands," *Trends in Pharmacological Sciences*, 424-427, Nov. 1980

Hindmarch et al, "The Effects of an Ergot Alkaloid Derivative (Hydergine) on Aspects of Psychomotor Performance, Arousal, and Cognitive Processing Ability," *J. Clin. Pharmacol.* 19 (11-12): 726-732, 1979

Stein et al, "Memory Enhancement by Central Administration of Norepinephrine," *Brain Res.* 84: 329-335, 1975

"Workshop on Advances in Experimental Pharmacology of Hydergine," *Gerontology* 24 (Suppl. 1): 1-154, 1978

Borison et al, "Metabolism of an Antidepressant Amino Acid [l-phenylalanine]," presented in poster session at April 7-14, 1978 Federation of American Societies for Experimental Biology (FASEB), Atlantic City, New Jersey

Drachman and Leavitt, "Human Memory and the Cholinergic System," *Arch. Neurol.* 30: 113, 1974

"Intermediary Metabolism" (4 wall charts of metabolic pathways, each 4-color, 23" x 35"), set of 4, $3.75, P.L. Biochemicals, 1037 West McKinley Ave., Milwaukee, WI 53205

Sachar et al, "Growth Hormone Responses to L-Dopa in Depressed Patients," *Science* 178: 1304-1305, 1972

Wurtman and Wurtman, *Nutrition and the Brain*, Vol. 1 (Pardridge, "Regulation of Amino Acid Availability to the Brain"): 141-204, Raven Press, 1977

Wurtman and Wurtman, *Nutrition and the Brain*, Vol. 3 (Growdon, "Neurotransmitter Precursors in the Diet: Their

Use in the Treatment of Brain Diseases," pp. 117-181; Sourkes, "Nutrients and the Cofactors Required for Monamine Synthesis in Nervous Tissue," pp. 265-299), Raven Press, 1979

Ehret, Dr. Charles and Lynne Waller Scanlon, *Overcoming Jet Lag*, Berkley Books, 1983, no references

Fernstrom and Wurtman, "Brain Serotonin Content: Increase Following Ingestion of Carbohydrate Diet," *Science* 174:1023-1025, 1971.

Sleep and Your Health

Although our understanding of the fundamental biochemical and physical processes underlying sleep is still rather crude, we now know enough to be able to modify some of them repeatably. Sleep is an altered state of consciousness from that of our everyday world. People whose brain functions resemble those of the sleep state during the day, when most of us are awake and alert, are considered to have a pathological physical condition or, at least, a psychological problem. Some hallucinogenic psychotropic drugs cause people to "dream" while awake, including drugs such as JB329 (an experimental anticholinergic, that is anti-acetylcholine, drug).

We are put to sleep by increased quantities of serotonin in the brain. Serotonin is an inhibitory neurotransmitter (chemical used for communication between nerve cells) that decreases the firing rate of certain nerve cells. This quantity depends on a day–night clock cycle that is maintained by the brain. Even in the absence of any external dark or light signal to establish the time of day, most people run on about a 25-hour daily rhythm. Serotonin is manufactured by the brain from the nutrient tryptophan, which may be obtained from the diet (e.g., bananas, milk) or purchased as a nutritional supplement in a drug or health food store. In order for the brain to convert the tryptophan to serotonin, vitamins C and

B-6 are required, so supplements of B-6 and C ought to be taken with tryptophan for best results. Reasonable doses are 1 gram of tryptophan, 100 milligrams of B-6, and 1 gram of vitamin C at bedtime. **WARNING:** We know of one case (a Chinese woman in her mid thirties) where, on three separate occasions, a 500 milligram dose of tryptophan caused excitation and insomnia rather than the expected sedation. Since we do not know the biochemistry of this rare excitatory effect, *prudence demands that one NOT use tryptophan supplements if one finds them excitatory rather than sedative.*

Animal studies by Fernstrom have shown that, after a large carbohydrate meal, more tryptophan enters the brain. This is because the insulin released in response to the carbo-

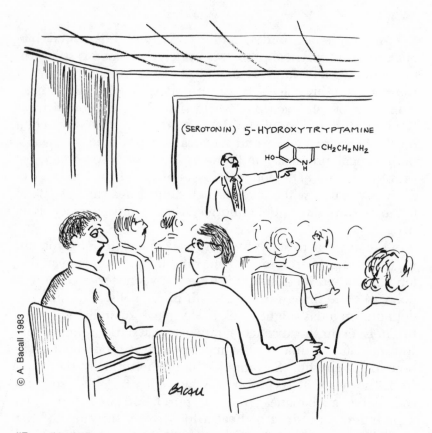

"Every time he lectures about serotonin, he puts me to sleep."

hydrates alters the binding properties of tryptophan to the protein that carries it in the bloodstream. This phenomenon explains, at least in part, why so many people fall asleep at lectures after lunch!

Another aspect of sleep is staying asleep, once serotonin has induced us to enter that state. The cholinergic nervous system in the brain uses the neurotransmitter acetylcholine for communication between its nerve cells, and is important to sleep. This system is responsible for regulating the input of stimuli from the outside world. When we sleep, this input is greatly reduced, allowing us to stop paying attention to our surroundings and enter the sleep state. Taking choline (along with vitamins B-1 and B-5, which are required for its conversion to acetylcholine by the brain) can help us to stay asleep. Lecithin (contains phosphatidyl choline) is also effective. Reasonable doses are 3 grams of choline, 100 milligrams of vitamin B-1, and 200 milligrams to a gram of vitamin B-5. Lecithin in doses of 20 to 80 grams per day is effective, too, especially with the B-1 and B-5. (For more information, see *Life Extension, A Practical Scientific Approach*, pages 189-195.)

WARNING: Much of the lecithin available to consumers is probably badly peroxidized (rancid). Polyunsaturated fats comprise much of the commercial lecithin, and these polyunsaturated fats can become hazardously peroxidized before a rancid odor can be smelled. Indeed, most store bought commercial lecithin we have smelled has been so badly peroxidized that the rancid odor was obvious. Dr. Harry Demopoulos of New York University Medical Center recently tested one bottle each of two major name brand lecithin consumer products. These samples were purchased off the shelf at two health food stores in high traffic locations. The analytical standard for good lecithin was provided by Sigma Chemical Company and was sealed in glass under dry nitrogen to prevent peroxidation.

Gas-liquid chromatography was used by Dr. Demopoulos to measure the arachidonic acid (an essential polyunsaturated fatty acid) content. *Both commercial lecithin products showed a loss of about 90%, indicating very extensive peroxidation. Another assay, the thiobarbituric acid (TBA) test,*

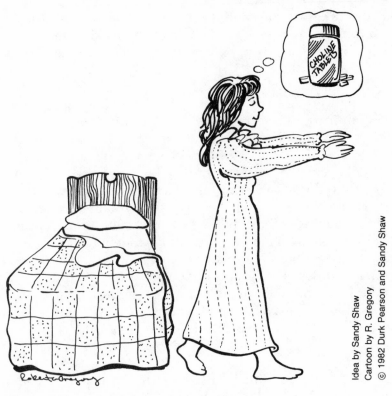

Idea by Sandy Shaw
Cartoon by R. Gregory
© 1982 Durk Pearson and Sandy Shaw

showed about 500 nanomoles per milliliter of TBA reactive organic peroxide decomposition products. The TBA test can be expected to understate the degree of peroxidation under these conditions. *DO NOT CONSUME PEROXIDIZED (RANCID) FATS, INCLUDING PEROXIDIZED LECI-THIN.* Peroxidized fats are mutagenic (damage DNA), carcinogenic (cause cancer), thrombogenic (cause abnormal blood clots), atherogenic (cause atherosclerosis), and suppress the immune system.

Regretfully, we must recommend *against* using lecithin until this problem is solved. We suggest that the manufacturers of these products make them available containing a carefully designed system of powerful natural or synthetic antioxidants and chelating agents.

Why do we need sleep? This is a question that has interested scientists and non-scientists alike since time immemorial. We still do not know, but we do have some hypotheses. An interesting hypothesis concerning our need for REM (rapid eye movement) sleep is that it may function to increase our brain's supplies of certain neurotransmitters, the catecholamines (dopamine, norepinephrine) which are important for learning, memory, long-term planning, emotions, primitive drives, motor activity (moving about), and others. An increase in these substances has been measured in the brains of experimental animals after REM sleep. A lack of REM sleep has been known for many years to reduce ability to concentrate and focus, and to cause increased aggressiveness and bad judgement.

REM is associated with dreaming, a fascinating altered state of consciousness. It is initiated in the brain by a release of the hormone vasopressin by the pituitary gland. Vasopressin is currently available as a prescription drug, Diapid® (Sandoz), used to treat a condition of excess urination caused by a deficit of vasopressin. We have experimented with this drug (because it has been shown to enhance intelligence and improve memory in animal studies, as well as in several human clinical trials) and found that it increases our ability to visualize. Thus, its connection with dreaming is not surprising. Indeed, vasopressin has been shown to increase theta brain wave activity which is associated with dreaming, creativity, and visualization. Dreams can be useful in the study of unconscious cognitive activity. They can be interpreted as free associations, using devices such as the play on words, the pun, allusions, and so on.

Another hypothesis concerning why we sleep is that it removes an individual from the relatively more dangerous night environment to the relative safety of his or her home territory, where he or she is put "on hold," so to speak.

One important event that takes place while we sleep is the release of growth hormone that occurs about 90 minutes or so after we begin to sleep. This release is triggered by serotonin and dopamine. Growth hormone is necessary for proper function of our immune system, the white blood cells, thymus gland (located behind the breastbone), spleen, bone marrow, and various chemicals, including antibodies, interferon, and complement. The thymus gland instructs certain white blood cells, called T-cells, what entities are foreign and which are you. When there is inadequate GH, the thymus shrinks in size and the white cells don't do as good a job of locating, killing, and eating bacteria, viruses, and cancer cells or they may attack you by mistake. Certain of these white cells instruct other white cells (called B-cells, that arise in bone marrow) to make antibodies. This, too, is performed less well when there is inadequate GH.

Older people release less growth hormone than younger people. It is possible to bring GH release back up to young adult levels by taking supplements of substances which cause a release of GH, including the nutrients L-tryptophan, L-arginine, and L-ornithine (amino acids) and the prescription drug L-Dopa (also an amino acid). Taking these just before bedtime increases GH release at a natural place in the daily cycle. Other stimulants of GH release include exercise and moderate fasting. The decline in GH output with age is suspected by some scientists studying aging, including ourselves, to be an important factor in the rapid decline in health that occurs after young adulthood.

Reducing sleep may be an effective strategy for life extension. If sleep time can be reduced without disturbing the brain's chemistry, even if we don't live any more years than is normal, we can increase our subjective life spans by up to about a third. There are reports of people who sleep as little as 15 minutes a night. On a NOVA science special shown during the last few years, some of these people were interviewed. They were studied by scientists, who put electrodes on their heads to detect whether they were sleeping in cat-naps or on their feet or, in some way, making up for their very short sleep time at night. They weren't, so we know that it is possible for at least some individuals to function with very small amounts of sleep. Data indicates, however, that for most of us, sleeping 6 to 8 hours a night is normal and any substantial deviation from that amount is usually associated with a reduced life span.

Staying awake for prolonged periods can result in a psychotic state (including hallucinations and paranoid delusions) which closely resembles that seen in chronic abusers of amphetamines. Both situations result in depletion of brain stores of norepinephrine, an important neurotransmitter. Staying awake for a couple of nights has been of benefit to some people with depression, possibly by a mechanism involving a resetting of day–night cycles. It is known that REM deprivation reduces the threshold for electrical shock convulsions. Thus, it may activate an overly inhibited (depressed) nervous system.

Finally, we'd like to close this chapter with a little sleep experiment you can try. Vitamin B-12 increases the manufacture of RNA by the brain's neurons (nerve cells). It also has other interesting properties. It promotes the appearance of

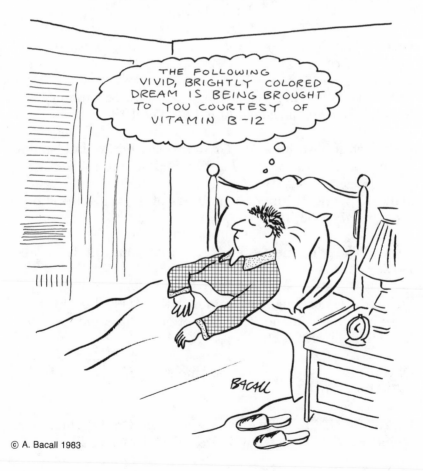

colored dreams! We and others have noted this when we have taken high doses of B-12 after a period of abstinence (you develop tolerance to the effect quickly). A dose of 1000 micrograms is a reasonable adult dose that often, but not always, produces vivid, brightly colored dreams. They may be so vivid that they wake you up. It must be taken *immediately* before going to sleep, and seems to work about half of the time.

Sweet dreams or, if you prefer, happy nocturnal hallucinations.

REFERENCES

Pearson and Shaw, *Life Extension, A Practical Scientific Approach*, Warner, 1982

Fernstrom, "Psychopharmacology of Brain Serotonin: Meal Effects," *Psychopharmacol Bull* 15(3): 59, 1979

Barbul et al, "Arginine: A Thymotropic and Wound-healing Promoting Agent," *Surgical Forum* 28:101-103, 1977

Marx, "Thymic Hormones: Inducers of T Cell Maturation," *Science* 187: 1183, 1975

Jerne, "The Immune System" *Sci. Amer.* offprint 1276, July 1973

Meites, "Role of Biogenic Amines in the Control of Prolactin and Growth Hormone (GH) Secretion," *Psychopharm Bull*, Oct. 1976, pp. 120-121

Oliveros et al, "Vasopressin in Amnesia," *The Lancet*, Jan. 7, 1978, Vol. 1, p. 42

Legros et al, "Influence of Vasopressin On Learning and Memory," *The Lancet*, Jan. 7, 1978, Vol. 1, pp. 41-42

Pardridge, "Regulation of Amino Acid Availability to the Brain," in Wurtman and Wurtman, eds., *Nutrition and the Brain*, Raven Press, 1977, p. 172

Walford, "Immunologic Theory of Aging: Current Status," *Fed. Proc.* 33(9): 2020-2027, 1974

Prinz et al, "Growth Hormone Levels During Sleep in Elderly Males," presented at the 29th annual Gerontological Society conference on Oct. 13, 1976

Boyd et al, "Stimulation of Human-Growth-Hormone Secretion by L-Dopa," *New Engl. J. Med.* 283(26): 1425-1429, 1970

Stern, "REM Sleep and Behavioral Plasticity: Evidence for Involvement of Brain Catecholamines," chapter 6 in *Sleep, Dreams and Memory*, Spectrum Publications, Inc., 1981

Tufik, "Changes of Response to Dopaminergic Drugs in Rats Submitted to REM-Sleep Deprivation," *Psychopharmacology* 72: 257-260, 1981

Gutheil, *The Handbook of Dream Analysis*, Washington Square Press, 1966

Moore-Ede, Sulzman, Fuller, *The Clocks That Time Us: Physiology of the Circadian Timing System*, Harvard University Press, 1982

DMSO: Its Uses and Mode of Action

DMSO (dimethyl sulfoxide) is one of those drugs caught up in the quagmire of FDA regulations. It is being "illegally" sold in many health food, hobby, and hardware stores in southern California. It is being offered via mail order, as well, through display ads in major newspapers and magazines. Judging from the prices at which it is offered, much of this quasi-illegal DMSO must be of industrial solvent grade (which contains undesirable impurities such as dimethylsulfone, dimethylsulfide, nitrogen oxides, and benzene) rather than the high purity reagent, spectrophotometric (very pure DMSO for use as a solvent for substances to be analyzed by the selective absorption of ultraviolet, infrared, and visible light), or pesticide quality (suitable for pesticide residue analysis) grades. DMSO is also available legally as an industrial solvent and as a prescription drug, RIMSO-50 (50% DMSO and 50% water). The prescription drug is approved by the FDA for the treatment of interstitial cystitis and they warn that use of DMSO for any other condition may be dangerous.

DMSO has an almost legendary public reputation as a treatment for arthritis and sports injuries. A recent *Science News* article stated that an estimated 5 to 10% of the U.S. population is using non-prescription DMSO. Yet, because so much of that reputation has stemmed from anecdotal accounts (which can provide leads but cannot be considered proof of anything), because there is no patent protection available for DMSO (and consequently little incentive for a private firm to invest in DMSO research), and because the mechanisms of its action were not known until recently, DMSO use has been considered controversial. Now, however, researchers have discovered a major mechanism of its action which explains much, if not most, of DMSO's beneficial effects in many cases of pain and swelling of arthritis and in reducing time required for the healing of injuries. At present, this drug is being used by millions of Americans, including sports teams, where injuries can represent a lot of lost income.

In 1974 McCord reported his studies indicating that free radicals are responsible for arthritis. Free radicals are molecules or atoms with an unpaired (free) electron, and they are extremely reactive. They are also ubiquitous in living organisms. All air-breathing organisms on this planet contain special protective enzymes (such as zinc-containing superoxide dismutase and selenium-containing glutathione peroxidase) and antioxidants (nutrient factors that both destroy free radicals and block uncontrolled oxidation reactions that result in their formation), including vitamins A, C, E, B-1, B-5, B-6, the amino acid cysteine, and the minerals zinc and selenium. Free radicals are now considered by many scientists to be major causative factors in aging, cardiovascular disease, cancer, certain epilepsies, emphysema, and many other conditions, including arthritis, bruises, dandruff, and acne pimples. (Note that we are *not* suggesting the use of DMSO for all of these conditions.)

Radiation sickness (except for that caused by neutrons) is an example of a pure free radical disease. Radiation kills by creating free radicals, which then attack cell membranes, fats, DNA, RNA, and proteins. Dr. Denham Harman of the University of Nebraska, who originated the free radical theory of aging, calls free radicals "internal radiation." Free radicals arising out of exposure to external radiation such as x-rays represent only a very small part of the total amount of free radicals to which we are exposed. The rest are created during normal metabolism (free radical reactions are a necessary part of energy production) and during the breakdown of peroxidized fats (rancid fats created in the body by exposure of these fats to oxygen or other oxidizers). Although we and other long-lived animals do contain a generous supply of protective enzymes, the protection is not perfect and, over time, much damage is done.

There are different types of free radicals. McCord found that superoxide radicals and hydrogen peroxide (a common byproduct of metabolism) must both be present in order to destroy the lubricating fluids and membranes in our joints. The enzyme superoxide dismutase (SOD) can protect our joints and other tissues against superoxide radicals; injections of SOD into arthritic joints have sometimes had dramatic effects. The enzyme catalase, which breaks down hydrogen peroxide to harmless products, also provides protection. According to McCord's studies, the agents that actually attack the lubricants in our joints are hydroxyl radicals, the nastiest type of free radical known. They are more reactive than fluorine and are so reactive that they can attack the "inert" or "noble" elemental gas xenon.

This is where DMSO comes in. DMSO is not a joint lubricant. DMSO is not an analgesic (pain deadener). Arthritis experiments based on these hypotheses were doomed to failure. DMSO *is* a powerful scavenger of hydroxyl free radicals. Inositol is another hydroxyl radical scavenger, though not as powerful as DMSO. By removing the hydroxyl radicals, DMSO provides excellent protection to joint-lubricating fluids and membranes. That isn't the end of the story, however. After chemically reacting with hydroxyl radicals, DMSO is itself converted to a sulfoxide free radical—not as dangerous as the hydroxyl radicals, but a free radical, nevertheless. Because of this, it is important to use DMSO in conjunction with other antioxidants, like vitamins C, E, and the others mentioned above. Large repeated doses of DMSO have caused cataracts in the eyes of experimental rabbits. Rabbits have relatively poor natural antioxidant enzyme protection compared to humans and, in experiments, could not adequately protect themselves from all those DMSO free radicals. The DMSO radicals oxidized the amino acids cysteine and methionine to their sulfoxide, sulfone, and disulfide forms, impairing the transparency of the lens and cornea in the rabbits. It is

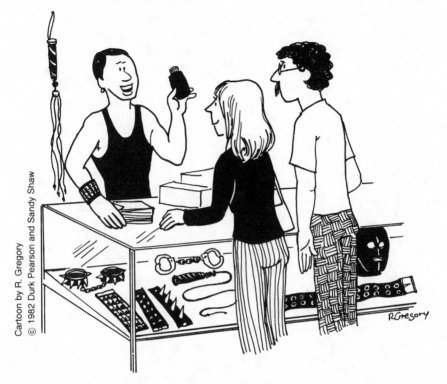

Cartoon by R. Gregory
© 1982 Durk Pearson and Sandy Shaw

"Whip . . . handcuffs . . . and for those telltale bruises, I recommend DMSO. . . ."

important, therefore, that if you choose to use DMSO, be sure it is very pure, dilute it with about 10 to 20% water before use and allow the evolved heat to dissipate, use it externally on limited areas of the body, and take plenty of supplemental antioxidant nutrients. Before using DMSO, consult with your physician.

Where do sports injuries come in? We now know that free radical damage is an important part of such injuries. When injuries occur, blood vessels leak blood into surrounding tissues. As the red blood cells hemolyze (that is, break down) they release copper and iron, which are very powerful catalysts of free radical reactions. The blue, black, yellow, and other colors you see in a crushing injury are a result of free radical attacks. The browning of freshly cut fruits such as apples and bananas is another example of free radical reactions, which also damage cell membranes and cause softening. We've found in our personal use that if you apply DMSO quickly enough (preferably in the first half hour, two to four hours at most) to a crushing injury, the colors never form and swelling is greatly reduced.

Dr. Dela Torre, formerly of Miami University, and Dr.

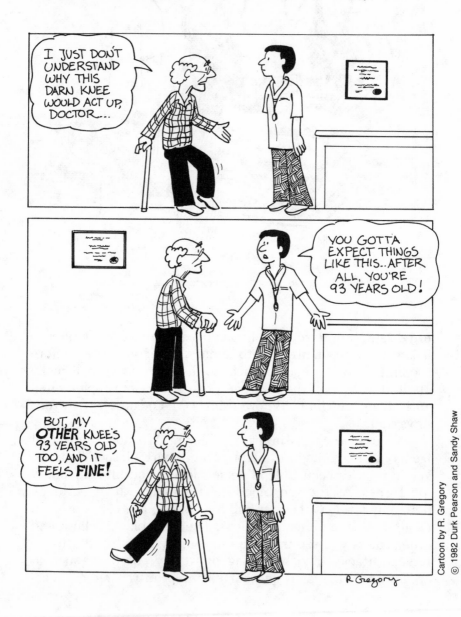

Harry Demopoulos of New York University and his coworkers found that prompt injection of DMSO reduced the degree of paraplegia occurring in cats that had been subjected to experimental crushing injuries of the spinal cord. Concussion damage to nerves is principally due to free radicals catalyzed by the leaking copper and iron. Using an electron spin resonance spectrometer (an electronic instrument that identifies and counts free radicals) and gas chromatography/mass spectrometry, they found that free radical activity increased to over 100,000 times normal several hours after the injury. Perhaps in the future, we will see DMSO in the emergency medical kits of paramedics. The San Francisco General Hospital Brain Trauma and Edema Center has recently begun the use of DMSO in treating brain injuries.

Before using DMSO for any purpose, whether FDA approved or not, and whether the DMSO is obtained by prescription or over the counter, we advise that you consult with a physician experienced in its use.

REFERENCES

McCord, "Superoxide Radical May Play a Role in Arthritis," paper presented at the Third Biennial Conference on Chemical Education, Pennsylvania State Univ., Aug. 1, 1974

Leake, "Dimethyl sulfoxide," *Science*, pp. 1646-1649, June 1966

"DMSO Cut Down to Size," *Nature* 247: 421, 1974

Szent-Gyorgyi, *Electronic Biology and Cancer*, Marcel Dekker, 1976

Harman, "Free Radical Theory of Aging," *J. Geront.* 23(4), Oct. 1968

Harman, "Free Radical Theory of Aging: Nutritional Implications," *AGE* 1(4): 145-152, 1978

Pryor, "Free Radicals in Biological Systems," *Scientific American*, August 1970

Tappel, "Selenium-glutathione Peroxidase and Vitamin E," *Amer. J. Clin. Nutr.* 27: 960-965, Sept. 1974

Demopoulos et al., "Further Studies on Free Radical Pathology in the Major Central Nervous System Disorders," *Canad. J. Physiol. & Pharmacol.* 60:1415-1424, 1982

Hydergine®, An Effective Treatment for Sickle Cell Anemia, Predicted by Free Radical Pathology Theory

This is an example of how an understanding of mechanisms that cause disease can lead to the prediction of possible therapies. Specifically, this is the story of how free radical pathology theory led to the very successful prediction that Hydergine® should be effective against sickle cell anemia crises.

Sickle cell anemia is an often devastating genetic disease in which its victims have an abnormally shaped hemoglobin, the molecule responsible for carrying oxygen to the body's tissues. Under conditions of hypoxia (inadequate oxygen available), the abnormal hemoglobin changes shape and converts the normally flexible, disc-shaped red blood cells to sickle-shaped cells that are rigid and cannot pass through capillaries. The result is hypoxia in the tissues served by these blocked capillaries, much like a large number of tiny strokes throughout the body, leading to severe pain and progressive damage, including severe cumulative damage to the brain. It is reported that over half the victims of sickle cell anemia die by the age of 21 and few reach 40.

About a year ago, Sandy was thinking about the problem. The damage of hypoxia is caused largely by free radicals, which are not controlled properly and are created in much larger numbers than usual under hypoxic conditions. Hydergine®, a drug usually prescribed for mild to moderate senility as well as Alzheimer's disease in the U. S., is a very powerful antioxidant. It has been shown in experimental animals and human subjects to provide substantial protection against hypoxic damage to the brain. Sandy thought that Hydergine® might be very beneficial to the victims of sickle cell anemia. (In fact, we included this as a research project idea in Chapter 12 of *Life Extension, A Practical Scientific Approach.*) We telephoned Bill Connelly, Director of Scientific Affairs for Sandoz Corporation (the manufacturer of Hydergine®). We suggested that Sandoz fund a small clinical trial. He replied that such trials had already been performed in hospitals in French-speaking Africa several years ago and the results published in obscure French-language medical journals. He offered to have several papers translated for us by an independent commercial scientific paper translating service.

The results were spectacular. Hydergine® can prevent most sickle cell crises when used prophylactically and can even reduce the duration of an attack already in progress at the time of administration by about 25%. The effective dosages were usually around 15 milligrams to 20 milligrams per day, about the same as we are taking for anti-aging effects. For example, in one study, homozygote children (who have two genes for the abnormal sickle cell hemoglobin) were treated with Hydergine® daily to test whether this would reduce the number of sickle cell crises. One child who, observed over two years, would have been expected (on the basis of his recent medical history) to suffer 48 attacks in this time, actually had only 4 attacks. A homozygote adult, who would have been expected to have 60 attacks in a 15-month period, had only 4. The study's heterozygote children and adults (who have one gene for the abnormal hemoglobin and one for the normal variety) would have had 1 to 8 crises during their periods of observation and almost all had no crises with Hydergine®.

We were delighted with this information and wanted to make it available to sickle cell anemia victims. It is illegal for Sandoz to inform physicians about this unapproved use, but no law says that we cannot do so. Sandy thought a good way to do that was to talk about it on "Tony Brown's Journal," a popular television show that reaches a large audience, including many blacks. We appeared on the show in December of 1982 and gave Tony Brown copies of three of the papers. We even mentioned during the program that doctors interested in trying Hydergine® therapy for sickle cell could contact Sandoz Corporation in East Hanover, New Jersey for information.

Research scientists are working on better treatments for sickle cell anemia, although the combination of a $50,000,000 or so cost for FDA approval combined with the limited potential market for such a treatment has undoubtedly chilled commercial R&D. In the future, genetic engineering will allow the abnormal hemoglobin gene to be removed or altered so that the disease can be truly cured. For years, scientists have been working on drugs to change the shape of the abnormal hemoglobin molecule so that it functions properly, but existing candidates so far have been too toxic or insufficiently effective. In the meantime, Hydergine® is available and is safe and effective. Hydergine® does not cure the fundamental biochemical problem of the abnormal hemoglobin molecule, but it certainly can reduce the severe suffering and brain and organ damage that accompanies it.

REFERENCES

Cuisinier, Ducloux, Lagarde, Barbotin, Darracq, "The Prevention of Painful Sickle Cell Anemia Crises by Hydergine," *Bull. Soc. Med. Afr. Noire Langue Franc.* 19:168-172, 1974

Pegue, Bertrand, Bonhomme, Coullet, David, Pierredon, Sankale, "The Efficacy of Dihydroergotoxine [Hydergine®] in the Treatment of Sickling Crises: Results of a Co-operative Double-blind Trial Carried Out in French-speaking Africa," *Nouv. Presse. med.* 7:2449-2452, 1978

Sanosho, Martin, Kuakuvi, Niang, "Sickle Cell Anemia in the Child: Role of Hydergine in the Treatment and Prophylaxis of

Crises," *Bull. Soc. Med. Afr. Noire Lang. Franc.* XX(1):83-89, 1975

Koreh, Seligman, Demopoulos, "The Effect of Dihydroergotoxine on Lipid Peroxidation in vitro," *Lipids* 17(10):724-726, 1982

Sex

Sex Play and Sexual Rejuvenation

The biochemistry of sex is complex and much remains to be determined. However, some aspects of sexual function have been discovered which allow individuals more volitional control of sexual expression and satisfaction. In this chapter, we discuss a few ways to augment sex experiences.

Areas of the brain which are involved in sex use the primitive neurotransmitters (substances nerve cells use to communicate with each other) acetylcholine, dopamine, norepinephrine, and serotonin. These same chemicals are found in the brains of amphibians and reptiles, as well as in mammals. When there are inadequate quantities of these neurotransmitters (or the nerve cell receptors are insensitive or too few in number), there can be a decrease in sexual interest and activity.

Depression is usually accompanied by a decline in sexual interest. In several clinical trials, depression often responded to small quantities of the amino acids phenylalanine and tyrosine, which are used by the brain to make both dopamine and norepinephrine. In one clinical trial, about 80% of depressions of a wide variety of types (endogenous, schizophrenic, the depressive phase of manic-depression, and others) were completely alleviated by 100 to 500 milligrams of phenylalanine a day for two weeks. Tyrosine has also been found effective in similar doses. Excess tyrosine or phenylalanine

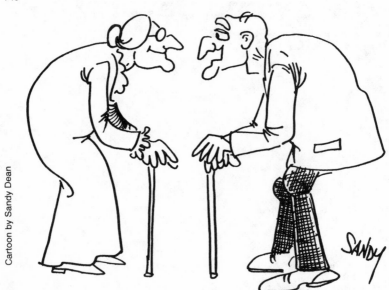

Cartoon by Sandy Dean

"But enough about *my* secret of longevity. Let's boogie."

can cause irritability, aggression, and insomnia. For best results, take on an empty stomach (some amino acids compete with each other to enter the brain). **CAUTION:** Persons with high blood pressure should use phenylalanine or tyrosine with caution because, at high doses, a small percentage of sensitive persons may experience higher blood pressure. Start at a low dose and increase slowly over a period of days to a few weeks, measuring blood pressure frequently while doing so. Tyrosine often seems to normalize blood pressure, decreasing it when it is too high and increasing it when it is too low.

WARNING: Tyrosine or phenylalanine should not be used together with MAO inhibitor antidepressant drugs because hazardous high blood pressure could result.

Dopaminergic stimulants (substances which activate parts of the brain using dopamine as a neurotransmitter) such as the amino acid prescription drug L-Dopa and the ergot derivative prescription drug bromocriptine frequently cause an increase in libido as a side-effect. Medical authorities often consider this a problem in institutionalized patients!

Sometimes depression can be alleviated by increasing brain supplies of acetylcholine (except in the depression of manic-depressive psychosis, which may be worsened). This may increase sexual activity as well; in our limited clinical experience, nobody under the age of 40 has had this experience, but it is common in people in their 50's and 60's. Choline and lecithin increase brain acetylcholine. In addition to mood elevations in those with inadequate acetylcholine (such as in some elderly persons), these nutrients also improved memory and learning (in tasks requiring concentration and focus) in several human clinical trials. Effective dosages were 3 grams a day of choline or 80 grams a day of lecithin. Vitamin B-5 is required for the conversion to acetylcholine, so a 200 milligram to 1 gram per day supplement of this vitamin should also be taken for best results. Vitamin B-1 is also required, so a 100 milligram per day B-1 supplement is helpful as well. In some clinical trials involving older persons, only a minority benefitted from choline, which we think may be due to, at least in part, inadequate availability of vitamin B-5 and possibly vitamin B-1. (It is well known that concentra-

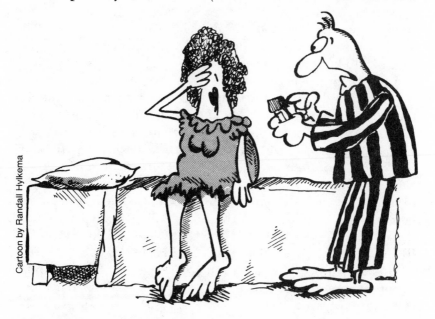

Cartoon by Randall Hylkema

"That's right, dear, for headache, take aspirin . . . but for *this* headache, try bromocriptine!"

tions of antioxidant vitamins such as B-1 and B-5 are decreased in the serum of older persons.)

Too much cholinergic stimulation results in aching or stiff muscles (excessively high muscle tone) or headache. A very recent study showed that choline given together with piracetam, an anti-senility drug available in Europe (over the counter in France), resulted in dramatic improvements in memory of aging animals. On one memory test, animals receiving both these substances performed four times better than controls (receiving no treatment) and three times better than animals receiving only choline or piracetam.

WARNING: Much of the lecithin available to consumers is probably badly peroxidized (rancid). Polyunsaturated fats comprise much of the commercial lecithin, and these polyunsaturated fats can become hazardously peroxidized before a rancid odor can be smelled. Indeed, most of the commercial store bought lecithin we have smelled has been so badly peroxidized that the rancid odor was obvious. Dr. Harry Demopoulos of New York University Medical Center recently tested one bottle each of two major name brand lecithin consumer products. These samples were purchased off the shelf at two health food stores in high traffic locations. The analytical standard for good lecithin was provided by Sigma Chemical Company and was sealed in glass under dry nitrogen to prevent peroxidation.

Gas-liquid chromatography was used by Dr. Demopoulos to measure the arachidonic acid (an essential polyunsaturated fatty acid) content. *Both commercial lecithin products showed a loss of about 90%, indicating very extensive peroxidation. Another assay, the thiobarbituric acid (TBA) test, showed about 500 nanomoles per milliliter of TBA reactive organic peroxide decomposition products.* The TBA test can be expected to understate the degree of peroxidation under these conditions. DO NOT CONSUME PEROXIDIZED (RANCID) FATS, INCLUDING PEROXIDIZED LECITHIN. Peroxidized fats are mutagenic (damage DNA), carcinogenic (cause cancer), thrombogenic (cause abnormal blood clots), atherogenic (cause atherosclerosis), and suppress the immune system. Lecithin producers should add a carefully designed synergistic system of synthetic or natural antioxidants and chelators.

The amino acid tryptophan has recently been found to be effective in alleviating some depressions, especially those involving excessive aggression and sometimes violent suicidal attempts. Tryptophan is converted in the brain to the inhibitory neurotransmitter (decreases nervous activity) serotonin. In some patients given tryptophan, hypersexuality developed. Typical human doses are 1 to 2 grams taken at bedtime on an empty stomach. Vitamins C and B-6 are required for this conversion of tryptophan to serotonin; 1 gram of C and 100 milligrams of B-6 can be taken with the tryptophan. Too much tryptophan can cause drowsiness, headache, and stuffy nose.

WARNING: We know of one case (a Chinese woman in her mid thirties) where, on three separate occasions, a 500 milligram dose of tryptophan caused excitation and insomnia rather than the expected sedation. Since we do not know the biochemistry of this rare excitatory effect, *prudence demands that one NOT use tryptophan supplements if one finds them excitatory rather than sedative.*

When serotonin is broken down in the body, a substance called 5-HIAA (5-hydroxyindoleacetic acid) is produced and then excreted in the urine. The presence of too little 5-HIAA in the urine has been found to be a very good predictor of possible suicide attempts. It would be a very good idea for suicide centers to perform routine analyses for 5-HIAA in urine of potential suicides.

One of the chemical events leading to orgasm is a release of histamine, a substance with many functions. For example, it is a growth promoter required for healing (it causes that itchy sensation in healing wounds). In people and animals having inadequate histamine release, orgasm may be difficult or even impossible to achieve. Histidine is an amino acid that is converted into histamine in the body. It is found in foods such as meats, dairy products, and some wines. In order for the histidine to be made into histamine, vitamin B-6 is required. Niacin is of interest because it causes the release of histamine. This release is what produces the flushing and itching some people complain of when they take large doses of niacin and that causes a niacin flush very similar to the sex flush described by Masters and Johnson. We often take a dose of niacin a half hour or so before having sex, because it augments the natural histamine release associated with orgasm. Acetylcholine, too, is involved in orgasm, being required for the buildup toward orgasm and the urethral and vaginal contractions during orgasm. The subjective perception of orgasm intensity and duration correlates fairly well with the measured strength and duration of these contractions.

About 20 to 25% of male impotence results from the pituitary gland's excess secretion of the hormone prolactin. Inadequate dopaminergic stimulation is one mechanism for the increase in pituitary release of prolactin. Dopaminergic stimulation generally declines with age. The prescription drug bromocriptine (Parlodel®, Sandoz) suppresses prolactin

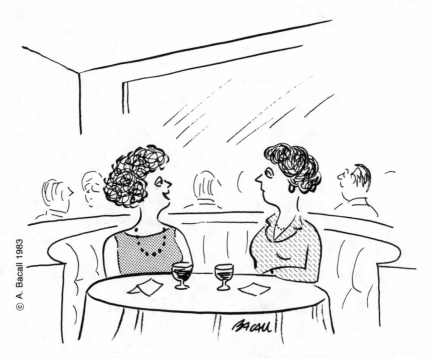

© A. Bacall 1983

"I think my relationship with Frank is getting serious. He asked me to take some niacin with him."

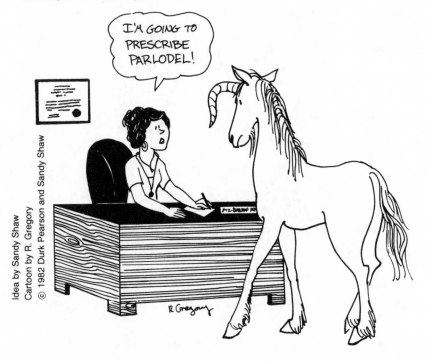

Idea by Sandy Shaw
Cartoon by R. Gregory
© 1982 Durk Pearson and Sandy Shaw

and is very effective in reversing this type of male impotency. In addition, bromocriptine increases libido in about 80% of those who take it, whether male or female. It has other unusual effects as well. Some postmenopausal women given bromocriptine for excess prolactin begin menstrual cycling again. This can happen to women in their 60's, 70's, or even older. The reversal of the ordinarily permanent event of menopause has interested us in the possible use of bromocriptine and related compounds for use against aging clocks (of which menopause is one).

Vasopressin is another pituitary hormone which has several functions, including regulation of urine volume. It is also involved in learning and memory. In a study of men in their 50's and 60's, 16 I.U. a day (about 8 snorts) of the intranasally administered prescription drug Diapid® (Sandoz), a synthetic version of vasopressin, caused a significant enhancement of memory and learning, as well as a faster reaction time. We have been using it for its intelligence boosting effects for a few years and also found that it prolongs and intensifies

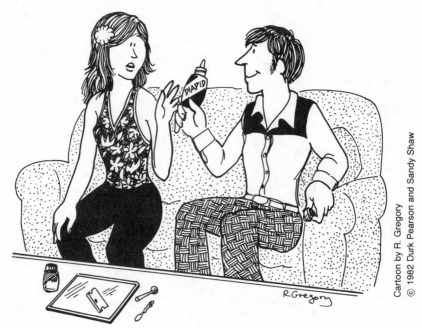

"This isn't exactly what I thought you had in mind when you said 'a few snorts.' "

orgasms, an effect not mentioned in the scientific literature! A subsequent literature search found that vasopressin is released from the mammalian pituitary during orgasm. Vasopressin has a short half life in vivo, less than two hours, and should therefore be used just before sex if it is to have the orgasm enhancing effect. At 16 I.U. a day, the men in their 50's and 60's did not have any side-effects.

CAUTION: Vasopressin should be avoided by those with angina pectoris because it may initiate an angina attack.

A vitamin may be able to increase your sexual stamina. Vitamin B-5 is part of the Krebs energy producing cycle in the body. In the process of oxidizing foodstuffs to carbon dioxide and water, energy is produced that is stored in high energy phosphate bonds of the molecule adenosine triphosphate (ATP). Vitamin B-5 (pantothenic acid or calcium pantothenate) is a part of the co-factor acetyl coenzyme A that is required to produce energy via the Krebs cycle, and also for the manufacture of acetylcholine; B-5 should be taken with choline or lecithin. (See lecithin warning earlier in this chapter.) In one experiment, rats were provided with diets either deficient, adequate or high in calcium pantothenate. They were then swum to exhaustion in 18 degrees C (64 degrees F) water. Swimming times were:

deficient	16 +/− 3 minutes
adequate	29 +/− 4 minutes
high	62 +/− 12 minutes

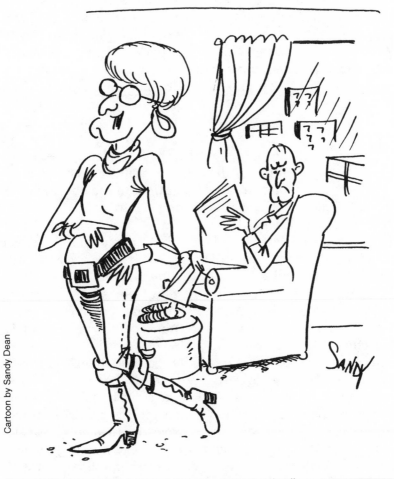

Cartoon by Sandy Dean

"I see nothing wrong in being a sensuous great-grandmother."

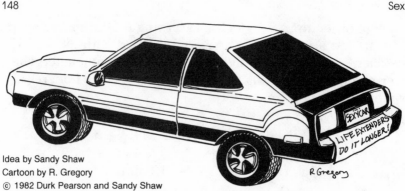

Idea by Sandy Shaw
Cartoon by R. Gregory
© 1982 Durk Pearson and Sandy Shaw

Human experiments with cold water stress are in agreement with these findings. Isolated perfused frog muscle preparations, in another experiment, had a doubled work output with calcium pantothenate added to the perfusing solution. A reasonable dose of calcium pantothenate (the most stable form of vitamin B-5) is 1 to 2 grams a day for a healthy adult. Start at a low dose and work up to the 1 to 2 grams over a period of a few days or so. Too much too soon may give you diarrhea or intestinal cramps due to excessive acetylcholine production in the gut. Vitamin B-5 is a peristaltic stimulant (due to its increasing the quantity of the neurotransmitter acetylcholine in the gut), so it will decrease transit time in the gut. It can be used as a very effective non-irritating laxative.

It has long been known that exposure to frequent changes of sexual partners seems to have a rejuvenating effect in humans. Some of this apparent effect may already have been noted in studies of experimental animals. In a study of old male rats given regular fresh female sexual partners, increased levels of the male sex hormone testosterone were measured, and the animals behaved more like young animals. (The study was conducted in order to see whether the frequent change of sex partners would increase their life span. It didn't, but their quality of life seemed to have been improved.) When male monkeys had the same female or females as their regular sexual partners, their interest in sex eventually diminished. However, upon exposure to a new female, their libido increased to levels more like those of young monkeys. Similar results occurred in female monkeys provided with new young male monkeys as sexual partners.

For more information on sex and aging, see *Life Extension, A Practical Scientific Approach*, especially pages 196-207.

REFERENCES

Pearson and Shaw, *Life Extension, A Practical Scientific Approach*, Warner, 1982

Debono et al, "Bromocriptine and Dopamine Receptor Stimulation," *Brit. J. Clin. Pharmacol.* 3:977-982, 1976

Malitz, ed., *L-Dopa and Behavior*, Raven Press, 1972

Ralli and Dumm, "Relation of Pantothenic Acid to Adrenal Cortical Function," *Vit. Horm.* 11:133-158, 1953

Myers, *Handbook of Drug and Chemical Stimulation of the Brain*, Medical Economics, 1974

Legros et al, "Influence of Vasopressin on Memory and Learning," *The Lancet*, 7 Jan. 1978, p. 41

Meites, "Role of Biogenic Amines in the Control of Prolactin and Growth-Hormone Secretion," *Psychopharm. Bull.*, Oct. 1976, pp. 120-121

Borison et al, "Metabolism of an Antidepressant Amino Acid [L-phenylalanine]," presented in poster session at the April 9-14 1978 meeting of the Federation of American Societies for Experimental Biology (FASEB), Atlantic City, New Jersey

The Herpes Epidemic:
A Possible Solution

Herpes viruses cause some of the most common of human diseases: herpes type 1 (cold sores) and herpes type 2 (genital herpes). Genital herpes is now an epidemic and is probably the most common form of venereal disease. Unfortunately, there are other even more serious conditions associated with herpes virus infections. Herpes viruses have been implicated as causative factors in several types of human cancers, including Burkitt's lymphoma, nasopharyngeal cancer, cervical carcinoma, and possibly colon cancer and some forms of breast and liver cancer. Herpes is a persistent virus; once a person is infected by herpes, he or she remains infected for life even if there are no symptoms most of the time.

The herpes virus inserts a few copies of its own genetic information into the DNA of many of your own cells. Once this information is inserted, there is no way available as yet to remove it. The herpes information seems to remain inactive until the cell's genetic material is damaged, when the herpes nucleic acid may become activated. This damage may occur as a result of ultraviolet light exposure, emotional stress, or illness, which reduce the ability of your immune system to control the newly created virus particles. The appearance of these newly made viruses is associated with symptoms such as cold sores or burning and itching genitalia.

Available approved treatments for herpes virus infections

have been highly toxic. The most frequently used is 2-deoxy-5-iodouridine (Idoxuridine), which interferes with normal incorporation of thymidine during DNA synthesis. It interferes with DNA synthesis in normal as well as in infected cells. Idoxuridine is a mutagen (causes mutations) and a carcinogen (can cause cancer). It is used in the treatment of herpes because of the absence of FDA approved safer systemic treatments and because, left untreated, herpes infections can have serious consequences, such as blindness or death by brain infection or, possibly, cancer. A new, less hazardous nucleic acid analog, Acyclovir®, has just been approved by the FDA, but only for topical treatment of new cases of herpes. While safer than Idoxuridine, Acyclovir®, nevertheless, works by interfering with DNA synthesis and can interfere with your own cells' DNA synthesis as well.

Herpes viruses belong to a class of viruses that have a lipid (fatty) coat surrounding their protein and nucleic acid core. This coat makes it difficult for immune system antibodies and white blood cells to recognize the virus as foreign because the fatty coat is made up of fats normally found in our tissues. Other lipid coated viruses are implicated in persistent virus degenerative diseases: for example, measles virus antibodies are found in far larger than normal numbers in victims of multiple sclerosis.

A new and apparently effective treatment for herpes viruses has recently been discovered. BHT, butylated hydroxytoluene, is a relatively low toxicity food preservative (antioxidant) which has been found to kill all small nucleic acid core diameter, lipid-coated viruses tested, including herpes. Dr. George Rouser at the City of Hope Hospital, a world renowned expert in fatty acid structures, explained to us that the molecules in the lipid coat surrounding herpes viruses are spirally arrayed very tightly about the nucleic acid core, like the spiral steps in a lighthouse staircase, with considerable steric strain. When BHT dissolves into this lipid coat, he thinks it likely that it destabilizes these hydrogen bonds so that the coat is stripped off. Once the lipid coat is gone, the white blood cells and antibodies and nucleases (enzymes that destroy unprotected DNA) recognize the foreign viral nucleic acid and accompanying foreign proteins and destroy it.

BHT's effectiveness has been demonstrated in vitro against several types of small nucleic acid core diameter, lipid-coated viruses. BHT has already undergone very extensive tests of toxicity, many conducted by companies selling it as a food preservative. Monkeys have been fed up to 30 grams a day in a short term test, an immense dose. (**Do not try this on yourself!**) The only adverse results reported at these doses were very elevated liver enzyme levels and an enlarged liver (BHT induces the synthesis of certain liver detoxification enzymes) which returned to normal after the animals were taken off the BHT. We started taking BHT (2 to 6 grams per day) in 1968 for its free radical controlling, life extension effects, which had been discovered several years earlier by Dr. Denham Harman, the creator of the free radical theory of aging. When we saw the Snipes paper on in vitro tissue culture studies of BHT and herpes in 1975, we immediately calculated that our experimental 2-gram-per-day life extension dose should be highly effective in treating herpes in man and other animals. Snipes had performed no animal experiments and expressed some doubt that enough BHT would be absorbed orally to be effective. We knew from the mild psychotropic (mind altering) effects of a large dose of BHT taken on an empty stomach that substantial amounts were rapidly absorbed from the gut and that it could easily penetrate the blood-brain barrier as well. We also knew that, according to our clinical test results, 2 grams of BHT per day was reasonably safe, at least for us.

When, in 1975, a medical cytologist friend with severe persistent genital herpes was told by her gynecologist to be celibate for six months and hope for improvement, we conducted the first (to our knowledge) human experiment on the effect of BHT on herpes. We supplied copies of the Snipes paper, toxicological data, our own clinical test results, BHT, and instructions. It worked perfectly (the herpes was completely suppressed) and our friend's clinical tests remained normal. The BHT also worked on all her infected friends. Indeed, although sexually active and exposed to plenty of ultraviolet light and assorted stresses, Durk has had no herpes infections since 1968 when we started taking BHT, except when he discontinued his BHT for about three months as an experiment involving lipids and liver enzymes, which resulted in a nasty attack of herpes-caused psoriasis. This vanished within a few days of his resuming regular BHT use. (Sandy has never had herpes attacks.) The three-month delay is in reasonable accord with the known half life of BHT in humans and the concentration of BHT found by Snipes to kill herpes viruses.

BHT has also been used in a doctor's uncontrolled clinical trial involving over 150 patients with herpes (involving cases with either or both type 1 and type 2), almost all of which achieved remission with BHT. We personally know several people who had genital herpes which had been considered untreatable by their doctors and which subsequently responded to BHT. The herpes patients used 2 grams per day to control their herpes. BHT use should be maintained (although

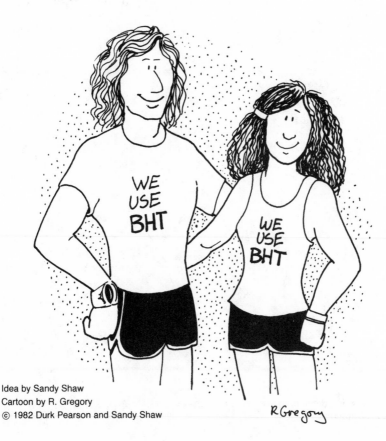

Idea by Sandy Shaw
Cartoon by R. Gregory
© 1982 Durk Pearson and Sandy Shaw

the dose may be reduced to as little as ¼ gram per day after about 10 days to two weeks in some cases) because the BHT kills only the free viral particles, not the viral information inserted into otherwise normal cells. So far, we do not have any way to destroy the inserted viral information.

We always take our daily dose of BHT at bedtime, generally on an empty stomach. This dosage schedule maximizes the amount of BHT that escapes destruction in the liver and is hence available to other tissues. A few uncontrolled observations suggest that herpes is substantially more difficult to control if small doses of BHT are taken throughout the day with food.

Few doctors know about BHT as a treatment for herpes because this is not an FDA approved therapy. BHT's patents have long ago expired, so there is no incentive for any company to spend the more than $50,000,000 (on the average) and 8

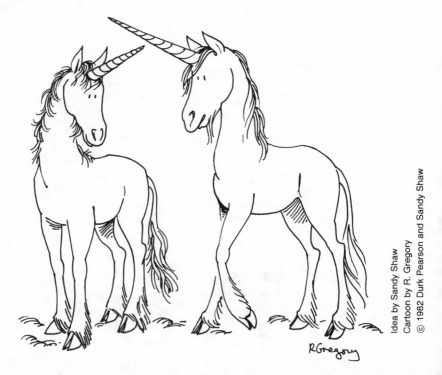

Idea by Sandy Shaw
Cartoon by R. Gregory
© 1982 Durk Pearson and Sandy Shaw

"That was an advanced questionnaire for the swinger's club. . . . It asked whether I used L-Dopa or BHT!"

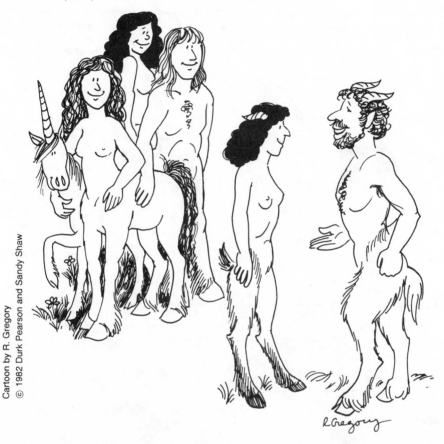

"At this orgy, we all use BHT!"

to 12 years to get BHT approved for this purpose. Even if FDA's approval could be obtained (far from a sure thing), the company spending this money could not charge any more for their BHT than any other company and, hence, could not recover their expenses. In the meantime, any doctor who uses BHT has to consider possible suits for malpractice, which are much more likely to occur when an FDA unapproved treatment is used.

WARNING: Remember that this FDA unapproved treatment is experimental, and pre-drug baseline and post-drug followup clinical tests for liver function, serum lipids, and a complete blood count should be performed.

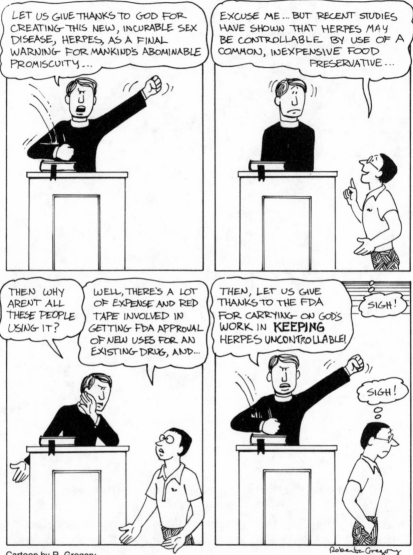

Cartoon by R. Gregory
© 1982 Durk Pearson and Sandy Shaw

WARNING: Do not use BHT if your liver is diseased or damaged, or if your pre-BHT liver tests are abnormal.

WARNING: BHT should not be used with barbiturates, other downers, or alcohol since it will increase their effects. BHT combined with alcohol is not likely to cause respiratory collapse, however, as alcohol and barbiturates and other combinations of sedatives can. When first using BHT, hypotension may occur, resulting in lightheadedness upon standing or arising in the morning. This is not a toxic side-effect, but when experiencing this, one should not operate an automobile or other hazardous equipment. This effect tends to go away after a few days. If the BHT is taken at bedtime, starting at ¼ gram and slowly increasing the dose, if necessary, this is rarely a problem.

REFERENCES

Branen, "Lipid and enzyme changes to organs of monkeys fed BHA and BHT," *Food Product Development*, April, 1973

Dr. George Rouser, City of Hope Hospital, Duarte, California, possible mechanism for BHT's disruption of lipid coat surrounding some viruses, personal communication

Snipes, Person, Keith, Cupp, "Butylated Hydroxytoluene Inactivates Lipid-Containing Viruses," *Science* 188: 64-66, 1975

Snipes and Keith, "Hydrophobic Alcohols and Di-tert-butyl Phenols as Antiviral Agents," in *Symposium on the Pharmacological Effect of Lipids*, edited by Jon J. Kabara, The American Oil Chemists' Society, 1978

Brugh, M., Jr., "BHT Protects Chickens Exposed to Newcastle Disease Virus," *Science* 197:1291, 1977

Kim, Moon, Sapienza, Pularkat, *J. Infect. Dis.* 138: 91-94, 1978

Cupp, Wanda, Keith, Snipes, *Antimicrob. Agents Chemother.* 8:698-706, 1975

Wanda, Cupp, Snipes, Keith, Rucinsky, Polish, Sands, *Antimicrob. Agents Chemother.* 10:96-101, 1976

Sex Hormones: Some Uses and Their Risks

The dangers associated with the use of birth control pills have been greatly exaggerated. Dr. Christopher Tietze has made a study of the annual number of deaths per 100,000 nonsterile women associated with the use of several fertility control techniques (including no control, the pill, IUDs, diaphragm or condom, diaphragm or condom and abortion, and abortion). In fact, the product insert in the oral contraceptives of Ortho Pharmaceutical Corp., and probably that of other manufacturers, contains a chart prepared by Dr. Tietze which summarizes his data. Dr. Tietze told us recently that he is about to publish a new chart, but he said that the differences between it and the older one, published in 1977 (which we describe here) are small.

The chart shows that risks of death for birth control pill users are low, lower than the risks for no birth control at every age except *smoking* users over 40. The risk for non-smoking pill users is comparable to that of diaphragm or condom users at all ages, though slightly higher over the age of 40. The risk for smokers who use the pill is elevated (but still lower than no birth control) between the ages of 35 and 39. Pill users over 40 who smoke have a greatly elevated risk of death compared to non-smoking pill users and to the other birth control methods evaluated.

Risks that have been associated with birth control pill use include blood clots. It is known that both smoking and the use of oral contraceptives reduces the serum concentrations of vitamins C and B-6. These vitamins are important antioxidants, which help prevent the formation of abnormal clots. Healthy arteries are lined with prostacyclin, an anti-clot hormone recently discovered by Vane and Moncada. Lipid peroxides (the products of the spontaneous, uncontrolled oxidation of fats in the body) prevent the manufacture of prostacyclin, greatly increasing the chances of abnormal clot formation. Antioxidants like vitamins C and B-6 block the formation of lipid peroxides and, consequently, help maintain prostacyclin levels. In one study of hospitalized subjects, 1 gram of vitamin C a day decreased the incidence of deep vein clotting (a significant danger for bedridden patients) by about half.

Another controversial use of sex hormones is to restore their levels in postmenopausal women. Without such treatment, a woman will probably have discomfort (pain, burning, and soreness) during intercourse because the vagina atrophies without adequate estrogenic stimulation. In addition, the vagina may be more subject to chronic infections. Far more importantly, however, within a few years after menopause, women who do not take hormone replacement have, on the average, a risk of heart attacks as high as that for a man their age. Moreover, the overall death rate for postmenopausal women who do not take hormone replacement is about two to three times, on the average, that of those women who do. The incidence of some types of cancer, such as uterine cancer, are lower for women taking balanced hormone replacement after menopause, with the exception of injected conjugated estrogens, which cause an increased cancer risk.

Orally administered sex hormones have significant systemic effects. They stimulate the breasts, ovaries, and uterus, in addition to the vagina; cancers of these sexually responsive female tissues are sometimes stimulated by estrogens. It is desirable to use replacement sex hormones topically in the vagina to avoid excess systemic concentrations of estrogens. There is a commercial vaginal suppository for the topical application of hormones, Test-Estrin Vaginal Inserts® (Marlyn Pharmaceuticals) which contains 5 milligrams of testosterone and 0.5 milligrams of estradiol. Only about half of what is applied is absorbed. This suppository exposes the rest of the body to about 4 to 8 times less of these sex hormones than the conventional hormone replacement tablets. In addition, the suppository supplies testosterone, which helps prevent excess estrogenic stimulation. Conventional replacement tablets supply only female sex hormones, no testosterone, even though postmenopausal women produce less testosterone as well as less of the estrogens. A relatively safe oral hormone replacement strategy involves the use of low total dose birth control pills with a moderately high ratio of progestin to estrogen. The cardiovascular risk is increased only for smokers, so non-smokers may want to consider this approach, since it reduces the incidence of female sexual cancers by 40 to 90%, with the greater levels of protection being for some of the most lethal types. Even if you don't smoke, we do recommend a total of 100 milligrams of B-6 and 3 grams of C in 3 or 4 divided doses each day. (For further details, see our book *Life Extension, a Practical, Scientific Approach*, Warner Books, 1982.)

REFERENCES

Tietze, "New Estimates of Mortality Associated with Fertility Control," *Family Planning Perspectives* 9(2):74-76, March/April 1977

Rosenberg, Shapiro, Slone, Kaufman, Helmrich, Miettinen, Stolley, Rosenshein, Schottenfeld, Engle, "Epithelial Ovarian Cancer and Combination Oral Contraceptives," *J. Amer. Med. Assoc.* 247: 3210, 18 June 1982

Hulka, Chambless, Kaufman, Fowler, Greenberg, "Protection Against Endometrial Carcinoma by Combination-Product Oral Contraceptives," *J. Amer. Med. Assoc.* 247: 475, 22/29 January 1982

Bush, Cowan, Barrett-Connor, Criqui, Karon, Wallace, Tyroler, Rifkind, "Estrogen Use and All-Cause Mortality," *J. Amer. Med. Assoc.* 249(7):903, 18 Feb. 1983

Purdy and Goldzieher, "Toward a Safer Estrogen in Aging," paper presented at the "Intervention in the Aging Process: Basic Research, Pre-Clinical Screening, and Clinical Programs" conference, sponsored by the Fund for Integrative Biomedical Research and Boston University School of Medicine, 5 & 6 November 1982 at the Boston Marriott Hotel, Long Wharf, Boston, Mass.

Fads and Fallacies

FDA Notice: Prescribing Approved Drugs for Unapproved Uses

(Reprinted from the *FDA Drug Bulletin* 12(1), 1982)

NOTICE

USE OF APPROVED DRUGS OF UNLABELED INDICATIONS

The appropriateness or the legality of prescribing approved drugs for uses not included in their official labeling is sometimes a cause of concern and confusion among practitioners.

Under the Federal Food, Drug, and Cosmetic (FD&C) Act, a drug approved for marketing may be labeled, promoted, and advertised by the manufacturer only for those uses for which the drug's safety and effectiveness have been established and which FDA has approved. These are commonly referred to as "approved uses." This means that adequate and well-controlled clinical trials have documented these uses, and the results of the trials have been reviewed and approved by FDA.

The FD&C Act does not, however, limit the manner in which a physician may use an approved drug. Once a product has been approved for marketing, a physician may prescribe it for uses or in treatment regimens of patient populations that are not included in approved labeling. Such "unapproved" or, more precisely, "unlabeled" uses may be appropriate and rational in certain circumstances and may, in fact, reflect approaches to drug therapy that have been extensively reported in medical literature.

The term "unapproved uses" is, to some extent, misleading. It includes a variety of situations ranging from unstudied to thoroughly investigated drug uses. Valid new uses for drugs already on the market are often first discovered through serendipitous observations and therapeutic innovations, subsequently confirmed by well-planned and executed clinical investigations. Before such advances can be added to the approved labeling, however, data substantiating the effectiveness of a new use or regimen must be submitted by the manufacturer to FDA for evaluation. This may take time and, without the initiative of the drug manufacturer whose product is involved, may never occur. For that reason, accepted medical practice often includes drug use that is not reflected in approved drug labeling.

With respect to its role in medical practice, the package insert is informational only. FDA tries to assure that prescription drug information in the package insert accurately and fully reflects that data on safety and effectiveness on which drug approval is based.

OUR COMMENTS

First, we are grateful to FDA for publishing this important clarification. We are confident that this will result in greater utilization of safe and effective modern therapies that have not yet received FDA approval. We would like to thank the individual or individuals at FDA responsible for making this information available.

Additional clarification: The establishment of a drug's being "safe and effective" by the FDA is a legal description, rather than a scientific one. Because a drug has *not* received

FDA approval does not necessarily mean that it is not safe and effective for a particular use. FDA approval is required, however, before one may legally market the drug for that use. The statement that FDA approval for a new use "may take time" puts it mildly. It may take as long as FDA approval for the original use, an average of 8 to 12 years and about $50 million for a truly new compound. This has a direct bearing on why manufacturers often fail to attempt to receive FDA approval for new uses.

The Fallacy of Perfect Safety

The Safety Occurrence Board (SOB) of the government agency was concerned that avid ping pong players might be suffering brain damage by being hit repeatedly on the head by ping pong balls. Even though one hit seems harmless, they thought, there might be cumulative damage. So, they dropped a four ton safe on the head of an experimental animal to test whether being hit on the head once every hour for fifty years would be dangerous! They called it an accelerated hazard test. As a result, ping pong was outlawed in the U.S. They laughed in Europe and Japan (and even in Russia). The black market started smuggling in ping pong balls and many health food stores offered them for sale as "Christmas tree ornaments."

This seemingly absurd hypothetical event is analogous to what are called accelerated tests for safety being conducted by some actual government agencies. The reasoning is this: Suppose there is a very weak carcinogen being added to foods as a coloring agent or a sweetener. If you test a reasonable number of animals, the carcinogen may be so weak that you can't detect any effect. In order to detect an effect, you can either increase the number of animals (which could be very expensive), or you can increase the dose of the carcinogen. There is a problem, however. Animals, like people, have protective enzymes and other systems that allow them to handle a certain amount of carcinogens. Beyond that, these protective systems become overloaded, and the animal is much more likely to get cancer. Exposing animals to immense doses of a weak carcinogen may have very little to do with what happens to animals chronically exposed to small quantities of a weak carcinogen. In fact, this is what happened to saccharin. Exposing experimental animals to immense doses of this very weak carcinogenic promoter caused cancer in a

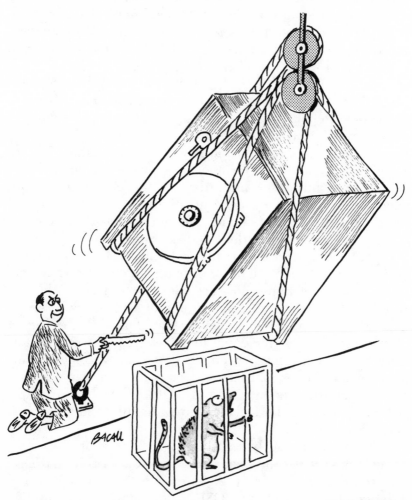

"Help! I volunteered for a Ping-Pong–ball study!"

Idea by Sandy Shaw
© A. Bacall 1983

small percentage of them. The dose was the equivalent of a human being drinking over 1,000 cans of saccharin-containing soft drinks a day! A widespread public outrage at the prospect of saccharin's being banned, however, led to Congressional action which prevented the FDA from removing saccharin from the market.

Can this sort of accelerated ultra-high dose hazard test ever be valid? Yes, it can under certain *very* special circumstances. To the best of our knowledge, none of the accelerated ultra-high dose hazard tests to date have included the validity verification experiments that are necessary. For ultra-high dose accelerated hazard tests to be valid, the following must be shown: the substance is metabolized and/or excreted in exactly the same way, regardless of dose (rarely true), and this is the same in both the test species and in humans (sometimes true). The damage done should be linearly related to the dose in both species (often untrue), or the dose-damage curve must be known quite precisely at low doses for both species (but if it was known at low levels, accelerated hazard testing would not be performed!). The protective and damage repair mechanisms of both the test species and humans should be qualitatively and quantitatively identical (rarely true), and the character and effectiveness of these mechanisms should be independent of dose (rarely true).

One can see that much accelerated hazard testing is political rather than scientific in nature. Political? The sugar lobby funded the hyper-dose accelerated hazard tests that led to the Delaney Amendment banning of artificial sweeteners. The same test animals exhibit an elevated incidence of cancer if they are given sugar equal in sweetening power to a few percent of the artificial sweetener dose they were given. The artificial sweetener lobby cannot use this sugar-can-be-a-carcinogen or carcinogen promoter data to try to ban sugar, however, because the Delaney Amendment excludes natural carcinogens!

Behind many of the safety requirements being enforced by agencies such as the Food and Drug Administration (FDA), Environmental Protection Agency (EPA), the Occupational Safety and Health Agency (OSHA), and others is the implicit premise that it is possible to mandate perfect safety. The requirement for zero tolerance for carcinogens (the Delaney Amendment of the FDA Act) is an explicit example. The regulations of OSHA and EPA require that control of certain substances be carried out regardless of cost, that is, regardless of whether the resources used for that purpose might have been better used for a different problem. The searchers for perfect safety first and foremost fail to consider that resources are limited while problems are virtually unlimited.

Nothing is perfectly safe! Let's consider some things we normally don't associate with danger. We breathe oxygen all the time and almost always take it for granted. Yet, oxygen is a potent poison at high enough concentrations. Oxygen causes damage to the eyes and other parts of the central nervous system via the creation of free radicals. In mice not given protective antioxidant supplements, exposure to 1 atmosphere of pure oxygen (that's five times normal) caused complete destruction of the thymus gland after four days and the animals died shortly afterward of pulmonary edema. Humans, however, have much better protection. At sufficiently high doses of oxygen for long enough, damage can occur. Deleterious eye changes can occur, for example. Air Force pilots breathing too much pure oxygen (as they did, years ago) would sometimes suddenly become paralyzed. Many premature infants in respirators breathing pure oxygen became blind, depending on the length of exposure, before prudent exposure limitations were developed. At a concentration fifteen times normal oxygen concentration, human beings die in convulsions after less than an hour. This damage is probably largely due to free radicals. Water can be harmful, too. Too much water given to infants can result in hyponatremia, a deficiency of sodium chloride, common salt, and even result in convulsions and death within a day. Even an inert gas such as helium can be lethal; high pressure helium will cause rapid death by convulsions even in the presence of the proper amount of oxygen.

Safety standards are also applied very unevenly. For example, people seem to be willing to accept relatively large risks from some forms of energy production, while, at the same time, expecting much more stringent safety from nuclear energy. A major hydroelectric (energy generating) dam has a failure risk of about $\frac{1}{10}$ of 1% to 1% per year on the basis of the actual historical record. Commercial nuclear power plants have never killed anybody. Dam failures have killed tens of thousands of people over the years. If the Oroville Dam failed, 200,000 people could be killed. In the 40's, a coal burning power plant explosion in the USA killed 143 people. About a year ago, an oil burning power plant in Venezuela blew up and incinerated over 200 people, with practically no media attention in the USA. The 1985 EPA coal-burning power plant standards for new plants—which no one has met —allow the release of more radiation (of a more dangerous sort, too) than even ancient nuclear power plants of the 50's. Modern nuclear power plants compare even more favorably. Polynuclear aromatic hydrocarbons, PAH, the combustion tar carcinogens that are created when almost anything (gasoline, cigarettes, wood, etc.) is burned, are a hazardous product of coal burning power plants. In fact, these PAH carcinogens are much more dangerous by themselves than the coal burning power plant's radiation release. Worse yet, there is strong evidence for a potent co-carcinogenic synergy (more cancer than the sum of either substance considered alone) between PAH and radioactive isotopes on the same particles of respirable fly ash. Nuclear plants do not create PAH pollutants. Yet, there are no EPA standards for PAH emissions from coal burning power plants. Coal burning power plants release more radioactive pollutants into the air than do nuclear power plants. Yet, there are no NRC or EPA radiation standards applied to the coal plants.

Why do so many people seem to perceive risks as greater if they derive from nuclear power plants and do not respond to much larger risks stemming from coal burning power plants? We think that the scores of cheap horror movies, Japanese and otherwise, that depicted the monster crawling out of the swamp after being exposed to radiation may have prejudiced many people. The association of nuclear power with nuclear bombs is another problem. Yet another may be a religious/philosophical problem stemming from a *feeling* that coal or water (dam) power is less dangerous than nuclear power. Such a nature worshiping religious feeling might be very resistant to evidence to the contrary. Few people actually read technical reports and attempt to evaluate the data regarding safety of energy sources. But that doesn't stop anyone from having feelings about these things, regardless of the facts. It is ironic that the ecologists' beloved tightly sealed, passively solar heated, energy efficient homes often have radon and polonium radiation levels inside that are higher than those permitted by OSHA for 40-hour-per-week exposure in a uranium mine. One solar heated home in Maine delivered radiation to the lungs of the occupants at a rate equal to several thousand chest x-rays per year. Rock, bricks, tiles, concrete, and glass all contain traces of uranium and thorium and release the radioactive gas radon. Radon can easily escape from a normal home, but not from a tightly sealed building.

REFERENCE

Gougerot-Pocidalo, Jacquet, Pocidalo, "Demonstration of the Depressive Effect of Normobaric Oxygen on the Mouse Lymphoid System," *C. R. Seances Acad. Sci.* Ser. 3 1982, 294(18): 925-7 (Fr.)

Synthetic Versus Natural: Which Is Better?

> "I just don't understand those health freaks. I
> mean, the ancient Greeks ate only natural foods
> and look at them, they're all dead!"
> —Goldie Hawn

Many products in the marketplace are promoted as being more healthful because they are more natural than competing products. Are natural nutrients really better than synthetic nutrients?

The function of a nutrient depends upon its chemical structure, not upon its source. A molecule of vitamin C is the same as any other molecule of vitamin C, whether it's made in a soft, green leafy biological factory or in a shiny, man-made stainless steel factory. However, advocates of natural vitamins and other nutrients suggest that these substances are often associated in plants with other valuable nutrients, such as bioflavonoids with vitamin C, so that it is better to use nutrients derived from natural sources.

Let's consider why a plant contains nutrients such as vitamins C and E. These vitamins and many other nutrients (e.g., vitamins B-1, B-5, B-6, PABA, the amino acid cysteine, the minerals zinc and selenium, and others) are antioxidants, that is, they block certain uncontrolled spontaneous oxidation reactions which, if left unchecked, would damage various plant structures, including the DNA, their genetic blueprints. Unsaturated fatty acids and structures containing large quantities of them (such as cell membranes and plant seeds) are particularly susceptible to these damaging spontaneous free radical oxidations. When these fatty acids become oxidized via exposure to air or to chemical oxidizers, they turn rancid. Both the uncontrolled oxidation of the fat and the further chemical degradation of these chemically unstable rancid fats leads to the creation of highly chemically reactive and dangerous entities: free radicals. Their chemical reactivity is very promiscuous; they can attack any molecule in your body and are implicated as a major cause of cancer, cardiovascular disease, and aging. A lethal dose of x-rays kills because the x-rays produce free radicals in matter. Some free radicals are more potent oxidizers than fluorine. These are so ubiquitous that every air breathing organism on this planet is equipped with a battery of special enzymes and antioxidant nutrients to protect itself from damage by free radicals. Without these enzymes and antioxidants, ordinary air would quickly kill us, as well as all plants and microbes.

In a scientific study, it was found that plant seeds that contained oxidized lipids (rancid fats and oils) were less likely to germinate. There was nearly a negative-slope, straight-line relation between the percent of seeds that germinated and the degree of oxidation of its fat content; almost all seeds germinated at low levels of fat oxidation, but none did so at high levels. The very high levels of antioxidants such as vitamins C and E contained by plant seeds are necessary so that the seeds can germinate. But plants also contain many other substances to protect themselves from other enemies, such as animals which might eat them. For example, wheat germ (the embryo in a seed of wheat) contains, not only high levels of vitamin E, but also high levels of estrogens, female hormones. These hormones act as birth control pills that interfere with the reproductive cycle of female animals and also reduce the libido of male animals eating too much wheat, thereby reducing the number of offspring such animals produce! Cold pressed wheat germ oil also contains considerable quantities of these hormones, so that if a man were to take large doses (say 2,000 I.U. a day) of natural vitamin E in the form of cold pressed wheat germ oil, he could suffer a reduced libido or even testicular degeneration. Indeed, there are more estrogens in a single slice of whole wheat bread than there are in a pound of DES (diethylstilbesterol) treated calf liver.

About 98% of the plant matter on the planet dies before it is eaten either by animals or insects or microbes because of contained toxins. Even plants which have been specially bred to be non-toxic, like potatoes and tomatoes, contain toxins which we can detoxify in small quantities at a time, but which could kill us in large amounts, such as if we were taking megadoses of potato or tomato extracts. Highly purified natural vitamins, such as vacuum-distilled vitamin E, are nearly free of such toxins, but then there can be no advantage from possible unknown co-factors accompanying these vitamins. In one study of the bioavailability of synthetic vitamin C versus natural vitamin C, the synthetic C turned out to be slightly more bioavailable. One reason for this is that the natural vitamin C is bound to certain plant structures it protects. In order for us to be able to get at this C, our digestive system must break down these plant structures. No such barriers exist in the use of synthetic vitamin C. Bioflavonoids, which are synergistic in function with vitamin C, are contained in only very small quantities in crude vitamin C plant extracts. These bioflavonoids are however available inexpensively as relatively pure bioflavonoid extracts which may also contain insignificant amounts of natural vitamin C.

Many people are allergic to plant substances contained in natural vitamins. We have heard of numerous cases of allergic reactions to products advertised as containing natural C, but never to pure synthetic C. About 20% of the population shows an allergic response to the soy, yeast, or wheat added as a tabletting component.

Finally, synthetic vitamins are less expensive than natural vitamins. Natural vitamin C is a very expensive laboratory curiosity; it costs over $1000 per kilogram. So called "natural vitamin C" sold in health food stores is really almost entirely synthetic vitamin C plus a trace of natural C and other plant extractables, sometimes including allergens and insignificant amounts of plant toxins. When you pay a premium for "natural" vitamin C, you are shelling out your money to pay for a

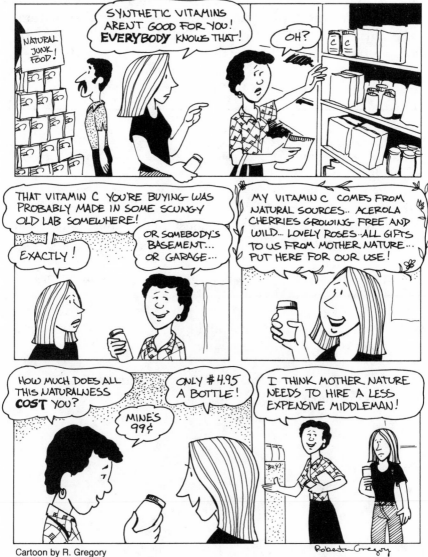

Cartoon by R. Gregory

fantasy. But don't worry about the slightly lower bioavailability of natural vitamin C extract; there is so little of it in so-called "natural" vitamin C that the impaired absorption is irrelevant. The scientific studies showing beneficial uses for vitamins have, in almost all cases, used synthetic vitamins so that it is possible to attribute the results to a single vitamin under study. As a result, we generally use synthetic vitamins and consider them to be far more cost-effective than natural vitamins. (Note, however, that B-12 is generally made by fermentation rather than by direct synthesis.)

REFERENCES

Pearson and Shaw, *Life Extension, A Practical Scientific Approach*, Warner, 1982

Today's Food and Additives, General Foods Corp. (For a free copy, write to General Foods Consumer Center, 250 North St., White Plains, NY 10625.)

Gregory and Kirk, "The Bioavailability of Vitamin B-6 in Foods," *Nutr. Rev.* 39(1): 1-8, 1981

Pelletier and Keith, "Bioavailability of Synthetic and Natural Ascorbic Acid," *J. Am. Diet. Assoc.* 64: 271-275, 1974

Harman and Mattick, "Association of Lipid Oxidation with Seed Aging and Death," *Nature* 260: 323-324, 1976

Natural Versus Synthetic Vitamin E: A Reply to Henkel Corporation

After the publication of *Life Extension, A Practical Scientific Approach*, in which we discussed the merits of synthetic versus natural vitamins, we received a long letter from Henkel Corporation. The letter had been sent to others, as well, including scores, perhaps hundreds, of people in the health food industry. However, we have not seen their mailing list. This firm is one of the major producers of "natural" vitamin E, which is encapsulated and sold under many different brand names. In their letter, written by Gerald G. Wilson, who used to be Vice President & General Manager of the company's Fine Chemicals Division, they disagreed with a number of our points. We consider this issue important and, hence, we are replying here.

Below, we reprint (except for a few minor and redundant points) the letter from Henkel. In brackets after each point, we give our reply. The page numbers indicated refer to *Life Extension, A Practical Scientific Approach*. We hope that this discussion will help clear the air about a very important scientific and philosophical matter.

This is not intended as a criticism of Henkel's vitamin E products, but only of some of the representations made about them. To avoid possible misunderstandings, we would like to emphasize these points:

We have no complaints about the quality of Henkel's vitamin E; we believe that it is a good product.

We believe that the comments made by Henkel's Gerald G. Wilson were made sincerely, though often in error.

We have had several constructive conversations with representatives of Henkel and Banner Gelatin (a major encapsulator of Henkel's vitamin E), and in our opinion, these people seem to be responsible, diligent and truly interested in investigating the incidence and severity of peroxidized oils in vitamin E capsules. We hope to report the results of their work in our next book.

Finally, we have an unsolicited recommendation for Henkel's marketing department. We think that they will sell more of their "natural" vitamin E, properly called natural form vitamin E and its esters, by emphasizing the virtues and quality of their products than by an ultimately hopeless and fallacious attack on the virtues and quality of synthetic vitamin E. Their "natural" product is indeed more expensive per International Unit of biological potency, but this price difference is no more than exists between some supermarket chain private label products and their successfully competing brand name counterparts. Moreover, many persons have a personal or aesthetic preference for "natural" vitamin E, just as we aesthetically prefer chocolate to vanilla ice cream. Far larger price spreads occur between functionally identical products in the cosmetic industry, price differences that are maintained by superior promotion of the more expensive product, not by knocking lower price competitors.

September 22, 1982

Mr. Durk Pearson   Henkel Corporation
Ms. Sandy Shaw   4620 West 77th St.
c/o Warner Books   Minneapolis, MN 55435
75 Rockefeller Plaza   612/828-8000
New York, NY 10019

Dear Authors,

We read with interest those portions of your "Life Extension" that dealt with vitamin E, since Henkel Corporation is the world's largest producer of natural-source vitamin E. Most of the information on vitamin E in the book is well written, but there are several major errors that need immediate correction:

pg. 31 " . . . vitamin E (dl-alpha tocopherol acetate) . . . " should read " . . . synthetic vitamin E (dl-alpha tocopheryl acetate) . . . "

[D&S: Both forms (dl-alpha tocopherol acetate and dl-alpha tocopheryl acetate) are correct, as indicated in major reference works such as the second edition of the *Food Chemicals Codex* and the ninth edition of the *Merck Index*. In fact, the use of the adjective "synthetic" in the "synthetic dl-alpha tocopheryl acetate" is redundant since "dl" identifies it as synthetic.]

pg. 54 All of the natural-source vitamin E sold in the USA is produced from unsaturated vegetable oils, primarily soybean oil. None is from wheat germ oil, so your comments about "vitamin E extracted from cold pressed wheat germ oil . . ." are incorrect and misleading. ". . . you don't hear loud outcries against this type of natural vitamin E" because there is none in the market place.

[D&S: Soybean oil also contains natural estrogenically active steroid hormones. As we pointed out in *Life Extension, A Practical Scientific Approach*, careful vacuum distillation removes these undesirable constituents, whereas they remain in cold pressed oil products. Many health food stores are selling cold pressed wheat germ oil as a natural nutritional supplement which is high in vitamin E. These crude natural preparations are also high in natural estrogens.]

pg. 407 "Synthetic vitamin E is a 50/50 mixture of the D and L forms. . . " Not true.

"The choice between this type of natural E and synthetic E should be made strictly on the basis of price." In the case of vitamin E, the choice is not that simple. As we indicate in our enclosed booklet "Human Needs for Vitamin E," natural vitamin E is d-alpha tocopherol. Synthetic vitamin E consists of 8 different isomers, only one of which is d-alpha tocopherol. The other seven isomers are not found in nature, and some have never been isolated and adequately tested in animals, let alone humans. Put another way, natural vitamin E is d-alpha tocopherol, one molecule. Synthetic vitamin E contains 8 different molecules, only one of which is d-alpha tocopherol, the other 7 being unnatural.

[D&S: The synthetic form of vitamin E is the form used in nearly all scientific experiments, including those investigating the effects of vitamin E on animals and humans. The booklet published by Henkel, which lists abstracts for scientific papers published in 1980 investigating vitamin E, even mentions the use of synthetic vitamin E in some of the listed papers. However, in most of the papers they list and discuss, Henkel does not state whether synthetic or natural vitamin E was used. It is completely untrue that commercial synthetic vitamin E has not been adequately tested in animals or humans. In fact, more is known about the effects of commercial dl-alpha tocopherol than d-alpha tocopherol, due to the use of the synthetic form of vitamin E in most scientific experiments. Synthetic vitamin E has been tested in humans at up to 65,000 I.U. per day, unlike natural vitamin E.

Many vitamins exist as a family of closely related chemicals, all of which exhibit significant vitamin activity. Vitamin B-3 is a simple example: nicotinic acid, nicotinyl alcohol, nicotinyl esters, and niacinamide are all biochemically acceptable forms of vitamin B-3.

Vitamin E is actually a very large family of molecules, both natural and synthetic. (We speak here about chemical structures, not FDA label regulations.) There are dozens of closely related compounds, natural and synthetic, in the vitamin E family which have varying degrees of biological potency. This is why experiments with vitamin E usually express the quantities in I.U., International Units of biological potency, rather than in milligrams of the vitamin.

The dl-alpha tocopherol of commerce is indeed a mixture of 8 isomers (geometric variations), only one of which is found in nature. Contrary to Henkel's claim, all 8 of these isomers have been tested and all have vitamin E activity. (See Weiser and Vecchi, "Stereoisomers of Alpha tocopherol acetate; Characterization of the Samples by Physico-Chemical Methods and Determination of Biological Activities in the Rat Resorption Gestation Test," *Int. J. Vitam. Nutr. Res.* 51: 100-113, 1981) In fact, there is evidence of strong positive synergy within the commercial 8 isomer product. Positive synergy is often exhibited by antioxidant mixtures. (Positive synergy means that the results of the combination are greater than the sum of the results of the components when tested one at a time. See Weber et al, *Biochemistry and Biophysics Res. Comm.* 14:186, 1964.)]

pg. 403 In unsaturated oils, it is the non-d-alpha forms of tocopherols that are the more effective antioxidants in preventing peroxidation of the oils. In most in vitro systems, the d-delta form is the most potent, followed in order by d-gamma, d-beta, and then d-alpha.

[D&S: In unsaturated oils in vitro (outside the body), it makes no difference in antioxidant potency whether the tocopherols are d, dl, or l. The d, dl, or l-delta and d, dl, or l-gamma tocopherols are indeed more potent antioxidants of unsaturated oils in vitro than are the d, dl, or l-alpha tocopherols. As we mentioned in *Life Extension, a Practical Scientific Approach*, however, the non-alpha isomers have relatively low in vivo (in the body) biological potency, probably because of their rapid metabolic destruction in animals.]

The original dl-alpha tocopherol which [their typo] did contain only the d- and l-forms. This type is no longer sold commercially. The above is one difference between natural-source and synthetic vitamin E.

[D&S: The original commercial dl-alpha tocopherol acetate which contained 2 isomers was used to define the I.U. as 1 I.U. = 1 milligram of dl-alpha tocopherol acetate. This was adopted by the National Institute for Medical Research of England for the World Health Organization. When the manufacturing process was changed to that which produces an 8-isomer product, the relative biological potencies of these two materials were compared and found to be equal within the limit of experimental error. This was reviewed in September 1982 by the WHO Expert Committee, and they reported no difference in bioactivity between these two alpha tocopherol products. Moreover, they reported that there was no need to change the 1 to 1.36 biological potency ratio of dl-alpha tocopherol to d-alpha tocopherol. This 1 to 1.36 international standard ratio was determined by averaging the experimental results found in 22 scientific papers using 8 different biopotency assay systems.]

Another difference is that natural-source vitamin E is derived from all-natural unsaturated vegetable oils primarily soybean oil. Synthetic or unnatural vitamin E is chemically synthesized from petroleum derivatives and turpentine.

[D&S: In Henkel's booklet, "Human Needs for Vitamin E," on page 37, it states that "Most natural Vitamin E sold in the U.S. is recovered from soybean oil. However, in soybean oil, the tocopherols occur in about the following proportions: d-alpha tocopherol, 9%; d-beta tocopherol and d-gamma tocopherol, 60%; d-delta tocopherol, 31%. **Accordingly, the d-beta, d-gamma, and d-delta tocopherols are normally methylated to the biologically active d-alpha form before being offered for sale.**" (Emphasis added by us) We see, therefore, that 91% of the "natural-source" vitamin E is produced synthetically by chemical methylation! This synthetic reaction is performed using formaldehyde, or methyl (wood) alcohol, or with chloromethylating agents or other alkylating chemicals. However, it is a chemical's structure that determines its function, not its chemical source. We think that it is a fine idea to chemically methylate the non-d-alpha tocopherols to produce the biologically more active d-alpha tocopherol. But this cannot be considered a natural process. Even though the product molecules are identical in structure and function to natural d-alpha tocopherol, we would describe Henkel's product as 9% natural and 91% synthetic d-alpha tocopherol.]

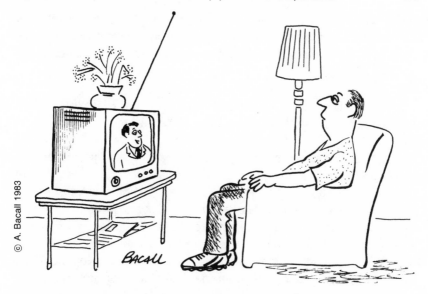

© A. Bacall 1983

"And remember, our vitamins are all-natural—synthesized in our own modern laboratories, from naturally occurring substances."

pg. 80 " . . . no difference between a synthetic molecule of a vitamin and a natural molecule of the same vitamin." Absolutely not true. See comments under pg. 54.

[D&S: The belief that the same molecule produced from a natural source is superior in biological effects to the same molecule produced synthetically is just that: a belief, a religion. We have no objection to people having any non-coercive personal beliefs they may choose, but it is very important to separate these feelings from scientifically valid statements. The idea that there was a special quality of naturally produced molecules was called vitalism in the nineteenth century and was destroyed (we thought) when urea was chemically synthesized by Frederick Wohler in 1828. Vitamin E is an important biochemical because it has a particular type of chemical structure which results in its biological antioxidant function.]

pg. 499 "Artificial vitamins are the same molecules as their natural counterparts." For vitamin E, not true, not true, not true!

[D&S: We have commented on this earlier. We can accept their feelings as a personal belief. But it cannot be demonstrated scientifically that the source of a chemical, rather than its structure, determines its function.]

Gram for gram, natural-source vitamin E is 36% more biologically active than the synthetic form.

[D&S: Yes, but it costs more than 36% more per gram than the synthetic form. The most economical buy, I.U. for I.U. (equivalent biological activity), is the synthetic vitamin E. For example, the 27 December 1982 Chemical Marketing Reporter stated that, as of that date, d-alpha tocopherol was being sold by U.S. producers for $48 to $50 per kilo. At the same time, the synthetic form of vitamin E, dl-alpha tocopherol, was selling in the range of $20 to $27 per kilo, about half the price per gram being asked for the natural form of vitamin E.]

pg. 78 "Vitamin E can be stored in the body for only a few days to weeks, depending on intake. . . " Not true. Vitamin E remains in the body for long periods of time.

[D&S: Vitamin E at high doses can be stored in the body and maintain the desirable unnaturally high serum levels for only a few days to weeks. At small intakes, it may remain in the body for long periods of time, but serum E levels are then in the normal range.]

pg. 114 The molecular structure for d-alpha tocopherol is incorrect. The end group should be $-CH_3$, not $-CH_2$.

[D&S: You are correct. Thank you for spotting a misprint.]

". . . Santoquin antioxidant acts like vitamin E in all known metabolic functions." Not true. Vitamin E has functions other than as an antioxidant in humans. For example, many researchers believe that vitamin E is an integral part of a number of enzyme systems.

[D&S: That quotation was taken from Monsanto's "Report No. 6 on Current Technology: Santoquin® Ethoxyquin Antioxidant, can it actually slow the process of aging?" which we reprinted in Life Extension, A

Practical Scientific Approach. On page 55, we say "Using a wide variety of metabolic tests, Monsanto's synthetic antioxidant ethoxyquin—which is not an exact copy of any known natural antioxidant—is able to replace dietary vitamin E in poultry (although not in people)." Monsanto should have been more explicit in the statement from its report, but this conclusion is based on work with ethoxyquin in poultry, as was apparent from the original context. We have not seen convincing evidence that vitamin E functions as a co-enzyme, though it certainly isn't impossible. If it does function as a co-enzyme, it could most plausibly be associated with controlling or facilitating mitochondrial single electron transfer reactions, that is, dealing with free radicals in the energy producing power plants in your cells.]

pg. 347 "Do not buy bottles of vitamin E oil; unless they contain very potent antioxidants such as BHT and BHA, the oil is apt to rapidly become badly autoxidized." This sentence is misleading: No vitamin E products on the market contain BHT or BHA. Why should they? Vitamin E is an antioxidant itself!

[D&S: Alpha tocopherol, whether synthetic or natural, is readily oxidized. That is why it is shipped by manufacturers such as Hoffmann-La Roche in aluminum bottles under dry nitrogen gas. Once the container is opened, it must be used rapidly or protected with antioxidants or quickly sealed into another airtight container.

Most vitamin E, whether natural or synthetic, is converted chemically to the unnatural synthetic ester form (for example, to alpha tocopheryl acetate), which is reasonably stable in the presence of air because it is not then an antioxidant. The ester group protects the otherwise oxidation-susceptible -OH group of the tocopherol. The body de-esterifies the vitamin E, converting it back to the alpha tocopherol which functions as an antioxidant. Henkel discusses their "natural" vitamin E acetates and acid succinates on page 17 of their booklet, "Vitamin E: Questions & Answers": "When exposed to air, d-alpha tocopherol will oxidize fairly rapidly. Its stability is greatly increased when converted to an oil, the acetate, or a powder form, the acid succinate. . . " "It is true that natural vitamin E acetates and acid succinates do not exist to any extent in nature. However, when ingested, these forms are converted in the body into d-alpha tocopherol, which is the form in which natural vitamin E functions in the body."

Henkel admits that they chemically convert their "natural-source" vitamin E to a non-natural substance to increase its chemical stability, but they do not think this disqualifies them from implying that their product is natural vitamin E in their promotional brochures. It has the chemical structure of natural vitamin E, but is only 9% natural. We applaud Henkel's esterification of the otherwise oxidation-sensitive d-alpha tocopherol (dl is just as sensitive), but we aren't as enthusiastic about the usual claims made in natural vitamin E promotional litera-ture. Henkel, unlike some of their competitors, has the honesty to correctly call their 9% natural 91% synthetic d-alpha tocopherol prod-ucts "natural source," but they should not imply that it is natural vitamin E. We suggest calling it "natural form" vitamin E and its esters. This designation refers to its chemical structure, which determines its biological function, the source of the starting materials being irrelevant.

One good reason to use TBHQ or other antioxidants (such as ascorbyl palmitate) in a vitamin E containing vegetable oil preparation is that the vegetable oil's stability is greatly enhanced by the presence of these much more potent, and in the case of TBHQ much less expensive, antioxidants.]

" . . . to avoid potentially oxidized filler oils. Do not buy vitamin E in safflower or other polyunsaturated oils." This is nonsense! Polyunsaturated oils themselves contain tocopher-ols which will give them some protection from peroxidation. The vitamin E, itself an antioxidant, in the capsule will offer complete protection.

[D&S: There is no such thing as "complete" protection. Every antioxi-dant has limits, vitamin E as alpha tocopherol is not an especially potent antioxidant by itself, and the esterified tocopherols are not antioxidants until de-esterified in your gut. Commercially refined vege-table oils have generally had much of their natural tocopherols re-moved in the refining process. Henkel obtains their raw tocopherols from the sludge residue remaining after refining soybean oil. These natural antioxidant tocopherols are in the oil refinery residue because they have been removed from the refined soy oil. Polyunsaturated oils are well known for how quickly they become rancid. One thing that is not as well known is that a vegetable oil will generally contain three times the level of hydroperoxides (mutagens, carcinogens, clot pro-moters, atherosclerosis promoters, immune system depressants) as animal fats before they can first be detected by a rancid odor. There have been about fifteen to twenty uncontrolled clinical reports of humans ingesting vitamin E purchased at local stores who had sudden unexpected clotting episodes soon after starting to take high doses of the "vitamin E." However, in all the scientific laboratory studies using pure vitamin E (mostly synthetic) and its esters (without polyunsaturated oils) there have never been reports of abnormally accelerated clot formation, even at 65,000 I.U. per day in humans; quite the contrary, vitamin E has been shown to decrease the likelihood of abnormal clot formation. The vitamin E esters do not provide antioxidant protection to the added polyunsaturated filler oils.

Dr. Harry Demopoulos, Associate Professor of Pathology at New York University School of Medicine, tested four brands of vitamin E capsules containing polyunsaturated oils and found they all contained potentially hazardous levels of vegetable oil peroxides and hydroperoxides. This test was the standard food industry thiobarbituric acid assay for the malonaldehyde breakdown product of the oil peroxide and hydroperoxide.

If you believe that the natural tocopherols in commercial polyunsaturated vegetable oils are adequate to protect it from autoxidation, try this simple experiment. Take a paper towel and soak it in pure commercial natural safflower oil. Squeeze out the excess oil, fluff up the towel, and put it in a wide mouth jelly jar with the cap on loosely. Smell every day until you can detect rancidity. Do you really think that safflower oil-filled vitamin E capsules go from the manufacturer, through the wholesalers, retailers, and finally into your stomach in less time? The gelatin capsule acts as an oxygen diffusion barrier and hence slows down the peroxidation reaction but cannot stop it. Nutritional supplement capsules may take as long as 1½ years (data from Banner Gelatin) to go from manufacturer to consumer, and another 6 months to use up the package.

Vitamin E manufacturers and encapsulators have been concerned about the stability and potency retention of the vitamin E in their capsules and have demonstrated that this is not a problem. In the past, however, they merely assumed that the polyunsaturated vegetable filler oils were stable. Both Henkel (which does not itself encapsulate vitamin E) and Banner Gelatin, an encapsulator of vitamin E purchased from Henkel and others, have said that they will try the experiment of performing tests to detect peroxidized filler oils. We applaud this responsible approach to this problem and hope to report

the results of these tests and tests that we will be performing ourselves in our next book, *The Life Extension Companion, Volume II*.]

"What is the reason that you mention d-alpha tocopheryl
acid succinate, a natural-source form of vitamin E, only once
in your book? Is it because there is no synthetic form of the
succinate readily available in the USA?"

[D&S: No. The succinate was not as readily absorbed in some experiments. Perhaps this is one reason why its use is relatively uncommon
nowadays in scientific experiments.]

"Be particularly wary of vitamin E esters in oil-filled
gelatin capsules. Many vitamin packagers add oil to their
capsules to make them larger." Nonsense. On an identical I.U.
basis, the larger capsule would obviously cost the manufacturer more to make. Small amounts of vegetable oils are sometimes added to capsules to adjust the international units to
meet label claims.

[D&S: Some consumers are willing to pay more for the larger capsules
than smaller ones. It looks as though you are getting more. Soft gelatin
capsules are quite elastic during the manufacturing process. If a
particular batch of natural vitamin E has an unusually high purity and
potency, we would rather see this batch of capsules turn out a little bit
smaller than usual than keep them the same size by adding a vegetable oil filler. We think that consumers will understand this if a note to
this effect is put on the product package, just as consumers generally
understand settling of breakfast cereals in their box before purchase.
We suggest that manufacturers of vitamin E gelatin capsules
including polyunsaturated vegetable oils institute strict quality controls
to detect peroxides and develop safer formulations, possibly using
special stabilized oils, such as those used by the food industry for
applications like deep fat frying, or with added antioxidants such as
TBHQ and ascorbyl palmitate. From our food industry scientific consulting experience, we know that this is possible, even using only
"natural" antioxidants and chelating agents. We ourselves are trying
to develop an inexpensive and easy-to-use peroxide test to be made
available to consumers concerned about peroxides in their vitamin E

capsules, foods and edible oils. If some suppliers are reluctant to do the necessary quality control, consumers will have to do it.]

pg. 403 "We use vitamin E acetate (an ester) on a dry, powdered, hydrolyzed protein carrier. . . It contains no oil fillers." In spreading the vitamin E throughout a powder capsule, you greatly increase its contact with oxygen. Chances for oxidation are greater than in an oil filled capsule, where the skin of gelatin prevents contact of the vitamin E and oil from air.

[D&S: In long-term tests, the acetate ester is quite stable either as a powder, in a capsule, in a tablet, or as the pure viscous fluid. The gelatin capsule provides a limited diffusion barrier, but oxygen slowly dissolves into it and attacks the vegetable oils inside. Banner Gelatin's stability tests of dl-alpha-tocopherol (no vegetable oils) in their gelatin capsules does show that vitamin E potency is retained very well over a few years under their storage conditions.]

pg. 465 "Vitamin E (dl-alpha tocopherol acetate)." Why not indicate that the natural-source forms of vitamin E could be used; d-alpha tocopherol, d-alpha tocopheryl acetate, d-alpha tocopheryl acid succinate, for those people who do not want to take unnatural forms of vitamin E?

[D&S: We have explicitly stated that an International Unit (I.U.) of vitamin E potency is a measure of biological effectiveness. Why should we advise people to waste their money? The synthetic vitamin E gives you more International Units of biological potency per dollar. For those people whose personal beliefs prohibit their using synthetic vitamins, our formulas are given in I.U.'s of vitamin E, rather than milligrams, to emphasize biological potency so as to make it easy for those who prefer to use d-alpha tocopherol esters to obtain the same biological potency. There is plenty of vitalistic nonsense in some of the popular health magazines, and we do not wish to encourage it.]

pg. 490 "It makes no difference biologically whether a nutrient is obtained from natural sources or is synthetic." For vitamin E, *not true.*

[D&S: We have already commented on this error before. We agree with our original statement. *An I.U. is a measure of biological potency!*]

"No matter what form of vitamin E you buy, an I.U. (International Unit) is the same standardized measure of biological activity." No longer true. See previous comments on WHO.

[D&S: Even if we were to take the most optimistic figure giving "natural-source" vitamin E the greatest advantage in biological activity per gram over synthetic vitamin E, the price differential would still show that synthetic vitamin E is easily the best buy. If Henkel can devise a process whereby they can provide the same biological activity of their vitamin E less expensively than synthetic vitamin E, we will be happy to inform our readers of this bargain. A good step in this direction might be to take the money Henkel spends publicly attacking synthetic vitamin E and instead invest it in their production process improvement research and development.]

pg. 631 Synthetic versus Natural Controversy: why not list "Consumer Guide to Natural-Source Vitamin E" by the Henkel Corporation.

[D&S: Because, in our opinion, it contains too many errors. Its major thrust is an attempt to persuade people that their "natural" product, which is not price competitive with synthetic vitamin E per international unit of biological activity, has superior vitalistic properties, which is not supported by experimental evidence. If Henkel confined its material to promoting the virtues of either vitamin E in general or even their product in particular (which, we repeat, is a good product in spite of their advertising practices) we would be delighted to recommend their booklet, because there really is a lot of good information in there, too.]

We would appreciate receiving a response to our letter.

[D&S: This is it. We would like to thank Henkel for having the integrity to send us a copy of their objections, which they also sent to many members of the nutritional supplement industry. This is an honest, ethical way of dealing with our disagreements. Unfortunately, this standard of integrity is not universal.]

We hope that the next edition of your book will include the corrections with respect to vitamin E that we have indicated.

[D&S: We hope that this section of the book accomplishes that purpose.]

Yours very truly,
HENKEL CORPORATION

Gerald G. Wilson
Vice President & General Manager
Fine Chemicals Division

[D&S: P.S.: Roche's vitamin E is synthesized from carbon, limestone, water, and air (an amazing accomplishment!). Surely these qualify as natural sources, since they occur in nature. Plants synthesize their vitamin E from carbon dioxide, water, and air, though it took hundreds of millions of years of evolutionary trial and error to do it.

It is interesting to note that over two dozen chemical manufacturing steps are required to extract, partially purify, methylate, and esterify the natural source soybean oil refinery sludge to produce the d-alpha tocopheryl acetate that is sold commercially. In contrast to this, synthesized vitamin E acetate requires fewer than half the steps. Word games about the "naturalness" of vitamin E obscure the much more important issue of *why* the structure of vitamin E provides the biological benefits it does.]

Back to Butter, or the Truth about Polyunsaturated Fats

For a long time, many medical authorities (including the American Heart Association until very recently) have recommended substituting polyunsaturated fats in the diet for saturated fats. This is because of the belief that, since polyunsaturated fats slightly reduce serum cholesterol levels, they reduce the risk of heart attack. The findings of several large studies indicate otherwise.

It is true that polyunsaturated fats can reduce serum cholesterol levels to a small degree, but studies have shown that heart attack deaths are not lowered. Not only that, but it appears that cancer deaths are increased in patients on high polyunsaturated fats diets, and cancer deaths are unquestionably increased in experimental animals on these diets. A new understanding about the biochemistry of fat production and destruction provides a theoretical framework for understanding these otherwise puzzling findings.

Polyunsaturated fats are fats in which there are double bonds between two or more pairs of the carbon atoms. Saturated fats do not have any of these available double bonds to act as chemical reaction sites. Monounsaturated fats have only one double bond, and are usually much less readily autoxidized. Polyunsaturated fats are much more susceptible to autoxidation, when oxygen or other oxidizers directly attack the double bond sites in the absence of enzymatic control, forming oxidized fats called organic peroxides.

The same chemical process results in what is commonly called rancid (peroxidized) fats. These peroxidized fats are toxic, mutagenic (damage DNA), thrombogenic (cause abnormal blood clots), atherogenic (cause atherosclerosis), immunosuppressive (impair the function of parts of the immune system) and carcinogenic (cause cancer) substances. Upon further breakdown, peroxidized fats form highly chemically reactive molecules with unpaired electrons. These dangerous entities are called free radicals. Free radicals are strongly implicated as causative agents in aging, cardiovascular disease, cancer, arthritis, cataracts, senility, plus a whole host of

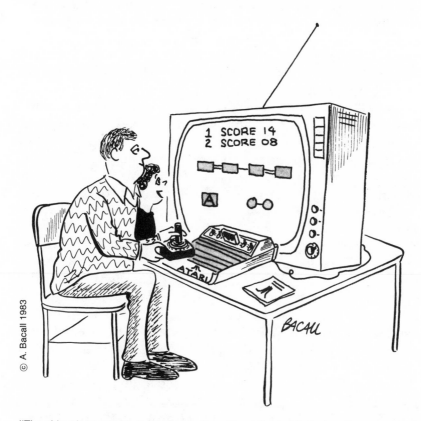

"The object is to get the antioxidant to the polyunsaturated fat before the oxygen does."

other conditions including such lowly ones as bruises and dandruff.

Dr. Denham Harman of the University of Nebraska, the originator of the free radical theory of aging (which emerged in the late 1950's), calls free radicals "internal radiation." That is a very good description of them because radiation sickness is a pure form of free radical disease. External radiation kills because it creates free radicals. "Internal radiation," free radicals created chemically within the body, can kill, too. And just as the prudent person avoids excess external radiation, he or she can minimize unnecessary "internal radiation" (free radical exposure) by decreasing consumption of fats, especially polyunsaturated ones, and increasing his or her consumption of antioxidants, substances which react with the free radicals, converting them to less harmful products. Common antioxidants include vitamins A, E, C, B-1, B-5, B-6, PABA, the amino acid cysteine, glutathione, the minerals zinc and selenium, and the synthetics BHT, BHA, propyl gallate, TBHQ, and DMSO.

Dr. Harman fed fatty acids of varying degrees of unsaturation, including the highly polyunsaturated safflower oil, menhaden oil, corn oil, olive oil, and the saturated fat lard to groups of rats beginning at the age of two months. Different groups of rats received the fats at 5%, 10%, or 20% by weight of their diet. At age 32-35 months, the rats were tested on a maze learning task. The amount or degree of unsaturation of the fat in the diet did not have an effect on the mortality rate. The number of maze errors generally increased both with an increase in the dietary percentage of fat and with an increase in the polyunsaturation of the fat. The ease with which the polyunsaturated fats are autoxidized (self-catalyzed oxidation that is not under enzymatic control) is the most probable explanation for this strange phenomenon. Autoxidized (rancid) fats break down to yield free radicals, which damage the surrounding tissues. These free radicals can damage other fats, DNA, RNA, and proteins. Since the brain and spinal cord contain a far higher content of polyunsaturated fats than any other tissue, they are far more susceptible to free radical damage.

Our brain and other tissues contain a complex system of

protective enzymes and antioxidants to control free radical activity. For example, the brain has two special vitamin C pumps—one in the blood-brain barrier (the selective barrier formed by the cells lining the insides of blood capillaries in the brain and spinal cord) and one in each nerve cell membrane—which concentrates vitamin C so that it ends up inside of brain cells at 100 times the blood plasma concentration! And during a heart attack, white blood cells carry vitamin C from other parts of the body to the injured heart, even when other areas of the body have to be depleted of 50% of their vitamin C.

Free radicals are a necessary part of certain metabolic reactions, such as those that metabolize food to create energy. Without free radical control enzymes, such as superoxide dismutase and glutathione peroxidase, and antioxidants such as vitamins C, E, B-1, B-5, B-6, PABA, the amino acid cysteine, glutathione, and the minerals zinc and selenium, we would quickly die. In fact, all air breathing organisms on this planet have very similar control enzymes and antioxidants, although relative proportions and total amounts vary. Radiodurans, a bacteria which lives inside of operating nuclear reactors, contains the highest levels of these protective antioxidant enzymes yet observed.

Cholesterol itself is an antioxidant. We think that the increases in serum cholesterol seen in some people is a bodily response to an increasing free radical load. It is interesting to note that some antioxidants taken singly in large doses, such as vitamins C and B-6, can sometimes reduce serum cholesterol by up to 40% percent or so. In our personal observations, combinations of antioxidants can reliably reduce serum cholesterol by up to 50%.

Scientists now know that the process of clotting is controlled via free radical reactions. A substance called thromboxane causes platelets in the blood to aggregate (which triggers the process of blood clotting), while another material called prostacyclin prevents platelet aggregation. Prostacyclin lines the walls in normal arteries, preventing abnormal clots (clots only form in a healthy artery when a hole is torn in it). Free radicals produced in the breakdown of autoxidized (rancid) fats can interfere with the normal production of prostacyclin, resulting in abnormal clot formation. In experiments, vitamin E has been shown to be an effective preventive of abnormal blood clots. Until recently, it was not understood how vitamin E could do this, but its basic biological function as a lipid (fat) antioxidant is the key. Vitamin E can protect the lipid membrane dependent enzymatic prostacyclin manufacturing apparatus from inhibition by free radical and organic peroxide damage, to which it is known to be very sensitive.

In another study, a small quantity of slightly peroxidized (rancid) polyunsaturated oil (where the rancidity could not be detected by nose) inhibited the activity of rabbit alveolar macrophages (white blood cells that patrol the lungs looking for invaders and foreign particles) by 50%. The rabbit's dose, if scaled up to human size, would be about one tablespoonful of slightly rancid (but with no perceptible rancid odor yet) polyunsaturated vegetable oil. One likely major factor why very overweight people often have depressed immune systems is that their bodies contain significant quantities of peroxidized fats.

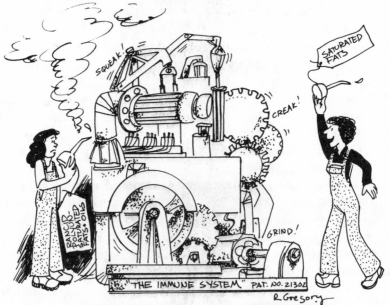

"Here, you may have better luck with *this*!"

Cartoon by R. Gregory
© 1982 Durk Pearson and Sandy Shaw

Rather than substituting polyunsaturated fats for saturated fats, we have radically (no pun intended) increased our intake of antioxidant supplements. It is probably also safest to eat a diet with only a moderate level of fat. Do not eat a lot of polyunsaturated fats, especially without antioxidant supplements added to your diet. The recent National Academy of Science report "Diet, Nutrition, and Cancer" (commissioned by the National Cancer Institute in 1980), which examined the role of nutrition in the causation of cancer, also concluded that dietary fat should be reduced and that data in animals suggest that when fat intake is low, polyunsaturated fats are more effective than saturated fats in enhancing tumorigeneses (the process of tumor formation). Even with the best of diets, the quantities of antioxidants you can get is limited. When we buy cooking oils, for example, we always add BHT (a synthetic antioxidant) to it, and we purchase oils which are *not* labelled as being high in polyunsaturates. Cooking oils often contain a high level of polyunsaturates and become autoxidized (rancid) very rapidly upon exposure to air. With added antioxidants, the shelf life may be many times as long.

The American Heart Association's 1983 dietary recommendations take cognizance of these findings. They very properly suggest a moderate reduction in total fat calories, with monounsaturated fats in greatest quantity, followed by saturated fats, with polyunsaturated fats being least. Bravo!

REFERENCES

Pearson and Shaw, *Life Extension, A Practical Scientific Approach*, Warner, 1982

Harman, Hendricks, Eddy, Seibold, "Free Radical Theory of Aging: Effect of Dietary Fat on Central Nervous System Function," *J. Am. Geriatr. Soc.* 24(7): 301-307, 1976

Harman, "Role of Free Radicals in Mutation, Cancer, Aging, and the Maintenance of Life," *Radiat. Res.* 16: 753-64, 1962

Tappel, "Vitamin E as the Biological Lipid Antioxidant," *Vit. Horm.* 20: 493-510, 1962

Slater and Alfin-Slater, "Effect of Dietary Cholesterol on Plasma Cholesterol, HDL Cholesterol, and Triglycerides in Human Subjects," *Fed. Proc.* Abstr. 2194, 1 Mar. 1978

Pryor, "Autoxidation of Polyunsaturated Fatty Acids," *Arch. Environ. Health*, pp. 201-210, July/Aug. 1976

Steiner and Anastasi, "Vitamin E: An inhibitor of the platelet release reaction," *J. Clin. Invest.* 57: 732-737, 1976

Shute, *Vitamin E for Ailing and Healthy Hearts*, Pyramid, New York, 1972

Hume et al, "Leukocyte Ascorbic Acid Levels after Acute Myocardial Infarction," *Brit. Heart J.* 34: 238-243, 1972

Nightingale et al, "Effect of Vitamin C and High Cholesterol Diet on Aortic Atherosclerosis in Dutch Belted Rabbits," paper presented at the 62nd Annual Meeting of the Federation of American Societies for Experimental Biology (FASEB), 9-14, April 1978

Charman et al, "Nicotinic Acid in the Treatment of Hypercholesterolemia," *J. Angiology*, Jan. 1973.

Spector, "Vitamin Homeostasis in the Central Nervous System," *N. Engl. J. Med.* 296:1393, 1977

Dix, Marnett, "Metabolism of Polycyclic Aromatic Hydrocarbon Derivatives to Ultimate Carcinogens During Lipid Peroxidation," *Science* 221(4605): 77-79, 1983

The Facts About Food Preservatives

"PRESERVATIVES MAY BE PRESERVING YOU
. . . I THINK THAT'S SOMETHING YOU
MISSED"
> —"Eat Starch, Mom,"
> lyrics by Grace Slick

[Food] preservatives may be preserving you, says the rock and roll singer. But what of all those others who just as vehemently believe that food preservatives should be avoided like the plague? What are the facts about food preservatives?

Food ages, just as living organisms do. The ways that food ages involve similar chemical processes, too. In order to understand why various types of preservatives are used, we have to know how food degrades with time. One of the most important of the food aging processes is the spontaneous oxidation of fats and oils.

Fats and oils contained in foods are subject to spontaneous, self-catalyzed oxidation (autoxidation) reactions when exposed to air. Both the creation and the breakdown of the oxidized fats result in the formation of chemically reactive and highly promiscuous entities called free radicals. Free radicals are mutagens (mutation causers), carcinogens (cancer causers), and a major cause of aging, both in food and in living organisms. In living plants and animals, special enzyme systems and antioxidants (substances which block uncontrolled oxidation reactions) control free radical reactions. Uncontrolled free radicals can do serious harm (they are implicated as causative factors in aging, cardiovascular disease, and cancer, as well as a host of less deadly but still unpleasant conditions). However, free radicals are necessary in some reactions of normal metabolism, such as the burning of food for energy. Without the free radical control enzymes (such as superoxide dismutase and glutathione peroxidase) and antioxidants (like vitamins C, E, B-1, B-5, B-6, the amino acid cysteine, glutathione, the minerals zinc and selenium), all air breathing organisms on this planet would quickly die.

Men used to risk their lives to trade in spices. When Magellan travelled around the world, one of his missions was to find and return with spices. And his crew was willing to face the risks that would kill most of them before the journey was over. In those days, spices were not just a way to make food taste good; they provided a form of food preservation that was very important to survival. Many spices, such as cloves, sage, oregano, and rosemary, contain potent antioxidants. In fact, a certain extract of rosemary is a stronger antioxidant than BHT. A ham studded with cloves not only tastes better, but the fats in the meat are protected against autoxidation.

Foods are tissues of dead animals or plants, or substances derived from them. The fats and oils in these tissues are still susceptible to oxidation. (Polyunsaturated fats are particularly easy to autoxidize.) Since the organism is no longer actively synthesizing the control enzymes and antioxidants, the fats and oils in these foods are especially vulnerable to oxidation (rancidity). Manufacturers of foods such as potato chips and cooking oils used to add antioxidants such as BHT (butylated hydroxytoluene) to protect the fats from oxidative degradation. But now, in response to misinformed public clamor for removal of preservatives, most such foods contain no antioxidant additives. In fact, food packages boast that they contain no preservatives. The sad fact is that such foods are much more dangerous to eat without added antioxidants than with

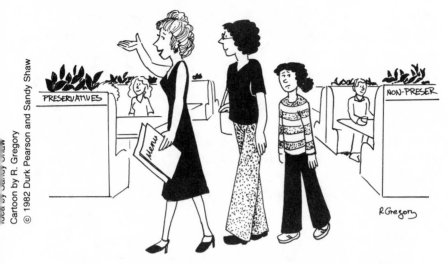

"And you have your choice of the 'Preservatives' or 'Non-preservatives' section. . . ."

them. The FDA itself has expressed concern about the removal of antioxidants from fats and oils.

Although BHT has been removed from many food products, a trend has recently started in the opposite direction. Shortly after the appearance of *Life Extension, A Practical Scientific Approach*, BHT began to be offered at health food stores. The BHT is usually supplied in the quantity required to preserve one quart of cooking oil. We hope people will use it for this purpose. If you insist on using a polyunsaturated cooking oil, another synthetic antioxidant called TBHQ (and mixtures containing it) is apt to be even more effective. In addition, BHT can be used to usually effectively and relatively safely control herpes infections. See "The Herpes Epidemic: A Possible Solution" elsewhere in this book.

An experiment in which oils were fed to rabbits showed that even oil that is only slightly oxidized, in which a rancid smell cannot yet be detected, contained enough oxidized fats to inhibit the rabbit alveolar macrophages (lung white blood cells, part of the immune system) from ingesting bacteria. If our white blood cells were as sensitive as a rabbit's (fortunately, they are not), it would take only about one tablespoon of these slightly oxidized oils to reduce the activity of these white blood cells by 50%! Our alveolar macrophages are an important defense against lung cancer; healthy active alveolar macrophages seek out, identify, kill, and eat cancer cells.

Manufacturers of foods have turned to other methods of protecting foods containing fats and oils. One successful method is to package the food in an airtight container such as a tin can, glass bottle, or plastic bag lined with aluminum foil. Of course, once the container is opened and the food exposed to air, it should be eaten immediately. Or you can immediately add your own antioxidants, such as BHT or ascorbyl palmitate.

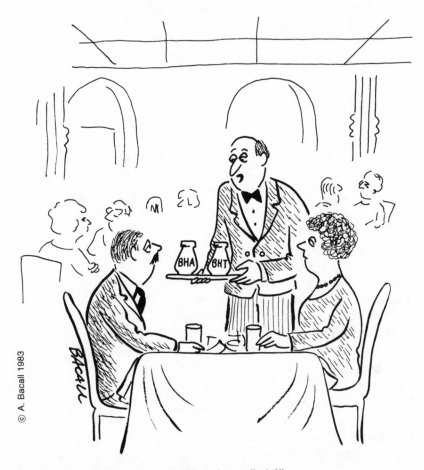

"Are you the party that's concerned about free radicals?"

Leftovers such as meats develop off flavors which are a reflection of the level of oxidized (rancid) fats they contain. Whenever we want to save these foods for later eating, we coat them with one of several antioxidants. Ascorbyl palmitate, a fat-soluble form of vitamin C, is particularly good for this because it is a powerful antioxidant and excellent synergist with other antioxidants and has little or no flavor of its own. The food is placed in a Ziploc® bag, ascorbyl palmitate powder is sprinkled generously over the food, the bag is shaken to disperse the powder, the excess air squeezed out, the bag zipped closed, and then the food is refrigerated. You can do a simple experiment comparing food stored in this manner to food stored without added antioxidant that will demonstrate how much longer it takes the treated food to develop a rancid odor.

Autoxidation of fats and oils takes place naturally in the bodies of living plants and animals such as ourselves. The brain and spinal cord are particularly susceptible to autoxidation because they contain a higher content of polyunsaturated fats than any other organs in the body. In one experiment with Sprague-Dawley rats, the animals fed semi-synthetic diets (which did not significantly affect the death rate) made more errors on a maze test when larger amounts of polyunsaturated fats were fed in place of saturated fats. Free radical damage resulting from the autoxidation of the excess polyunsaturated fats is a likely explanation.

Many people have strong negative feelings about food preservatives, especially synthetic ones. BHT is a good example. BHT has long been accused of causing cancer. Yet the fact is that numerous experiments in both animals and cell tissue cultures have demonstrated that BHT inhibits the development of many different types of cancers. It reduced the number of DNA-damage chromosome breaks in cells exposed to benzoalphapyrene, a powerful carcinogen (one of the polynuclear aromatic hydrocarbons, product of almost any type of combustion). In another study, nude (hairless) mice exposed to ultraviolet light but fed antioxidants (including BHT, which was later found to provide most of the protection) developed far fewer skin tumors than control mice.

There are many more examples. In the Soviet Union,

BHT is sometimes used as part of cancer therapy. Some scientists believe that the drop in stomach cancer that has taken place in the U.S. since WWII is largely due to antioxidants such as BHT added to the food supply. Under unrealistic dietary conditions (exposure to certain carcinogens before exposure to BHT) in strains of test animals that have been chosen to be cancer sensitive, an increased incidence of cancer can sometimes be observed. These conditions are not applicable to the American diet, due to the ubiquity of BHT in food stuffs. Your "all natural" cookies are likely to have some of it as an incidental additive added by the primary raw ingredients producers.

Moreover, in this same type of test for carcinogenicity, cruciform vegetables such as brussels sprouts give results like BHT because they have natural compounds in them which biochemically activate certain enzyme systems like BHT. Note that the 1982 report of the National Research Council of the National Academy of Science on human cancer and diet

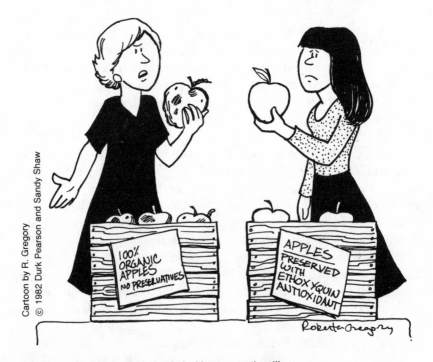

Cartoon by R. Gregory © 1982 Durk Pearson and Sandy Shaw

"How can you eat that? It's loaded with preservatives!"

recommends increased consumption of cruciform vegetables to reduce ones risk of cancer.

BHT has also increased the life spans of several species of experimental animals. Cancer-resistant strains of mice lived about 25% longer when given BHT, while a cancer-prone strain lived about 50% longer than normal. BHT given to pregnant mice, in one study, increased the lifespan of their offspring by about 20%, even though the young mice received no BHT after weaning. This is thought to be due to BHT's ability to prevent mutations. (However, we are *NOT* suggesting that pregnant women take BHT.)

So the next time you see a package of food in your supermarket bragging that it contains no preservatives, remember that preservatives may be preserving you and that unpreserved fats and oils spontaneously turn into immune system suppressive carcinogens when exposed to air. We hope that a more widespread public knowledge of these facts will lead to the return of routine antioxidant preservative use and to the development of even more effective new antioxidants. With the new scientific equipment we have acquired with royalties from our first book, such as an Altech laboratory computer-controlled Perkin-Elmer high pressure liquid chromatograph, we will be looking at plant material to find new, more potent antioxidants. Plants to be examined will include bristlecone pines (which live for about 4,000 years), creosote bush (which may live to 10,000 years), redwood trees, plants alleged to have anti-cancer activity, spices, jojoba, olive trees, and many others.

REFERENCES

Pearson and Shaw, *Life Extension, A Practical Scientific Approach*, Warner Books, June 1982

Khandwala and Gee, "Linoleic Acid Hydroperoxide: Impaired Bacterial Uptake by Alveolar Macrophages, a Mechanism of Oxidant Lung Injury," *Science* 182: 1364-65, 1973

Georgieff, "Free Radical Inhibitory Effect of Some Anticancer Compounds," *Science* 173: 537-39, 1971

Sherwin, "Antioxidants for Food Fats and Oils," *J. Amer. Oil Chem. Soc.* 49(8): 468-472, 1972

Harman, "Free Radical Theory of Aging: Nutritional Implications," *AGE Journal* 1(4): 145-152, 1978

Black and Chan, "Suppression of Ultraviolet Light Induced Tumor Formation by Dietary Antioxidants," *J. Inv. Derm.* 65: 412-414, 1975

Sato and Herring, "Chemistry of Warmed-over Flavor in Cooked Meats," *Food Product Dev.*, Nov. 1973

Harman, Hendricks, Eddy, Seibold, "Free Radical Theory of Aging: Effect of Dietary Fat on Central Nervous System Function," *J. Am. Geriat. Soc.* 24(7): 301-307, 1976

Harman, "Free Radical Theory of Aging: Effect of Adding Antioxidants to Maternal Mouse Diets on the Lifespan of Their Offspring—Second Experiment," paper presented at the 8th Annual Meeting of the American Aging Association, Oct. 5-7, 1978

Hydergine® Is *Not* a Vasoconstrictor

Some physicians are unwilling to prescribe Hydergine® for their patients because of a simple misunderstanding. Natural ergot alkaloids, such as ergotamine, have potentially hazardous vasoconstrictor properties. As a result, ergotamine, for example, is contraindicated for patients with peripheral vascular disease, coronary heart disease, and hypertension, among other conditions (*Physician's Desk Reference*, 35th edition, page 1575). Hydergine® is an ergot derivative and, therefore, some physicians have assumed that it has the same potential complications. This is untrue. "Hydergine tablets and sublingual tablets do not possess the vasoconstrictor properties of the natural ergot alkaloids." (*Physician's Desk Reference*, 35th edition, page 1575.) In fact, the results of both clinical and laboratory studies show that Hydergine® increases cerebral blood flow and oxygen consumption in people with cerebral insufficiency. Hydergine® is a powerful antioxidant that protects the brain from free radicals, the major source of damage resulting from hypoxia (inadequate oxygen available) in the brain. Hydergine® doesn't cause strokes; it provides substantial protection against stroke damage and probably helps to prevent them directly through its antioxidant, anti-free radical, and anti-clotting effects.

The contraindications to the use of Hydergine® are individual sensitivity to it or, possibly, acute psychosis. It also intensifies the stimulant effects of caffeine.

Hydergine® has an enviable safety record. No one has ever died from using it, even though a few attempts have been made to commit suicide with it. If a person ingested a whole bottle of 1000 1 milligram Hydergine® tablets, he or she would become nauseated and vomit and get a terrible headache, but they would live to regret choosing such an ineffective and expensive way of poisoning themselves. Most drugs and even some nutrients (e.g., water, oxygen, salt) would be fatal if taken at a level over 300 times the usual dose (which, for Hydergine® is 3 milligrams per day in the U.S. and 9 to 12 milligrams per day in many European countries).

REFERENCES

Venn, "Clinical Pharmacology of Ergot Alkaloids in Senile Cerebral Insufficiency," *Ergot Alkaloids and Related Compounds*, Berde and Schild, eds., Springer-Verlag, 1978

Koreh, Seligman, Demopoulos, "Effect of Dihydroergotoxine on Lipid Peroxidation in vitro," *Lipids* 17(10): 724-26, 1982

More Life Extension Information

How to Use
Case Histories and
Anecdotal Evidence

Anecdotes (individual case histories) should not be considered proof of anything. First, they are not statistically representative. Second, people are subject to biases which render their subjective impressions suspect in the absence of controlled experimental conditions. If you provide an inert substance (placebo) to people in pain and tell them it is morphine, about 40% will temporarily be relieved of their pain. At the end of a week, only about 10% will still respond to placebo. At the end of a year, only 1% respond. People will often respond favorably to any alteration in their environment which suggests that higher ups are concerned about them (Hawthorne Effect). For example, in one study at an electric equipment manufacturing company, increased lighting resulted in improved production within the group which, later, also responded favorably to a decrease in lighting.

Double blind control conditions (where neither the patients nor the doctors know which medication is the active and which the placebo) can enable us to get around the problem of human biases in evaluating medications. But this does not mean that non-controlled experiments (such as self-experiments) cannot provide valuable and interesting leads. **(Such self-experiments should be performed under the supervision of a physician.)** As Newton pointed out, all great scientific advances started out with a good guess. The results of

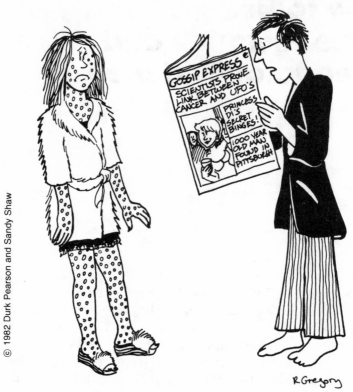

" 'Woman Gives Birth to Siamese Cats' . . . 'I Married an Extraterrestrial.' . . . Here it is: 'All About Spots.' "

uncontrolled experiments must be interpreted within a theoretical framework provided by properly performed scientific research, but they may lead to new insights.

THE EFFECT OF STATISTICAL VARIATION IN THE INTERPRETATION OF SCIENTIFIC STUDIES

Every time you flip a coin, you have a 50% chance of getting "heads" and a 50% chance of getting "tails." After you've flipped the coin 1,000 times, you will have gotten "heads" about 500 times and "tails" about 500 times. If, however, you flip the coin only 100 times, you will find that chance variation will change the results: they are likely to vary from the strictly 50% "heads"/50% "tails" result you'll get if you flip the coin enough times. If you flip the coin only 10 times, you will be even more likely to get something other than 5 "heads" and 5 "tails." And if you flip the coin only once, you will get either a "head" or a "tail."

Suppose you wanted to know what ratio of "heads" to "tails" you would get if you flipped a coin 1,000,000 times and used the results of these experiments to predict the answer. On the basis of 1,000 flips, you would say that you would get very nearly equal numbers of "heads" and "tails." On the basis of 100 flips, you would probably guess more "heads" than "tails" or vice versa, but the difference would not be great. On the basis of 10 flips, your answer would be an even

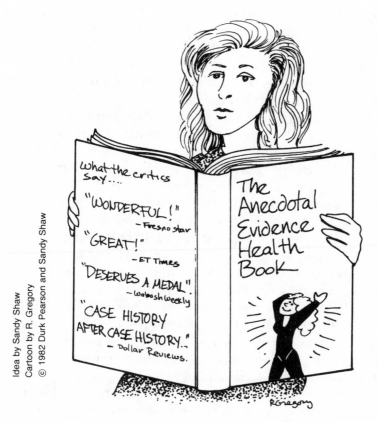

Idea by Sandy Shaw
Cartoon by R. Gregory
© 1982 Durk Pearson and Sandy Shaw

Check the bibliography!

greater inequality between "heads" and "tails." And, on the basis of only 1 flip, you'd have to say they would all be "heads" (or "tails")!

What we have demonstrated here is statistical variation, the tendency of measured values in experiments to differ, usually in a predictable manner. If we flip a coin 10 times, we won't get the right answer (usually) that "heads" will be essentially equal to "tails" in 1,000,000 coin flips. If, however, we repeat the 10 coin flips many times, each 10 coin flip result will be as unlikely to give the true ratio, but the average of the many 10 coin flip results is likely to give us much more accurate results. The single flipping of the coin ten times can give a varying result, ranging from ten "heads" and no "tails" all the way to ten "tails" and no "heads" and everything in between.

Suppose we treat a large group of mice (group A) with a possible life-extending substance and compare it to another large group of mice (group B) which is not given this substance. We find that the group A mice lived for 600 days, while the group B mice lived 500 days. Should we conclude that the treatment extended the life span of group A mice?

If all the mice in group A lived 600 days and all the mice in group B lived 500 days, we could confidently say that the treatment had worked. But, experiments don't work that way. There is a distribution of different life spans, with some mice living longer than the average and others shorter. Some mice in group B lived longer than some mice in group A. Is there really a difference between their life spans?

You can't answer this question simply by comparing the average life spans, 500 and 600 days. You have to consider the *variation* in their life spans in order to distinguish between a true difference and a chance variation between two groups of mice which really have the same average life span. If we had looked at 1,000,000 mice in the two groups, the difference is likely to be a real one. And if we looked at just two mice, we couldn't tell at all. Generally, though, experiments involve more than two mice and considerably fewer than a million!

Experiments in which averages alone are reported without a measure of the variation of the measured values (usually the standard deviation) are very difficult, even impossible, to interpret. We can't be sure the difference is real or a result of variation in a relatively small number of animals. Once the standard deviation (the amount of random noise or error) has been measured, the scientist can calculate whether the differences in the two groups are random or really caused by the experiment. This is called the statistical significance. For example, if the standard deviation were 200 days, the difference between the 500-day and 600-day life span groups would not be significant unless both groups were quite large. There would be no proof of life extension even though the treated mice lived 600 days compared to the 500 days of the untreated mice.

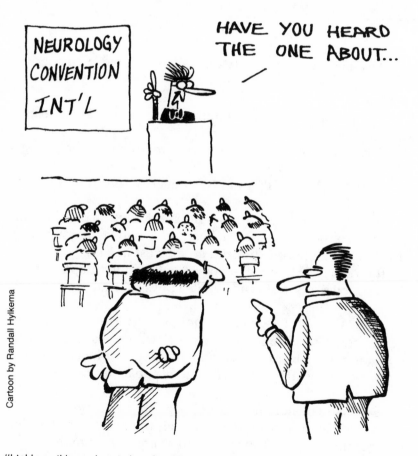

Cartoon by Randall Hylkema

"I told you this guy is notorious for citing anecdotal evidence!"

If, however, the standard deviation (roughly the average variation in life span within a group) were 10 days, the difference between the 600-day and 500-day groups would be 10 times the random error and these results would be highly significant. In fact, the odds would be over 1,000,000 to 1 that the life span difference between these groups was due to chance, even if the groups were relatively small!

SAVES	DATA
Study of Aging Volunteer Experimental Subjects	Doctors' Registry for the Treatment of the Aging

SAVES DATA SUMMARY

This book will initiate two data bases of our own conception:

SAVES: Study of Aging Volunteer Experimental Subjects.
and
DATA: Doctors' Registry for the Treatment of the Aging

SAVES DATA has two major purposes:

1. SAVES DATA enables self-experimenters in nutritional life extension to locate a licensed personal physician or physicians who have expressed an interest in closely monitoring the results of their self-experimentation with appropriate clinical laboratory tests and regular physical exams.

2. SAVES DATA saves the unique and irreplaceable biomedical data resulting from *existing* widespread self-experimentation with nutrients which laboratory evidence suggests can beneficially affect at least some of the aging processes.

SAVES does not advocate either self-experimentation or the use of these nutrients. **SAVES** simply saves this data for science, instead of letting it go to waste. The physicians in DATA will be collecting case histories and administering comprehensive physical exams and clinical laboratory tests to their self-experimenting patients. These examinations and tests are requested by and paid for by the self-experimenters. **SAVES DATA** merely collects these data, keypunches it into a computerized data base, and makes copies of the data base available to all researchers at reproduction cost. **SAVES DATA** pays for *no* tests or medical services, nor makes any medical recommendations.

SAVES: Study of Aging Volunteer Experimental Subjects: THE **SAVES** SUBJECT REGISTER

SUBJECTS NEEDED FOR LONG-TERM STUDY OF EFFECTS OF ANTIOXIDANT AND NUTRITIONAL SUPPLEMENTS

SUBJECTS WANTED to participate in a multiyear study of the effects of regularly self-administered doses of antioxidants and nutrient supplements. If at least 20,000 volunteer experimental subjects can be found, it may be possible to detect potential differences in rates of cardiovascular disease, cancer, other illness, and also of overall deaths in comparison to a similar population not taking such supplements.

The **SAVES** Subject Register data base system is designed to collect medical data on the very large group of people who are currently engaging in self-experimentation using doses of nutrients (especially the antioxidants and growth hormone releasing nutrients) which exceed the FDA's RDAs, and in some cases, non-nutrient antioxidants, too. It must be stressed that the **SAVES** Subject Register will *not* be encouraging these self-experiments. The purpose of **SAVES** is not advocacy; its purpose is to *save* the biomedical data derived from these self-experiments and make these data available to all legitimate researchers.

There are millions of people already engaging in nutritional self-experimentation. The **SAVES** Subject Register data base system can help assure that these self-selected and self-medicated human guinea pigs (or self-selected, self-medicated biomedical volunteer subjects, if you prefer) receive responsible medical supervision by providing an institutional framework within which subjects are more likely to request regular clinical laboratory tests from their own personal physician and keep him or her informed of their activities.

SAVES saves the unique and irreplaceable biomedical data resulting from *existing* widespread self-experimentation with nutrients and antioxidants which laboratory evidence suggests can beneficially affect at least some of the aging processes. In general, these experiments would never be

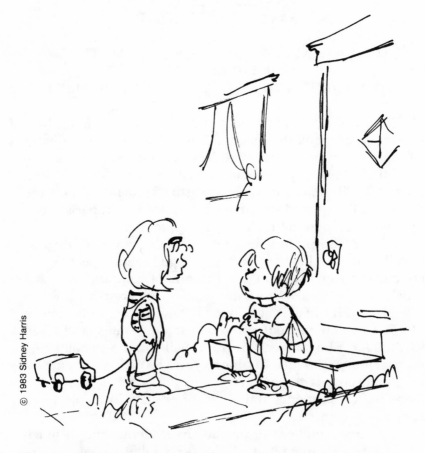

© 1983 Sidney Harris

"Sure, I'm depressed. According to the latest actuarial figures, I've only got 63.27 years to live."

funded by a government agency, nor would they usually be approved by a hospital experimental subject ethics committee. It would be a great loss to science to lose this unique and irreplaceable human epidemiological data.

The **SAVES** study that will use data contributed by the subjects registering in response to this announcement should be large enough to be able to report possible benefits, as well as much more reliably detect possible harm. Such a study set up in the conventional manner, with the experimental subjects receiving their supplements from the research doctors conducting the study, would require extensive cooperation from institutions such as government, hospitals, and universities. Judging from past experiences, it probably could not be done. This **SAVES** Subject Register simply recognizes that people will be self-administering nutritional supplements and antioxidants whether or not a study is made of the effects. Rather than waste this valuable information, we propose to collect it and make it available to any research scientist.

SUBJECTS WANTED to participate in this study should see their personal physician fairly regularly and have periodic clinical tests. **SAVES** is *not* looking for careless persons who take large quantities of various substances and do not have medical supervision. **SAVES** does *not* provide nutritional supplements, funds for clinical tests, or personal medical advice.

HOW TO REGISTER

Fill out the two short forms on the following pages. Give one to your doctor (to authorize him or her to send medical records and clinical test results to the **SAVES** Subject Register, where research scientists can access them). Send the other to:

SAVES SUBJECT REGISTER
2835 Hollywood Blvd.
Hollywood, FL 33020

WHAT HAPPENS TO YOUR DATA

1. It is the intent of the Subject Register management that all personal information be kept confidential. Your medical data is stored with data about thousands of other people, but your name and personal data (such as your street address and telephone number) is never released with that medical data. Legitimate researchers may, on request and for good reason, obtain your individual case history; however, even in this case, your name, telephone number, and street or PO box address will be replaced with a secret coded identification number to protect your privacy, and the researchers will not be informed of these personal identifiers.

2. You will *not* receive medical advice from the **SAVES** Subject Register as a response to medical data sent in about you. The Register is simply a way of collecting a vast amount of medical information that would otherwise be wasted. Data will be reported on a statistical basis in the scientific literature.

3. Any research scientist who wishes to use the pooled data can get a copy of it for the price of the copying media, e.g. the copy of the magnetic tape or whatever. The **SAVES** Subject Register is not intended to make money in providing this service.

4. Medical records including a participant's name and address will not be released to a researcher or anyone else without the participant's explicit written permission, and we anticipate that such permission would rarely be sought. Of course, you are under no obligation to give such permission, even if it is requested.

5. Participants' names and addresses, *without their medical records,* may be used for mailings by Saul Kent's Life Extension Foundation, Dr. Denham Harman's AGE, Dr. Linus Pauling's Institute of Science and Medicine, and other legitimate research organizations. Copies of this mailing list

will be available at media cost to biomedical research organizations for use in their research, public education, and fund raising programs. Participants may, however, request that their names not be included in these (or other) mailing lists.

SAVES: Study of Aging Volunteer Experimental Subjects

SUBJECT REGISTRATION FORM

INSTRUCTIONS: Photocopy this form, fill it out, and send it to the address below. Additional forms may also be obtained by phoning toll-free 1-800-327-6110 or (in Florida) 305-925-2500

       Send to: Neil A. Ahner, M.D.
                Life Extension Foundation
                2835 Hollywood Blvd.
                Hollywood, FL 33020

NAME _____

ADDRESS _____
           street   city, state   ZIP code

AGE _____ SEX _____ HEIGHT _____ WEIGHT _____

I have been taking nutritional supplements for _____ years.

I am currently taking the following supplements, at these doses and times of day: _____

_____

_____

_____

(Use a separate sheet of paper to continue list if necessary.)

I am currently using the following prescription drugs for these purposes, taken at these doses and times of day: _____

_____

_____

_____

I have a personal physician who I see reasonably regularly.

yes [ ]   no [ ]

I use tobacco. yes [ ]   no [ ]

I use alcohol. yes [ ]   no [ ]

If yes, what type and how much of alcohol and/or tobacco _____

_____

I have had the following major illnesses in the indicated years: ____

_____

_____

_____

My general health is: excellent [ ]   very good [ ]   average [ ]

fair [ ]   poor [ ]

My highest level of education attained is:

elementary school graduate [ ]   some high school [ ]

high school graduate [ ]   some college [ ]

college graduate [ ]   some postgrad work [ ]

postgraduate degree [ ]

I am married or partnered   yes [ ]   no [ ]

I usually buckle up my car seatbelt.   yes [ ]   no [ ]

I understand that I will receive no nutritional supplements, lab tests, or medical advice as a "SAVES" research subject.

yes [ ]   no [ ]

I have read and fully understand and agree with the **SAVES DATA SUMMARY** material in *The Life Extension Companion* by Pearson and Shaw, published by Warner Books, 1984. I will hold the authors, publishers, and distributors blameless for any inconveniences arising from my participation.   yes [ ]   no [ ]

I request that my name not be included in any mailing lists. [ ]

I hereby authorize my physician _____
name

_____
address, city, state, ZIP

to send a copy of my medical records to: Neil A. Ahner, M.D., at the "SAVES" Subject Register address above.

_____   _____
signature of self-selected,   date
self-medicated volunteer subject

SAVES: Study of Aging Volunteer
Experimental Subjects
Research Subject Physician Authorization Form

I hereby request and authorize you, as my physician, to send a copy of my medical records to:

Neil A. Ahner, M.D.
The Life Extension Foundation
2835 Hollywood Blvd.
Hollywood, FL 33020

I have notified Dr. Ahner to expect these records, which will be used in long-term clinical and preventive gerontology research studies.

The data about me and other subjects who are self-administering nutritional supplements (in doses higher than the RDA's, the Recommended Dietary Allowances) will be made available to any legitimate research scientist. (Personal data, however, will be coded so my privacy is maintained.)

signed _____ date _____

DATA: Doctors' Registry for the Treatment of the Aging

THE DATA PHYSICIANS' REGISTER

DATA is a registry of physicians with an interest in geriatrics and clinical gerontology. Geriatricians are physicians who treat the aged. Clinical gerontologists are doctors who attempt to treat aging, rather than merely treating the aged after the damage has occurred, as well as treating older individuals.

Clinical gerontologists are physicians who will order clinical tests for preventive purposes on a patient who is not yet ill, and will probably agree to reasonable suggestions for additional tests from well-informed individuals.

And, of course, they are physicians who will find new patients among those persons who ask DATA for a list of local physicians with a strong interest in geriatrics and clinical gerontology.

We described DATA to Dr. Denham Harman (the originator of the free radical theory of aging and one of the founders of AGE, the American Aging Association), a scientist, physician, and professor at the University of Nebraska School of Medicine. He was delighted with the idea and offered to operate and maintain DATA as a function of AGE. We gladly accepted his offer.

DATA: Doctors' Registry for the Treatment of the Aging

THE **DATA** PHYSICIANS' REGISTER

HOW TO REGISTER

This is an invitation to doctors practicing geriatrics and clinical gerontology to be listed in this Physicians' Registry.

This registry will be managed by the American Aging Association (**AGE**), whose present Executive Director is Denham Harman, M.D. (the University of Nebraska research scientist who created the free radical theory of aging).

Patients seeking a physician may write the American Aging Association for the office addresses and phone numbers of registered physicians in their area.

The American Aging Association
University of Nebraska College of Medicine
42nd & Dewey Ave.
Omaha, NB 68105
Attention: Denham Harman, M.D.

Telephone **AGE** at 1-(402) 559-4416 or, for a toll-free 800 number, call 800 information at 1-(800)-555-1212 and ask for the number of the American Aging Association.

December 20, 1982

John Doe, M.D.
University of Nebraska Medical Center
42nd & Dewey Avenue
Omaha, Nebraska, 68105

Dear Dr. Doe:

The American Aging Association (AGE) frequently receives requests for the names of physicians interested in the care of older individuals. Usually the inquiries come from sons and daughters concerned about their elderly parents' confusion, nursing home placement, etc.

Recently individuals have contacted the office for the names of physicians who have an interest in the application of our growing knowledge of aging to the problem of extending the healthy life span. Many of these individuals take self-selected dietary supplements and wish to be monitored medically to reduce the chance of possible adverse effects.

In order to more readily respond to these requests, the American Aging Association plans to establish a data bank with the names of physicians in the United States interested in the care of the elderly, as well as those concerned with the broader field of clinical gerontology. If you would like to be included on one or both of these lists, please fill out and return the enclosed brief questionnaire.

The American Aging Association (AGE) was founded in 1970 as a national, non-profit, lay-scientific health organization patterned after the American Heart Association. The formation of AGE was largely prompted by the pressing need for more biomedical aging research.

AGE holds a meeting once a year. The program for the 12th annual meeting, held last September in San Francisco, is enclosed. Beginning in 1974, a day to day and a half of the annual meeting has been devoted to a symposium; these symposiums are published by the Raven Press as a volume in the series, Aging. In 1978 the American Aging Association began publication of the journal, *Age*. This journal is devoted to biomedical aging research and is published 4 times a year.

We hope that you will elect to join with AGE in meeting the need for geriatrics and clinical gerontology referral services.

Cordially,

Denham Harman, M.D.
Executive Director
American Aging Association

DH:bmc

American Aging Association
DATA
Data Bank of Geriatrics and Clinical Gerontology Physicians

1) If you would like to have your name listed in the data bank for possible referrals in geriatrics and/or clinical gerontology please mark one or both of the boxes below:

[ ] Geriatrics

[ ] Clinical Gerontology

2) Approximately what percent of the patients in your current practice are over 65 years of age? (PLEASE CHECK ONE)

_____ 0–25%   _____ 51–75%

_____ 26–50%   _____ 76–100%

3) In the past month, how many nursing home patients have you seen? (PLEASE CHECK ONE)

_____ 0–15   _____ 46–60

_____ 16–30   _____ 61–75

_____ 31–45   _____ more than 75

4) Are you currently a member of:

A) The American Aging Association   [ ] Yes   [ ] No

B) The American Geriatrics Society   [ ] Yes   [ ] No

C) The Gerontological Society of America   [ ] Yes   [ ] No

Please type or print your name, office address and telephone number below and mail this form in the enclosed business envelope. Thanks.

Name: _____

Address: _____

_____

_____

Telephone: Area Code (   ) _____

Sources of Information About Aging and Maintaining Your Health

The recent increase of public interest in aging processes and means of intervention has been reflected in a tremendous outpouring of articles and books in the marketplace. Most of these writings contain a good deal of misinformation (such as "avoid food preservatives at all costs") and must be read very selectively. Without prior knowledge of what to look for, it is not very likely that reading these works would result in an increase of understanding. There are, however, some excellent publications available on this subject. In this chapter, we review a selection of books that can prepare a careful reader of above average intelligence (but not necessarily a college graduate) to plan his or her own rational life extension program.

Scientific information can be derived from primary sources (the original scientific papers, usually appearing in peer-reviewed journals), secondary sources (popular scientific books and publications which interpret the original scientific papers, for example *Scientific American* and *Science News*), or lay sources (popular books). Lay sources tend to contain faddist or ideological thinking and, in our experience, may contain as much as 50% incorrect information.

Few people will want to read original scientific papers, for which some scientific background is usually required. For those who do, there is a search service available at many large university medical libraries across the country for the National Library of Medicine's MEDLARS computerized data base. For a low price (as little as $10), you can have the over 3,000 different journals in the data base searched and receive a printout listing references to scientific papers that involve your area of interest. Suppose you want to know what type of treatments have been tried in a particular type of rare cancer. You have a search done for treatments of this cancer and receive a printout (in the mail) of references. You can then follow up by going to a medical library and obtaining the papers of most interest. The references to papers of recent years usually have a summary of the study's findings, which is of great help in determining which papers you should follow up on. Ask for abstracts with the citations when they are available.

There are a large number of excellent secondary sources about aging and its attendant health problems, as well as how to improve your health status regardless of your age. We recommend the following enthusiastically (but just because a book or publication is not listed here does not mean that we disapprove of it or that it is no good). **NOTE:** The listing of a book here does not mean we agree with everything in it or that the techniques described will work for everyone. Anyone seriously interested in intervening in their own aging processes should have their own shelf of reliable references. We wholeheartedly recommend the purchase of *all* of the following books, but they are *not* meant to replace your physician. Isn't your health too valuable to trust to hearsay and popular delusions?

Life Extension, A Practical Scientific Approach, Durk Pearson and Sandy Shaw, Warner Books, June 1982, hardback, 858 pages.

This book, aimed at scientists, physicians, and the intelligent lay public, offers two different types of information. First, a great deal of primary scientific information is reviewed (including hundreds of references). This provides the basis for a theoretical understanding of how aging works, with particular emphasis on free radical pathology, and the mechanisms underlying successful intervention in aging processes in both experimental animals and humans. The other type of information is an examination and evaluation of different interventions in human aging, including self-experiments of Sandy, Durk, and other self-selected human guinea pigs. Sandy and Durk's complete experimental nutrient and antioxidant regimens are included, as well as clinical laboratory test results.

Total Fitness in 30 Minutes a Week, Morehouse and Gross, Simon and Schuster, 1975, paperback, $2.95.

Dr. Lawrence Morehouse was the head of NASA's astronaut physiological testing program. He wanted to find out what exercise schedule would provide the greatest benefits for the least amount of time. He found that the exercise that produced the most benefits in terms of cardiovascular conditioning was peak-effort exercise done for only a short time. Morehouse and Gross suggest ten minutes every other day of any exercise you like, as long as you work sufficiently hard for the ten minutes. Jogging will not do it. This book has a chart showing the heart rate you should try to achieve, depending on your age, and how quickly you should work up to it.

Physician's Desk Reference, Medical Economics Co., Oradell, NJ 07649, annual, hardback, $17.95, 2049 pages.

We were surprised recently to hear that this is the third best selling hardback book in the country. It is very good news because there is a great deal of vital information in this book for anyone attempting a life extension program. Here is where you will find out the side-effects to drugs you may be using; unfortunately, doctors do not always inform their patients of side-effects. You can find out about undesirable drug interactions. You can learn what dosage ranges are typically used and how fast you can increase (or decrease) your dose. One thing you won't find mentioned in here are unapproved uses. For example, if you look at the entry for Diapid® nasal spray (Sandoz), you will find information only for its approved use (treatment for a condition of excessive urination), not for a recently discovered unapproved use (improving memory and learning, and decreasing reaction time). The FDA forbids manufacturers from providing this data to doctors, including merely sending out copies of legitimate scientific papers.

The Life Extension Revolution, Saul Kent, Morrow, 1980, available in paperback, 467 pages; and *Secrets of Life Extension*, John A. Mann, Harbor Publ., And/Or Press, 1980, paperback, $7.95, 180 pages.

Both of these books are excellent introductions to theoretical and practical aspects of current aging science. The Mann book is more oriented to practical application. It contains hundreds of references, a large percentage of which are to the primary scientific literature. Kent's bibliography contains an amazing 750 references, well worth the price of the book by themselves. He is a veteran medical writer with a long list of articles published, many of them in a geriatrics magazine for doctors. His articles are almost invariably impeccably researched and he rarely draws conclusions that go beyond the data. Both these books have much data on free radicals.

This is the foreword we wrote to the Spring 1983 paperback edition of Saul Kent's *The Life Extension Revolution*:

> We are delighted that *The Life Extension Revolution* is now available in a paperback edition. This is one of the few books on the subject of life extension that contains scientifically accurate information and is also written in an easily readable style. We consider it *must* reading for anyone seriously interested in living a longer, more healthful life. *The Life Extension Revolution* provides a lively guided tour to a wide variety of possible life extension techniques under current investigation. The book is clearly written and comprehensible to interested laypersons, as well as to physicians and scientists. Although *The Life Extension Revolution* is not a how-to book, its contents provide considerable data to help readers who are interested in investigating the use of experimental life extension techniques in their own

lives. The book is divided into short sections on various aspects of theory and experiment. Each topic is carefully discussed, including both positive and negative results. Of course, one should not attempt to use any of these experimental techniques on oneself without careful investigation and the advice of a physician practicing preventive gerontology.

Saul Kent, the author of *The Life Extension Revolution*, is a scientist and author who has been actively studying aging processes since 1964. He has been writing articles on biological gerontology for *Geriatrics*, a professional publication for physicians, for seven years. In addition, Saul is the publisher and editor of *The Anti-Aging News*, a newsletter available by subscription that we highly recommend. Like us, Saul plans to put most of the money he makes from sales of his book into more aging research, to the benefit of himself, of us, and of you, the reader.

A truly outstanding feature of this book is its extensive bibliography of over 750 references, most to the primary scientific literature (original scientific papers, usually published in refereed journals). This book is a tremendous bargain for these references alone! The author has shown excellent judgement in his selection of references and in his interpretation of the research reports. Saul's enthusiasm for life extension is boundless, but he has not allowed this emotion to replace a dispassionate scientific judgement in reporting experimental results.

We applaud the addition of a glossary to the paperback version of *The Life Extension Revolution*. It makes this excellent book even more useful, particularly to the layperson.

Life extension is a rapidly growing field, with the amount of information doubling roughly every five years. Many books on this subject are being offered in the marketplace now, and many more can be expected in the near future. It is important to choose carefully among these available books, because misinformation is far more common than is accurate information. The basis of a scientific book is original scientific studies. This book provides references to the studies that are the basis of the information it contains. Like us, the author of *The Life Extension Revolution* would prefer that readers check his sources and investigate his ideas, rather than blindly accepting or rejecting them. Many books provide no references or refer largely to newspapers or popular health magazines, which are frequently unreliable guides to rational action.

Among the many health books about aging being offered today, this book stands out. We hope that you will buy and read it; you will be glad that you did. Live long and prosper!

Durk Pearson
Sandy Shaw

Los Angeles
November 2, 1982

Maximum Life Span, Roy L. Walford, M.D., W. W. Norton & Co., 1983

Roy Walford is the creator of the immunological theory of aging and is an outstanding gerontologist. This book will make a valuable new addition to your life extension library. It is a good overview of the field, although not a how-to book. It is written in a friendly personal style that is a pleasure to read. See pages 140 and 147 for a partial list of Walford's daily supplements, which includes 250 milligrams of BHT, in addition to quantities of vitamin E, selenium, cysteine, methionine, ascorbyl palmitate, vitamin C, calcium pantothenate (vitamin B-5), DMAE (Deaner) and bioflavonoids. This book emphasizes Walford's work on life extension in animals using dietary restriction and reduction of body temperature, two techniques that reduce free radical activity, as well as altering aging and development clocks in the case of dietary restriction.

Vitamin C, the Common Cold, and the Flu, Linus Pauling, Freeman, 1976, paperback, $3.45, 230 pages; *Cancer and*

Vitamin C, Cameron and Pauling, Pauling Institute of Science and Medicine, 1979, hardback, $9.95, 238 pages

Both these books are musts for anyone seriously interested in improving his health. Vitamin C is an important antioxidant nutrient that does have anticancer properties, as well as performing myriad other functions in the body: stimulating healing (it is required for the synthesis of the protein collagen in connective tissue), stimulates the activity of certain white blood cells, protects the brain and spinal cord from damaging oxidation (these structures use active transport, requiring considerable energy, to increase the vitamin C content within individual nerve cells to 100 times that in the general circulation), and others. Many of these are discussed in the two books on vitamin C. These books are well documented and cover vastly more subject matter than their titles suggest.

Prolongevity, Albert Rosenfeld, Knopf, 1976, paperback, $2.50; *Slowing Down the Aging Process,* Kugler, Pyramid, 1974, paperback, $1.50, 236 pages.

Both of these books were written for a wider public audience than *Life Extension, A Practical Scientific Approach, The Life Extension Revolution,* or *Secrets of Life Extension.* Both of them are excellent introductions to the subject of aging processes and means of intervention. Neither is a how-to book, but they do provide generally clear and accurate information concerning reasonably current thinking in gerontology. Since these were published a few years ago, we believe that they lag behind, particularly in the greatly increased recognition of the importance of free radical pathology in aging and in newer forms of anti-aging therapy. Many good references are given to the primary scientific literature. We understand that *Prolongevity* has been updated by Mr. Rosenfeld and will be available in late 1983.

Regulating New Drugs, edited by Richard L. Landau, The University of Chicago Center for Policy Study, 1973, paperback, $5.50, 297 pages.

This economic study provides an excellent analysis of the effects of regulations on drug innovation and production in this country. Of particular interest is Dr. Sam Peltzman's section entitled "The Benefits and Costs of New Drug Regulation." He found that, considering costs and benefits, consumers were losing at least $250,000,000 per year (in late 1960's dollars), mostly in terms of reduced health, as a result of drug regulations requiring proof of efficacy (the 1962 Kefauver amendments) using a set of assumptions that are incredibly charitable to the FDA. Dr. Peltzman has shown that these amendments (which have increased the costs of drug approval to an average of $50-80 million dollars and 8-12 years delay) have provided *no* significant increase in either safety or efficacy. He has also demonstrated that the adverse health costs of a *three-month* increased delay in new drug introduction exceed the health costs of a West German thalidomide maxi-disaster scaled up to U.S. size once each decade! This book is a real eye opener.

The following two references are to medical journals, however these papers are relatively easy for the layperson to understand.

Spector, "Vitamin Homeostasis in the Central Nervous System," *New Engl. J. Med.* 296: 1393, 1977 [Vitamin C pumps in blood-brain barrier and in neuronal membranes maintain vitamin C concentration about 100 times as high as in bloodstream.]

Legros et al, "Influence of Vasopressin on Memory and Learning," *The Lancet*, 7 Jan. 1978, p. 41

Kelner, *Searching the MEDLARS Database: A Practical Guide for Profilers*, published by Bibliographic Retrieval Services, 702 Corporation Park, Scotia, NY 12302

A list of libraries and medical centers offering MEDLARS Searches in the United States and foreign countries can be found on page 1767 of *Remington's Pharmaceutical Sciences,* Mack Publishing Company, 15th ed., 1975

Supernutrition, Richard Passwater, Dial Press, 1975, 224 pp.
This book is six years old and, consequently, we feel it is somewhat out of date. However, it was a bit ahead of its time,

so there is much of value remaining. For example, it contains cogent explanations for the layman of what free radicals are and how they cause much of the damage that produces aging, cardiovascular disease, and cancer, to name a few. This alone is worth the price of the book. There is also an informative discussion of why cholesterol reducing diets usually do little, if any, good in preventing heart attacks. There are recommended nutrient regimens (somewhat conservative by our standards) and uses for individual nutrients are generally well explained. One complaint we have is the rather dry, dull style in which the book is written. Two pages of references are included.

Vitamin E for Ailing & Healthy Hearts, Wilfrid E. Shute, M.D., Pyramid Books, 1972, 208 pp.

Anyone planning to use doses of vitamin E of 200 I.U. per day or more or who plans to use vitamin E and has a damaged (particularly rheumatic) heart, should read this book. The famous Shute clinic in Canada has treated about 40,000 patients with vitamin E and much of their experience is reported here. The book explains how to use the vitamin and possible side-effects that may be encountered. For example, when vitamin E is first used, there may be a transitory blood pressure elevation. That could be important if a person taking vitamin E has high blood pressure. Also, it is possible to get differential benefits in damaged heart, so that some parts become stronger sooner than other parts, resulting in a strain on the weaker areas. It's all here in this book. There are 5 pages of references. Highly recommended.

The Healing Factor, Irwin Stone, Grosset & Dunlap, 1972, 258 pp.

This is an excellent book on vitamin C and its many uses. The bibliography is a good one, with many references to the primary scientific literature. Stone even explains in the beginning how man and all other primates came to be dependent on the environment for their vitamin C (through the loss of an enzyme necessary to manufacture C in our bodies). Dr. Stone, who first interested Linus Pauling in vitamin C, explains how to use vitamin C for herpes and other viral infections, bacterial infections, cancer, heart attacks and strokes, aging, arthritis and rheumatism, allergies, ulcers, diabetes, hypoglycemia, stress, pollution, poisons, wounds, pregnancy, and even mental diseases. Vitamin C, for example, has been found of value in the treatment of schizophrenia. And vitamin C is required in the brain's manufacture of many neurotransmitters (substances used by brain cells to communicate with each other). The book contains 53 pages of references! Highly recommended.

Nutrition Against Disease, Dr. Roger J. Williams, Bantam Books, 1973, 276 pp.

This is an excellent introduction to the field of nutrition, with many references to original scientific papers, written by the scientist who first identified, isolated, and synthesized pantothenic acid, vitamin B-5. He also did pioneer work on folic acid, and gave it its name. There are 31 pages of references! Highly recommended.

Vitamins & You, Robert J. Benowicz, Grosset & Dunlap, 1979, 186 pp.; *Non-Prescription Drugs and Their Side Effects*, Robert J. Benowicz, Berkley Books, 1982

Robert J. Benowicz used to work for the FDA. He believed their claim that most people could get all the nutrition they required with a knife and fork (in their diet). Benowicz decided to write a book exposing the use of vitamin supplements as a hoax. However, being a real scientist, he did extensive literature searching on the subject and found, to his surprise, that the scientific literature didn't support the notion that all nutritional needs can be obtained in even a good diet. When Benowicz tried to bring these facts to the attention of his superiors, he was rebuffed. He quit the agency in disgust after that, calling it a "Kafkaesque organization." *Vitamins & You* is a good survey of vitamins, as found in the diet and in supplementation. It has 1½ pages of references. *Non-Prescription Drugs and Their Side Effects* is a useful guide concerning the use of common (and not so common) over the counter remedies.

You Can Use the National Library of Medicine: MEDLARS and MEDLINE: Computer Searches by Mail

The latest developments in medicine can save your life—but only if you are aware of them. The National Cancer Institute has estimated that *twice as many* cancer patients would bring their cancers under control or be cured if the most effective forms of conventional treatments for cancer available right now were used. Information about these better ways to utilize conventional cancer treatments can usually be found in many biomedical journals. But even if you subscribed to the top 3,000 biomedical journals in the world, you would still have to extract the information of interest to you and your physician.

There is an inexpensive biomedical data search service that will look through the top 3,000 biomedical journals in the world for you, and find just that information in which you and your physician are interested. This data retrieval service is called MEDLARS. It was set up by the National Library of Medicine to provide rapid access to current literature to health professionals. The information is made available to anyone willing to pay the modest fee for the search.

Why is MEDLARS underutilized by physicians? First, MEDLARS was set up after most physicians had already received their medical training. Second, since MEDLARS is not a commercial information service, it does not advertise and, as a result, very few physicians have heard of it. We expect physicians to quickly become more frequent users of this valuable service as soon as significant numbers of them learn of its benefits. MEDLARS can also function as a comprehensive second opinion for physicians, both improving patient care and reducing the probability of malpractice suits. In the meantime, you can help yourself and your physician by investigating what MEDLARS can do for you.

What can MEDLARS be used for? MEDLARS can tell you the most effective reported conventional treatments for diseases, even rare ones. No physician, no matter how experienced, can be reasonably expected to know all of this. Sometimes the order in which drugs are used to treat a disease, such as in chemotherapy of cancer, can be very important in the overall effectiveness of therapy. MEDLARS can also be very useful to the professional health researcher by providing information about newly developing therapies and theoretical understanding of disease processes and the maintenance of health.

There are a number of specific medical school libraries that perform the MEDLARS search service. A list of these

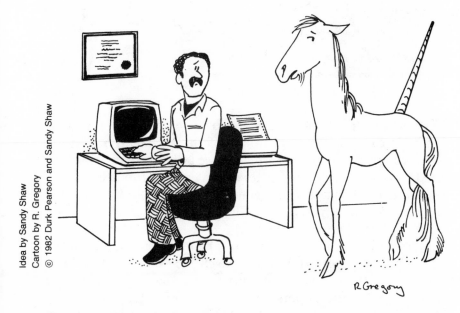

Idea by Sandy Shaw
Cartoon by R. Gregory
© 1982 Durk Pearson and Sandy Shaw

R Gregory

"Doctor, does Medlars have any references to unicorn diseases?"

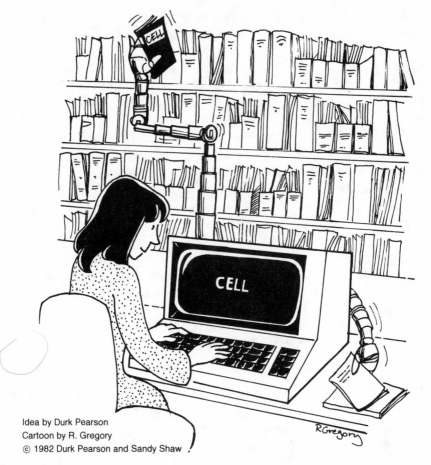

Idea by Durk Pearson
Cartoon by R. Gregory
© 1982 Durk Pearson and Sandy Shaw

centers appears at the end of this chapter. However, you do
not have to actually travel to any of the MEDLARS centers;
they will perform the information search by mail. You will
need to write one of the centers for a copy of the MEDLARS
search form, or make a photocopy of the sample form in this
chapter. We show you how to fill out the form in *Example of
a Search Request.*

Your physician can help you formulate the statement of
what you want MEDLARS to search for. The result, which
you may wish to have sent directly to your physician, is a
listing of scientific papers containing information you asked
MEDLARS to look for. Most of the recent paper references

will also include (if requested) abstracts, which are a brief summary of the paper's contents, making it much easier to decide which papers are relevant to your particular requirements. You and your physician will have to decide which of these papers should be obtained (by your going to any medical school library or large university life sciences library (these need not be MEDLARS centers) and making photocopies of the desired information). With an investment of $10 to $30 and a reasonable amount of effort, you can have access to the latest information from 3,000 biomedical journals about your health question.

REGIONAL MEDICAL LIBRARIES OFFERING MEDLARS SERVICES

1. GREATER NORTHEASTERN REGIONAL MEDICAL LIBRARY PROGRAM
The New York Academy of Medicine
2 East 103rd Street
New York, NY 10029
Phone: 212-876-8763
States served: CT, DE, MA, ME, NH, NJ, NY, PA, RI, VT, and Puerto Rico

2. SOUTHEASTERN/ATLANTIC REGIONAL MEDICAL LIBRARY SERVICES (STARS)
University of Maryland
Health Sciences Library
111 South Greene Street
Baltimore, Maryland, 21201
Phone 301-528-7637
States served: AL, FL, GA, MD, MS, NC, SC, TN, VA, WV, and the District of Columbia

3. REGION 3: REGIONAL MEDICAL LIBRARY
University of Illinois at Chicago
Library of the Health Sciences
Health Sciences Center

P.O. Box 7509
Chicago, Illinois, 60680
Phone 312-996-2464
States served: IA, IL, IN, KY, MI, MN, ND, OH, SD, WI

4. MIDCONTINENTAL REGIONAL MEDICAL LIBRARY
PROGRAM (MCRML)
University of Nebraska
Medical Center Library
42nd and Dewey Avenue
Omaha, Nebraska, 68105
Phone 402-559-4326
States served: CO, KS, MO, NE, UT, WY

5. SOUTH CENTRAL REGIONAL MEDICAL LIBRARY
PROGRAM (TALON)
University of Texas
Health Science Center at Dallas
5323 Harry Hines Blvd.
Dallas, Texas, 75235
Phone: 214-688-2085
States served: AR, LA, NM, OK, TX

6. PACIFIC NORTHWEST REGIONAL HEALTH
SCIENCES LIBRARY SERVICE (PNRHSLS)
Health Sciences Library
University of Washington
Seattle, Washington, 98195
Phone: 206-543-8262
States served: AK, ID, MT, OR, WA

7. PACIFIC SOUTHWEST REGIONAL MEDICAL
LIBRARY SERVICE (PSRMLS)
UCLA Biomedical Library
Center for the Health Sciences
Los Angeles, California, 90024
Phone: 213-825-1200
States served: AZ, CA, HI, NV

BIBLIOGRAPHIC SEARCH REQUEST   DATABASE(S)   YEARS

Name (Please Print)_____ Date_____
Mailing Address_____
  City_____ State_____Zip_____
Position or Title_____ Telephone_____
Department/Organization/School_____
Submitted by (if different from above)_____Telephone_____

1. **DETAILED STATEMENT OF QUESTION:** Please describe your search topic as specifically as possible. Indicate any points NOT to be included.

2. **ABSTRACTS:** Do you want abstracts included with the citations? Yes_____ No_____

3. **SCOPE OF SEARCH:** Do you wish your search to be:
   _____ Comprehensive: include all articles discussing topic regardless of emphasis
   _____ Selective: limit to major articles

4. RETRIEVAL ESTIMATION: Please estimate the number of articles you expect to be retrieved in the last three years (e.g. 25, 100, 200)._____

5. DEADLINE: Please indicate if you have a deadline (it usually takes 7 to 10 working days after the search is run to receive the printout)._____

OFFICE USE ONLY

Received		Disposition		Released	
Date	_____	Mail	_____	Mailed on	_____
Amount	_____	Pick up:	_____	Called for pick up:	
Payment mech.	_____	1st 25 citations	_____	1st 25 citations on	_____
Initials	_____	all citations	_____	all citations	_____

6. SEARCH PURPOSE:

____patient care ____teaching ____course

____talk/grand ____basic research assignment

rounds ____book or ____dissertation/

____cancer journal thesis

therapy/ publication ____other (specify)

research ____site review _____

____clinical _____

research

7. SEARCH SPECIFICATIONS:

Languages

_____ Accept English and foreign language articles with English summaries

_____ Accept only English

_____ Accept all languages

_____ Accept certain languages only (please specify): _____

Research subjects

____ Human   ____ Female   ____ Male
____ Animal experiments; if only certain animals or
animal groups are of interest, please list these:

Age groups

___0 to 1 month   ____ 6 to 12 years   ___45 to 64 years
___1 to 23 months ___13 to 18 years   ___65 years and
                                          over
___2 to 5 years   ___19 to 44 years

8. COST LIMITATIONS:

___Maximum number without additional cost
___All citations, regardless of cost
___Limit to ___citations or ___dollars

9. RELEVANT PAPERS PUBLISHED WITHIN THE LAST THREE YEARS:

I hereby authorize the Library to perform the online
search(es) specified on the reverse side and agree to pay the
charges incurred for computer time, telecommunications,
printing, and service fee (when applicable).

_____
Signature

Example of a Search Request:
Growth Hormone Secretion

We became interested in the life extension potential of substances that stimulate growth hormone secretion back in 1976. In order to find out what had been published about this, we paid $26 at that time for a search of the National Library of Medicine's database, called MEDLARS. The MEDLARS database covers over 3,000 different biomedical journals from all over the world. In order to facilitate your preparing a search request of your own, we show here the actual search request form as we filled it in and sent it to MEDLARS to be processed. In the next section, "Example of a Search Printout: Growth Hormone Secretion," we show you a few of the many references we got back from MEDLARS. If you have read the athletics, exercise, weight control, or immune system maintenance and stimulation sections of our *Life Extension, A Practical Scientific Approach*, you know how we made use of some of these growth hormone secretion studies.

BIBLIOGRAPHIC SEARCH REQUEST

REFERENCE DIVISION
BIOMEDICAL LIBRARY

Name (Please Print)__D.J. Pearson____ Date ____13 Feb. 1977____

Title or Position_____ Telephone _____

Organization/Department/School_____

Submitted by (if different from above) _____ Telephone _____

Mailing Address_____

City_____ State_____ Zip_____

Please check: On-campus user_____ Off-campus user_____X_____

1. FILES(S) to be searched:
   Medline and *all* Backfiles

2. DETAILED STATEMENT OF QUESTION: Please describe in your own words, the subject matter for which the
   search is to be conducted. Please be as specific as possible.
   Define any terms that may have any special meaning in
   your request. Also, if there are points NOT to be included,
   please state these.

   We want to find out which drugs cause an increase in
   growth hormone release from the pituitary, and how much.
   (Other terms for growth hormone include: pituitary growth
   hormone, adenohypophyseal growth hormone, hypophyseal
   growth hormone, anterior pituitary growth hormone,
   phyone, somatotrophic hormone, STH, somatotropin, human
   growth hormone, Antuitrin-Growth, Crescormon, Phyol, So-
   macton, HGH (not to be confused with human chorionic
   gonadotropin)).
   Drugs known to do this include: L-DOPA, apomorphine,
   Ritalin, (methylphenidate), and piribedil, all of which are
   dopaminergic (DA) stimulants of the pituitary. It is thought
   that serotonin (5-HT) and perhaps nor-epinephrine (NE) stimulation of the pituitary can also cause an increase in growth
   hormone (GH) output. We are interested in any drugs (regardless of the neurotransmitters involved) which increase
   GH output. We are particularly interested in any papers
   describing the effects on GH of lysergic acid compounds,
   isolysergic acid compounds, and dihydrolysergic acid compounds; examples include Hydergine (dihydroergotoxine,
   dihydroergocornine, dihydroergocristine, dihydroergokryp-
   tine).
   If the number of citations exceeds 300, please phone me
   so that we can arrange for additional funding.

3. SEARCH PURPOSE (i.e. research, talk, grand rounds, paper, chapter in book, etc.):

                              research

4. SEARCH SPECIFICATIONS:
    __X__ Human   _____ Male
                              _____ Female
    __X__ Animal experiments; if only certain animals or
          animal groups are of interest, please list these:
                  _____ ALL

Age groups (Please specify if only certain groups are of interest): _____ ALL
    _____ 0 to 1 month   _____ 13 to 18 years
    _____ 1 to 23 months   _____ 19 to 44 years
    _____ 2 to 5 years   _____ 45 to 64 years
    _____ 6 to 12 years   _____ 65 years and over

Languages:
    _____ Accept all languages
    _____ Accept only English
    __X__ Accept English and English abstracts only
    _____ Accept certain languages only (please specify)
    __X__ Would like abstracts included when available

5. KNOWN RELEVANT PAPERS:

Prinz et al, "Growth Hormone Levels during Sleep in Elderly Males," presented at the 29th Annual Gerontological Society Conference, Oct 13, 1976

Boyd et al, "Stimulation of Human-Growth-Hormone Secretion by L-Dopa," *New Engl. J. Med.* 183(26): 1425-1429, 1970

Meites, "Role of Biogenic Amines in the Control of Prolactin and Growth Hormone Secretion," *Psychopharm. Bull.*, Oct. 1976, pp. 120-121

EXAMPLE OF A SEARCH PRINTOUT:
GROWTH HORMONE SECRETION

Back in 1976, we became interested in the life extension potential of growth hormone releasing substances. The following references are a few of the 567 references we received from MEDLARS as a result of our 13 February 1977 "Growth Hormone Secretion" search request (see "Example of a Search Request" in this book). They are shown just as they appeared in the printouts sent to us. AU means the author or authors of the paper listed. TI is the title of the paper. AB is the abstract or summary of the paper's contents. About half the references we received in this search had abstracts.

If you have read our *Life Extension, A Practical Scientific Approach*, you will know of some revolutionary, practical, and readily applicable results of this study in the areas of athletics, exercise, weight control, immune system stimulation and maintenance, and wound healing.

AU— is the author(s)
TI— is the title
AB— is the abstract
SO— is the source

AU— Sutton J; Lazarus L
TI— Growth hormone in exercise: comparison of physiological and pharmacological stimuli.
AB— This study was designed to compare the serum growth hormone (GH) response with quantified exercise to that obtained with other stimuli. In eight normal males, aged 21-24 yr, we studied the serum GH response to 20 min cycle ergometer exercise at 300, 600, and 900 kpm/min on three separate occasions and compared the results with those found during sleep, insulin hypoglycemia, arginine infusion, and L-DOPA. Exercise at 900 kpm/min and insulin hypoglycemia resulted in the greatest elevations in serum GH which were significantly greater than those found with sleep, arginine, or L-

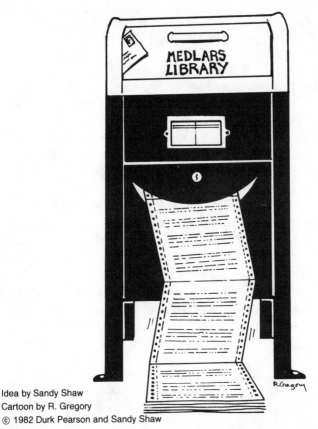

Idea by Sandy Shaw
Cartoon by R. Gregory
© 1982 Durk Pearson and Sandy Shaw

DOPA. The 20-min exercise at 900 kpm/min represented 75-90% of the subjects' maximal oxygen uptake and is a suitable provocative test for GH secretion. As a screening test for pituitary GH reserve, exercise compares favorably with insulin hypoglycemia and is superior to sleep, arginine, and L-DOPA.
SO— Biochem J 157(3):523-7, 1 Sep 76

AU— Verde G; Oppizzi G; Colussi G; Cremascoli G; Botalla L
AU— Müller EE; Silvestrini F; Chiodini PG; Liuzzi A
TI— Effect of dopamine infusion on plasma levels of growth hormone in normal subjects and in acromegalic patients.
AB— In ten normal subjects and in twenty acromegalic patients plasma levels of growth hormone were studied after administration of L-dopa and a dopamine infusion. In the ten

normal subjects L-dopa, but not dopamine, increased plasma levels of GH. In the acromegalic patients both L-dopa and dopamine were followed by an inhibition of GH release. Since dopamine does not cross the blood-brain barrier, these results, although not excluding a site of action at median eminence level, support the thesis that the inhibitory effect of dopaminergic stimulation on GH release in acromegaly possibly involves receptors present on GH-secreting cells.

SO— Clin Endocrinol (Oxf) 5(4):419-23, Jul 76

AU— Machlin LJ

TI— Role of growth hormone in improving animal production

AB— Pituitary growth hormone (GH) has considerable potential as an anabolic agent in animal production. For example, pigs treated with GH will grow faster (i.e. deposit protein), require less feed per unit of body weight gain, and will have less carcass fat than untreated animals. Lactating cows will produce more milk with less feed. It is likely, though not completely established, that young cattle will also respond to GH treatments. Most of the information on the mode of action of GH has been obtained with laboratory rather than farm animals. The hormone affects almost all aspects of metabolism although the specific mechanism for these effects is still not understood. Stimulation of protein accretion is reflected by increased nitrogen retention and incorporation of radioactive amino-acids into tissue proteins. An increased rate of protein synthesis is thought to be a result of enhanced ability of ribosomes to translate messenger RNA. GH increases polyamine synthesis by increased ornithine decarboxylase activity; RNA synthesis by increasing RNA polymerase and DNA synthesis by increased DNA polymerase. Cell division is stimulated in several tissues (e.g. muscle and lymphoid tissue). In vivo GH lowers the respiratory quotient indicating an increased oxidation of fatty acids. The numbers of fat cells do not change but the fat cells are reduced in size. The stimulating effects of GH on skeletal tissue, and perhaps other tissues as well, is mediated by the formation of at least three peptides called somatomedins. GH is a protein with a molecular weight of about 22,000 and contains 191 amino-acid resi-

dues. The amino-acid sequence varies with the species. GH isolated from one species is not always effective in a different species. Use of GH isolated from pituitaries does not appear to be economically feasible. A chemical synthesis for human GH has been accomplished. However, biological activity equivalent to the native hormone has not been unequivocally established. Synthesis of bovine or porcine GH is feasible but will be expensive. A partial sequence of GH with 39 amino-acid residues has some biological activity. Synthesis of this shorter peptide would be considerably less expensive. Since proteins generally are not active orally, an economic procedure for prolonged parenteral administration would have to be devised. Alternative approaches would be the stimulation of endogenous production of GH with hypothalmic GH releasing factor. This factor has not been identified but is probably a small peptide. Agents such as arginine, DOPA, and prostaglandins, which are known to stimulate GH release under some conditions, could also be considered. Another approach would be the implantation of sparganum from the spirometra family (a flatworm). This treatment is known to mimic GH effects in the rat. Implantation of a GH producing tumour could also be considered. Clearly these latter suggestions are quite speculative and would present some obvious problems. . .
SO— Environ Qual Saf [Suppl] (5):43-55, 1976

AU— Pinter EJ; Tolis G; Friesen HG
TI— L-dopa, growth hormone and adipokinesis in the lean and the obese.
AB— Fourteen human volunteers (5 lean of both sexes, 4 grossly obese male, 4 grossly obese female and one patient suffering from hypopituitarism) were given 500 mg of L-dopa orally, and growth hormone (HGH), cortisol, prolactin (hPRL), insulin, FSH, LH, free fatty acids (FFA) and blood glucose were determined up to 30 minutes following the drug. The lean group showed a uniformly marked increase in HGH followed by a significant FFA rise. The obese females exhibited blunted HGH and a somewhat reduced FFA response. In the obese male, there were no HGH and FFA increments. Unstimulated levels of HGH were lower and

FFA markedly higher in both obese male and female vs the lean group. The patient with hypopituitarism showed no significant HGH and FFA response. In all groups, hPRL decreased, while Cortisol, LH, FSH and blood glucose levels remained uninfluenced.

SO— Int J Clin Pharmacol Biopharm 12(1-2):277-80, Jul 75

AU— Ajlouni K; Martinson DR; Hagen TC
TI— Effect of glucose on the growth hormone response to L-dopa in normal and diabetic subjects.
AB— The effect of hyperglycemia on the growth hormone response to oral L-dopa (500 mg.) was assessed in eight normal and eight insulin-dependent diabetic subjects. A peak growth hormone response of 21.0 $+/-$ 4.0 ng./ml. (mean $+/-$ S.E.M.), significantly above baseline (p less than 0.01), was achieved in the normal group following oral L-dopa. Glucose concentrations did not change and were approximately 80 mg./100 ml. throughout. Administration of 100 gm. oral glucose with the L-dopa, or thirty minutes thereafter, totally suppressed the growth hormone response in all eight and six of the subjects, respectively. A peak growth hormone response of 20.0 $+/-$ 1.7 ng./ml. (mean $+/-$ S.E.M.), significantly above baseline (p less than 0.001), was obtained in eight nonobese, insulin-dependent diabetics, in spite of prevailing hyperglycemia (mean plasma glucose 243-258 mg./100 ml.) throughout the test. Endogenous hyperglycemia was achieved in these patients by lessening the usual strict adherence to plasma glucose control for the purpose of the study. These results suggest an abnormality in the hypothalamus or pituitary of diabetic subjects allowing growth hormone responsiveness in spite of hyperglycemia.

SO— Diabetes 24(7):633-6, Jul 75
AU— Müller EE
TI— Nervous control of growth hormone secretion.
SO— Neuroendocrinology 11(6):338-69, 1973

AU— Kato Y; Lian KO; Dupre J; Beck JC
TI— Observations on the control and release of growth hormone in plasma.
SO— Mt Sinai J Med NY 40(3):382-401, May-Jun 73

AU— Martin JB
TI— Neural regulation of growth hormone secretion.
SO— N Engl J Med 288(26):1384-93, 28 Jun 73

AU— Turner MR
TI— Dietary effects on the secretion and actions of growth
    hormone.
SO— Proc Nutr Soc 31(2):205-12, Sep 72

AU— Hunter WM
TI— Secretion of human growth hormone
SO— Proc Nutr Soc 31(2):119-203, Sep 72

AU— Tanner JM
TI— Human growth hormone
SO— Nature 237(356):433-9, 23 Jun 72

Some Original
Scientific Literature

Letter to the Editor
reprinted from THE LANCET, Nov. 30, 1957, pp. 1116–1117

ATHEROSCLEROSIS: POSSIBLE ILL-EFFECTS OF THE USE OF HIGHLY UNSATURATED FATS TO LOWER SERUM-CHOLESTEROL LEVELS

Sir,—Substitution of vegetable and marine fats for animal fats in the diet of humans may be accompanied by a lowering of serum-cholesterol levels. It is believed that this effect is related to the fact that vegetable and marine oils are more unsaturated than animal fats.[1] [2] This effect has been noted in rabbits, and the lowered serum-cholesterol levels were correlated with a lesser degree of atherosclerosis at the end of the experiment.[3]

At present there is an increasing interest in the clinical use of such unsaturated acids as linoleic acid to lower serum-cholesterol levels, and thus presumably to slow down the rate of progression of atherosclerosis. Unfortunately, the use of

1. Malmros, H., Wigand, G. *Lancet,* July 6, 1957, p. 1.
2. Ahrens, E. H., Jr., Insull, W., Jr., Blomstrand, R., Hirsch, J., Tsaltas, T. T., Petersen, M. L. *ibid.* 1957, i, 943.
3. Kritchevsky, D., Meyer, A. W., Tesar, W. C., Logan, J. B., Baron, R. H., Davier, N. C., Cox, H. R. *Amer J. Physiol.* 1954, **178**, 30.

highly unsaturated fats in the diet may lead to side-effects
that would outweigh any benefit they have in atherosclerosis.

In general, the more unsaturated a fat is, the more readily is it oxidised—peroxides and compounds of higher molecular weight are among the products.[4] Thus, increasing the
degree of unsaturation of dietary fats—particularly of those
containing two or more double bonds—will increase the intake of fat oxidation products.

> In rats oxidised dietary fats produced gastric
> ulcers,[5] and even gastric carcinomas.[6] In Japan, car-
> cinoma of the stomach is the leading cause of death
> from cancer.[7] Is this related to the fact that fish,
> which is rich in unsaturated fat, is an important part
> of the Japanese diet? Similarly, in Sweden, another
> country with a high consumption of fish, the death-
> rate of white males from gastric carcinoma in the
> age-range 55–64 is two to three times as high as it is
> among the comparable population in the United
> States—and this in spite of the fact that the death-
> rate in the 55–64 age-group in Sweden is less than in
> the United States.[8]
>
> Highly oxidised hog fat added to the diet of rats
> caused a weight-loss that could be explained neither
> by lack of unsaturated acids nor by lessened food
> intake. The degree of weight-loss was parallel to the
> degree of oxidation of the fat.[9] In another study the
> toxicity of highly unsaturated fatty acids was found
> to be due to the peroxide present; the peroxide was
> found in liver and muscle fats when the oxidised fats
> were fed.[10]

4. Holman, R. T., Lundberg, W. D., Malkin, T. Progress in the Chemistry of Fats
   and Other Lipids; vol. 2. London, 1954.
5. Morris, H. P. Biological Antioxidants. Transactions of the Second Conference,
   Josiah Macy, Jr., Foundation; p. 96. New York, 1947.
6. Roffo, A. H. Bol. Inst. med. exp. Cancer, B. Aires, 1939, 15, 407.
7. Takeda, K. Gann, 1955, 46, suppl.
8. Calculated from the vital statistics for the United States, 1949–51, and for
   Sweden, 1951.
9. Kaunitz, H. Arch. exp. Path. Pharmak. 1953, 220, 16.
10. Kanedi, T., Sakai, H., Ishi, S. J. Biochem., Tokyo, 1955, 42, 561.

In in-vitro studies, the number of metachondria separated from rat livers was decreased when oxidised fatty acids were added to the metachondria solution.[10] Ethyl oleate peroxide has been shown to oxidise slowly the mercaptan groups of proteins, first to disulphide, then, with an excess, irreversibly to a higher state of oxidation.[11] Oxidised fatty acids have been shown to have an adverse effect on a number of oxidative enzymes.[12]

Unsaturated fatty acids increase the body's demand for vitamin E.[13] This may be the result of an increased susceptibility to oxidation of the fat stores in individuals on a diet rich in unsaturated fat, as indicated by an experiment[14] in which cod-liver oil was fed to pigs—the fat laid down was abnormally susceptible to oxidation. Thus, even though dietary unsaturated fats such as linoleic acid are free of oxidation products, they would be expected to have an adverse effect on the organism.

The deleterious action of fatty acid peroxides on the body is probably related to the fact that they are strong oxidising agents; many important enzymes and vitamins are easily oxidised.[15] In the course of the action of an organic peroxide on a reducing agent, peroxy (RO) and hydroxy (HO) radicals may be produced. The mutagenic and carcinogenic actions of X rays are attributed to the formation of HO and HO_2 radicals, and recently it has been suggested that spontaneous cancer arises through the side-effects of HO and HO_2 radicals produced in the normal course of metabolism.[16] Thus the production of gastric carcinoma by oxidised fats, as observed by Roffo, is not too surprising.

Further, one of the initiating steps in atherosclerosis may be the oxidative polymerisation of some of the constituents of

11. Duboulog, P., Fondarai, J. *Bull. soc. Chim. biol.*, *Paris*, 1953, **35**, 819.
12. Bernheim, F., Wilbur, K. M., Kenastan, C. B. *Arch. Biochem. Biophys.* 1952, **38**, 177.
13. *Annu. Rev. Med.* 1953, **4**, 157.
14. Lea, C. H. *Rep. Fd Invest. Bd, Lond.* 1936, **73**, 5.
15. Barron, E. S. G. Biological Antioxidants. Transactions of 5th Conference, Josiah Macy, Jr., Foundation; p. 81. New York, 1950.
16. Harman, D. *J. Gerontol.* 1956, **11**, 298.

the lipoproteins.[17] If this is true, an increase in the degree of unsaturation of the dietary fats may, over a long term, actually increase the severity of atherosclerosis.

For these experimental and theoretical reasons, it is urged that the present enthusiasm for increasing the degree of unsaturation of dietary fats (to combat atherosclerosis) be curbed, pending additional study of the possible adverse effects of this dietary change, lest the "cure be worse than the disease."

Veterans Administration Hospital,
    San Francisco, California.   DENHAM HARMAN.

17. Harman, D. *ibid.* 1957, **12**, 199

Printed   The Lancet Office,
Great Britain   7, Adam Street, Adelphi, London, W.C.2

Dietary Carcinogens

In this issue of *Science,* Bruce Ames reviews the increasing body of evidence that large numbers of potent carcinogens arise from natural processes. Mutagens are present in substantial quantities in fruits and vegetables. Carcinogens are formed in cooking as a result of reactions involving proteins or fats. Dietary practices may be an important determinant of current cancer risks.

Ames describes the role of plant materials as follows: Plants in nature synthesize toxic chemicals in large amounts, apparently as a primary defense against the hordes of bacterial, fungal, and insect and other animal predators. Plants in the human diet are no exception. The variety of toxic chemicals is so great that organic chemists have been characterizing them for over 100 years, and new plant chemicals are still being discovered. Recent widespread use of short-term tests for detecting mutagens and the increased testing of plant substances for carcinogenicity in animals have contributed to the identification of many natural mutagens, teratogens, and carcinogens in the human diet.

Safrole and related compounds are present in many edible plants. Safrole is a carcinogen in rodents and some of its metabolites are mutagens. Oil of sassafras, once used to flavor some root beer, is about 75 percent safrole. Black pepper contains about 10 percent by weight of a closely related compound, piperine. Extracts of black pepper at a dose equivalent to 4 milligrams of dried pepper per day cause tumors in mice at many sites. Many hydrazines are carcinogens and mutagens, and large amounts of them are found in edible mushrooms. One carcinogenic hydrazine is present in the false morel at a concentration of 50 milligrams per 100 grams. It causes lung tumors in mice at a level of 20 micrograms per mouse per day.

Carcinogens and mutagens are present in mold-contaminated foods such as corn, nuts, peanut butter, bread, cheese, and fruit. Some of these contaminants, such as aflatoxin, are among the most potent known carcinogens and mutagens. Nitrosamines and nitroso compounds are suspect as causative agents of stomach and esophageal cancer in humans. In the digestive system these nitrogen compounds are formed from nitrate and nitrite. Beets, celery, lettuce, spinach, radishes, and rhubarb all contain about 200 milligrams of nitrate per 100-gram portion.

Rancid fats are possible causative agents of colon and breast cancer in humans. These forms account for a substantial fraction of all the cancer deaths in the United States. Unsaturated fats are easily oxidized on standing and in cooking to form mutagens, promoters, and carcinogens. Among the numerous products of such oxidations are fatty acid hydroperoxides and cholesterol epoxide. Thus the colon and digestive tract are exposed to many fat-derived carcinogens. Human breast fluid can contain high levels of cholesterol epoxide.

Burnt and browned materials formed by heating proteins during cooking are highly mutagenic. Chemicals isolated from such products have been found to be carcinogenic when fed to rodents. In addition, the browning reaction products from caramelization of sugars or the reaction of amino acids and sugars during cooking contain a large variety of DNA-damaging agents.

The view that dietary practices might be a causative factor in cancer is not new. Epidemiologists have noted marked differences in cancer rates between population groups. Effects from changes in diet following migration have also been observed. Results of current studies are beginning to delineate more sharply specific causative agents. When more definitive information is available, it should be possible for prudent people to choose fruits and vegetables that present minimal hazards. In the meantime, there is persuasive evidence that charred meats and rancid fats should not be part of the diet.

—PHILIP H. ABELSON

Dietary Carcinogens and Anticarcinogens

Oxygen radicals and degenerative diseases

Bruce N. Ames

Comparison of data from different countries reveals wide differences in the rates of many types of cancer. This leads to hope that each major type of cancer may be largely avoidable, as is the case for cancers due to tobacco, which constitute 30 percent of the cancer deaths in the United States and the United Kingdom (*1*). Despite numerous suggestions to the contrary, there is no convincing evidence of any generalized increase in U.S. (or U.K.) cancer rates other than what could plausibly be ascribed to the delayed effects of previous increases in tobacco usage (*1–3*). Thus, whether or not any recent changes in life-style or pollution in industrialized countries will substantially affect future cancer risks, some important determinants of current risks remain to be discovered among long-established aspects of our way of life. Epidemiologic studies have indicated that dietary practices are the most promising area to explore (*1, 4*). These studies suggest that a general increase in consumption of fiber-rich cereals, vegetables, and fruits and decrease in consumption of fat-rich products and excessive alcohol would be prudent (*1, 4*). There is still a lack of definitive evidence about the dietary components that are critical for humans and about their mechanisms of action. Laboratory studies of natural foodstuffs and cooked food are beginning to uncover an extraordinary variety of mutagens and possible carcinogens and anticarcinogens. In this article I discuss dietary mutagens and carcinogens and anticarcinogens that seem of importance and speculate on relevant biochemical mechanisms, particularly the role of oxygen radicals and their inhibitors in the fat-cancer relationship, promotion, anticarcinogenesis, and aging.

The author is chairman of the Department of Biochemistry, University of California, Berkeley 94720.

Summary. The human diet contains a great variety of mutagens and carcinogens, as well as many natural antimutagens and anticarcinogens. Many of these mutagens and carcinogens may act through the generation of oxygen radicals. Oxygen radicals may also play a major role as endogenous initiators of degenerative processes, such as DNA damage and mutation (and promotion), that may be related to cancer, heart disease, and aging. Dietary intake of natural antioxidants could be an important aspect of the body's defense mechanism against these agents. Many antioxidants are being identified as anticarcinogens. Characterizing and optimizing such defense systems may be an important part of a strategy of minimizing cancer and other age-related diseases.

Natural Mutagens and Carcinogens in Food

Plant material. Plants in nature synthesize toxic chemicals in large amounts, apparently as a primary defense against the hordes of bacterial, fungal, and insect and other animal predators (*5–40*). Plants in the human diet are no exception. The variety of these toxic chemicals is so great that organic chemists have been characterizing them for over 100 years, and new plant chemicals are still being discovered (*12, 24, 25*). However, toxicological studies have been completed for only a very small percentage of them. Recent widespread use of short-term tests for detecting mutagens (*41, 42*) and the increased number of animal cancer tests on plant substances (*6*) have contributed to the identification of many natural mutagens, teratogens, and carcinogens in the human diet (*5–40*). Sixteen examples are discussed below.

1) *Safrole, estragole, methyleugenol,* and related compounds are present in many edible plants (*5*). Safrole, estragole, and methyleugenol are carcinogens in rodents, and several of their metabolites are mutagens (*5*). Oil of sassafras, which had been used in "natural" sarsaparilla root beer, is about 75 percent safrole. Black pepper contains small amounts of safrole and large amounts (close to 10 percent by weight) of the closely related compound *piperine* (*26*). Extracts of black pepper cause tumors in mice at a variety of sites at a dose of extract equivalent to 4 mg of dried pepper

per day (about 160 mg/kg per day) for 3 months; an estimate of the average human intake of black pepper is over 140 mg per day (about 2 mg/kg per day) for life (26).

2) Most *hydrazines* that have been tested are carcinogens and mutagens, and large amounts of carcinogenic hydrazines are present in edible mushrooms. The widely eaten false morel (*Gyromitra esculenta*) contains 11 hydrazines, three of which are known carcinogens (28). One of these, *N*-methyl-*N*-formylhydrazine, is present at a concentration of 50 mg per 100 g and causes lung tumors in mice at the extremely low dietary level of 20 μg per mouse per day (28). The most common commercial mushroom, *Agaricus bisporus,* contains about 300 mg of *agaritine,* the δ-glutamyl derivative of the mutagen 4-hydroxymethylphenylhydrazine, per 100 g of mushrooms, as well as smaller amounts of the closely related carcinogen *N*-acetyl - 4 - hydroxymethylphenylhydrazine (28). Some agaritine is metabolized by the mushroom to a diazonium derivative which is a very potent carcinogen (a single dose of 400 ng/g gave 30 percent of mice stomach tumors) and which is also present in the mushroom in smaller amounts (28). Many hydrazine carcinogens may act by producing oxygen radicals (43).

3) Linear *furocoumarins* such as *psoralen derivatives* are potent light-activated carcinogens and mutagens and are widespread in plants of the Umbelliferae family, such as celery, parsnips, figs, and parsley (for instance, 4 mg per 100 g of parsnip) (17, 19, 44). The level in celery (about 100 μg per 100 g) can increase about 100-fold if the celery is stressed or diseased (19). Celery pickers and handlers commonly develop skin rashes on their arms when exposed to diseased celery (19). Oil of bergamot, a citrus oil, is very rich in a psoralen and was used in the leading suntan lotion in France (17). Psoralens, when activated by sunlight, damage DNA and induce tanning more rapidly than the ultraviolet component of sunlight, which is also a carcinogen (17). Psoralens (plus light) are also effective in producing oxygen radicals (18).

4) The potato glycoalkaloids *solanine* and *chaconine* are strong cholinesterase inhibitors and possible teratogens and are present at about 15 mg per 200 g of potato (12, 13). When

potatoes are diseased, bruised, or exposed to light, these and other (24) glycoalkaloids reach levels that can be lethal to humans (12). Plants typically respond to damage by making more (and often different) toxic chemicals as a defense against insects and fungi (19, 24, 25). The different cultivars of potatoes vary in the concentration of these toxic glycoalkaloids (the concentration is a major determinant of insect and disease resistance); one cultivar bred for insect resistance had to be withdrawn from use because of its toxicity to humans (> 40 mg of glycoalkaloids in a 200-g potato is considered to be a toxic level) (12).

5) *Quercetin* and several similar flavonoids are mutagens in a number of short-term test systems. Flavonoids are extremely widespread (daily levels close to 1 g) in the human diet (8, 16, 20, 21). There is evidence for the carcinogenicity of quercetin in two strains of rats (8), although it was negative in other experiments (21).

6) *Quinones* and their phenol precursors (9, 14, 16, 23, 45) are widespread in the human diet. Quinones are quite toxic as they can act as electrophiles or accept a single electron to yield the semiquinone radical, which can either react directly with DNA (14, 46) or participate in a redox cycle of superoxide radical generation by transferring the electron to O_2 (47). The superoxide radical and its metabolic product H_2O_2 can, in turn, lead to the oxidation of fat in cellular membranes by a lipid peroxidation chain reaction, thus generating mutagens and carcinogens, as discussed below. A number of quinones and dietary phenols have been shown to be mutagens (7, 9, 16, 23, 44). Mutagenic anthraquinone derivatives are found in plants such as rhubarb and in mold toxins (7, 16, 48). Many dietary phenols can spontaneously autoxidize to quinones, generating hydrogen peroxide at the same time [examples are catechol derivatives such as the caffeic acid component of chlorogenic acid (9), which is present at about 250 mg per cup of coffee]. The amounts of these phenols in human urine (and in the diet) are appreciable (45). Catechol, for example, is excreted in urine at about 10 mg per day and appears to be mainly derived from metabolism of plant substances (45). Catechol is a potent promoter of carci-

nogenesis (45), an inducer of DNA damage, a likely active metabolite of the carcinogen benzene (46), and a toxic agent in cigarette smoke (45). Catecholamine induction of cardio-myopathy is thought to occur through generation of oxygen radicals (49).

7) *Theobromine*, a relative of caffeine, has been shown to be genotoxic in a variety of tests, to potentiate (as does caffeine) DNA damage by various carcinogens in human cells, and to cause testicular atrophy and spermatogenic cell abnormalities in rats (27). Cocoa powder is about 2 percent theobromine, and therefore humans may consume hundreds of milligrams of theobromine a day from chocolate. Theobromine is also present in tea.

8) *Pyrrolizidine* alkaloids are carcinogenic, mutagenic, and teratogenic and are present in thousands of plant species (often at > 1 percent by weight), some of which are ingested by humans, particularly in herbs and herbal teas and occasionally in honey (7, 29). Pyrrolizidine alkaloid poisonings in humans (as well as in other mammals) cause lung and liver lesions and are commonly misdiagnosed (29).

9) The broad (fava) bean *(Vicia faba)*, a common food of the Mediterranean region, contains the toxins *vicine* and *convicine* at a level of about 2 percent of the dry weight (30). Pythagoras forbade his followers to eat the beans, presumably because he was one of the millions of Mediterranean people with a deficiency of glucose-6-phosphate dehydrogenase. This deficiency results in a low glutathione concentration in blood cells, which causes increased resistance to the malarial parasite, probably accounting for the widespread occurrence of the mutant gene in malarial regions. However, the low glutathione concentration also results in a marked sensitivity to agents that cause oxidative damage, such as the fava bean toxins and a variety of drugs and viruses. Sensitive individuals who ingest fava beans develop a severe hemolytic anemia caused by the enzymatic hydrolysis of vicine to its aglycone, *divicine*, which forms a quinone that generates oxygen radicals (30).

10) *Allyl isothiocyanate*, a major flavor ingredient in oil of mustard and horseradish, is one of the main toxins of the

mustard seed and has been shown to cause chromosome aberrations in hamster cells at low concentration (*50*) and to be a carcinogen in rats (*31*).

11) *Gossypol* is a major toxin in cottonseed and accounts for about 1 percent of its dry weight (*32*). Gossypol causes pathological changes in rat and human testes, abnormal sperm, and male sterility (*32, 33*). Genetic damage has been observed in embryos sired by gossypoltreated male rats: dominant lethal mutations in embryos were measured after males were taken off gossypol treatment and allowed to mate (*33*). Gossypol appears to be a carcinogen as well: it has been reported to be a potent initiator and also a promoter of carcinogenesis in skin painting studies with mice (*34*). Crude, unrefined cottonseed oil contains considerable amounts of gossypol (100 to 750 mg per 100 ml). Thus human consumption may be appreciable in countries, such as Egypt, where fairly crude cottonseed oil is commonly used in cooking. Gossypol is being tested as a male contraceptive in over 10,000 people in China (at an oral dose of about 10 mg per person per day), as it is inexpensive and causes sterility during use (*33*). Gossypol's mode of action as a spermicide may be through the production of oxygen radicals (*35*).

Plant breeders have developed "glandless cotton," a new strain with low levels of gossypol, but seeds from this strain are much more susceptible to attack by the fungus *Aspergillus flavus,* which produces the potent carcinogen aflatoxin (*36*).

12) *Sterculic acid and malvalic acid* are widespread in the human diet. They are toxic cyclopropenoid fatty acids present in cottonseed oil and other oils from seeds of plants in the family Malvaceal (for instance, cotton, kapok, okra, and durian) (*51*). Another possible source of human exposure is consumption of fish, poultry, eggs, and milk from animals fed on cottonseed (*51*). Cyclopropenoid fatty acids are carcinogens in trout, markedly potentiate the carcinogenicity of aflatoxin in trout, cause atherosclerosis in rabbits, are mitogenic in rats, and have a variety of toxic effects in farm animals (*51*). The toxicity of these fatty acids could be due to their ease of oxidation to form peroxides and radicals (*51*).

13) Leguminous plants such as lupine contain very potent teratogens (22). When cows and goats forage on these plants, their offspring may have severe teratogenic abnormalities; an example is the characteristic "crooked calf" abnormality due to the ingestion of *anagyrine* from lupine (22). In addition, significant amounts of these teratogens are transferred to the animals' milk, so that drinking the milk during pregnancy is a serious teratogenic hazard (22). In one rural California family, a baby boy, a litter of puppies, and goat kids all had "crooked" bone birth-defect abnormalities. The pregnant mother and the dog had both been drinking milk obtained from the family goats, which had been foraging on lupine (the main forage in winter) (22). It was at first mistakenly thought that the birth defects were caused by spraying of 2,4-D.

14) *Sesquiterpene lactones* are widespread in many plants (37), although because they are bitter they are not eaten in large amounts. Some have been shown to be mutagenic (37). They are a major toxin in the white sap of *Lactuca virosa* (poison lettuce), which has been used as a folk remedy. Plant breeders are now transferring genes from this species to commercial lettuce to increase insect resistance (38).

15) The *phorbol esters* present in the Euphorbiacea, some of which are used as folk remedies or herb teas, are potent promoters of carcinogenesis and may have been a cause of nasopharyngeal cancer in China and esophageal cancer in Curaçao (39).

16) Alfalfa sprouts contain *canavanine*, a highly toxic arginine analog that is incorporated into protein in place of arginine. Canavanine, which occurs in alfalfa sprouts at about 1.5 percent of their dry weight (40), appears to be the active agent in causing the severe lupus erythematosus–like syndrome seen when monkeys are fed alfalfa sprouts (40). Lupus in man is characterized by a defect in the immune system which is associated with autoimmunity, antinuclear antibodies, chromosome breaks, and various types of pathology (40). The chromosome breaks appear to be due to oxygen radicals as they are prevented by superoxide dismutase (52). The canavanine–alfalfa sprout pathology could be due in part to

the production of oxygen radicals during phagocytization of antibody complexes with canavanine-containing protein.

The 16 examples above, plus coffee (discussed below), illustrate that the human dietary intake of "nature's pesticides" is likely to be several grams per day—probably at least 10,000 times higher than the dietary intake of man-made pesticides (53).

Levels of plant toxins that confer insect and fungal resistance are being increased or decreased by plant breeders (38). There are health costs for the use of these natural pesticides, just as there are for man-made pesticides (41, 54), and these must be balanced against the costs of producing food. However, little information is available about the toxicology of most of the natural plant toxins in our diet, despite the large doses we are exposed to. Many, if not most, of these plant toxins may be "new" to humans in the sense that the human diet has changed drastically with historic times. By comparison, our knowledge of the toxicological effects of new man-made pesticides is extensive, and general exposure is exceedingly low (53).

Plants also contain a variety of anticarcinogens (55), which are discussed below.

Alcohol. Alcohol has long been associated with cancer of the mouth, esophagus, pharynx, larynx, and, to a lesser extent, liver (1, 56), and it appears to be an important human teratogen, causing a variety of physical and mental defects in babies of mothers who drink (57). Alcohol drinking causes abnormalities in mice (57a) and is a synergist for chromosome damage in humans (58). Alcohol metabolism generates acetaldehyde, which is a mutagen and teratogen (59), a cocarcinogen, and possibly a carcinogen (60), and also radicals that produce lipid hydroperoxides (61) and other mutagens and carcinogens (62; see below). In some epidemiologic studies on alcohol (56), it has been suggested that dietary green vegetables are a modifying factor in the reduction of cancer risk.

Mold carcinogens. A variety of mold carcinogens and mutagens are present in mold-contaminated food such as corn, grain, nuts, peanut butter, bread, cheese, fruit, and apple juice (15, 63). Some of these, such as sterigmatocystin and aflatoxin, are among the most potent carcinogens and mutagens known (*15, 63*). Dietary glutathione has been reported to counteract aflatoxin carcinogenicity.

Nitrite, nitrate, and nitrosamines. A number of human cancers, such as stomach and esophageal cancer, may be related to nitrosamines and other nitroso compounds formed from nitrate and nitrite in the diet (*64, 65*). Beets, celery, lettuce, spinach, radishes, and rhubarb all contain about 200 mg of nitrate per 100-g portion (*65*). Anticarcinogens in the diet may be important in this context as well (*66*).

Fat and cancer: possible oxidative mechanisms. Epidemiologic studies of cancer in humans suggest, but do not prove, that high fat intake is associated with colon and breast cancer (*1, 4, 67*). A number of animal studies have shown that high dietary fat is a promoter and a presumptive carcinogen (*4, 67, 68*). Colon and breast cancer and lung cancer (which is almost entirely due to cigarette smoking) account for about half of all U.S. cancer deaths. In addition to the cyclopropenoid fatty acids already discussed, two other plausible mechanisms involving oxidative processes could account for the relation (*69*) between high fat and both cancer and heart disease.

1) *Rancid fat.* Fat accounts for over 40 percent of the calories in the U.S. diet (*67*), and the amount of ingested oxidized fat may be appreciable (*70, 71*). Unsaturated fatty acids and cholesterol in fat are easily oxidized, particularly during cooking (*70, 71*). The lipid peroxidation chain reaction (rancidity) yields a variety (*71–73*) of mutagens, promoters, and carcinogens such as fatty acid hydroperoxides (*62*), cholesterol hydroperoxide (*74*), endoperoxides, cholesterol and fatty acid epoxides (*74–77*), enals and other aldehydes (*44, 59, 78*), and alkoxy and hydroperoxy radicals (*44, 72*). Thus the colon and digestive tract are exposed to a variety of fat-derived carcinogens. Human breast fluid can contain enormous levels (up to 780 μM (*75*)) of cholesterol epoxide (an oxidation product of cholesterol), which could originate from either ingested oxidized fat or oxidative processes in body lipids. Rodent feeding studies with oxidized fat (*79*) have not yielded definitive results.

2) *Peroxisomes* oxidize an appreciable percentage of dietary fatty acids, and removal of each two-carbon unit generates one molecule of hydrogen peroxide (a mutagen,

promoter, and carcinogen) (80, 81). Some hydrogen peroxide escapes the catalase in the peroxisome (80, 82, 83), thus contributing to the supply of oxygen radicals, which also come from other metabolic sources (72, 83–85). Hydroperoxides generate oxygen radicals in the presence of iron-containing compounds in the cell (72). Oxygen radicals, in turn, can damage DNA and can start the rancidity chain reaction which leads to the production of the mutagens and carcinogens listed above (72). Drugs such as clofibrate, which cause lowering of serum lipids and proliferation of peroxisomes in rodents, result in age pigment (lipofuscin) accumulation (a sign of lipid peroxidation in tissues) and liver tumors in animals (80). Some fatty acids, such as $C_{22:1}$ and certain *trans* fatty acids, appear to cause peroxisomal proliferation because they are poorly oxidized in mitochondria and are preferentially oxidized in the peroxisomes, although they may be selective for heart or liver (86). There has been controversy about the role of *trans* fatty acids in cancer and heart disease, and recent evidence suggests that *trans* fatty acids might not be a risk factor for atherosclerosis in experimental animals (87). Americans consume about 12 g of *trans* fatty acids a day (87) and a similar amount of unnatural *cis* isomers [which need further study (88)], mainly from hydrogenated vegetable fats. Dietary $C_{22:1}$ fatty acids are also obtained from rapeseed oil and fish oils (86). Thus oxidation of certain fatty acids might generate grams of hydrogen peroxide per day within the peroxisome (86). Another source of fat toxicity could be perturbations in the mitochondrial or peroxisomal membranes caused by abnormal fatty acids, yielding an increased flux of superoxide and hydrogen peroxide. Mitochondrial structure is altered when rats are fed some abnormal fatty acids from partially hydrogenated fish oil (89). Dietary $C_{22:1}$ fatty acids and clofibrate also induce ornithine decarboxylase (86), a common attribute of promoters.

A recent National Academy of Sciences committee report suggests that a reduction of fat consumption in the American diet would be prudent (4), although other scientists argue that, until we know more about the mechanism of the fat-cancer relation and about which types of fat are dangerous, it is premature to recommend dietary changes (90).

Cooked Food as a Source of Ingested Burnt and Browned Material

Work of Sugimura and others has indicated that the burnt and browned material from heating protein during cooking is highly mutagenic (21, 91). Several chemicals isolated on the basis of their mutagenicity from heated protein or pyrolyzed amino acids were found to be carcinogenic when fed to rodents (21). In addition, the browning reaction products from the caramelization of sugars or the reaction of amino acids and sugars during cooking (for instance, the brown material on bread crusts and toasted bread) contain a large variety of DNA-damaging agents and presumptive carcinogens (3, 38, 92). The amount of burnt and browned material in the human diet may be several grams per day. By comparison about 500 mg of burnt material is inhaled each day by a smoker using two packs of cigarettes (at 20 mg of tar per cigarette) a day. Smokers have more easily detectable levels of mutagens in their urine than nonsmokers (93), but so do people who have consumed a meal of fried pork or bacon (94). In the evaluation of risk from burnt material it may be useful (in addition to carrying out epidemiologic studies) to compare the activity of cigarette tar to that of the burnt material from cooked food (or polluted air) in short-term tests and animal carcinogenicity tests involving relevant routes of exposure. Route of exposure and composition of the burnt material are critical variables. The risk from inhaled cigarette smoke can be one reference standard: an average life shortening of about 8 years for a two-pack-a-day smoker. The amount of burnt material inhaled from severely polluted city air, on the other hand, is relatively small: it would be necessary to breathe smoggy Los Angeles air ($111 \mu g/m^3$ total particulates; $31 \mu g/m^3$ soluble organic matter) for 1 to 2 weeks to equal the soluble organic matter of the particulates or the mutagenicity from one cigarette (20 mg of tar) (95). Epidemiologic studies have not shown significant risks from city air pollution alone (1, 96). Air in the houses of smokers is considerably more polluted than city air outside (97).

Coffee, which contains a considerable amount of burnt material, including the mutagenic pyrolysis product methyglyoxal, is mutagenic (*21, 98*). However, one cup of coffee also contains about 250 mg of the natural mutagen chlorogenic acid (*9*) [which is also an antinitrosating agent (*66*)], highly toxic atractylosides (*10*), the glutathione transferase inducers kahweal palmitate and cafestol palmitate (*11*), and about 100 mg of caffeine [which inhibits a DNA-repair system and can increase tumor yield (*99*) and cause birth defects at high levels in several experimental species (*100*)]. There is preliminary, but not conclusive, epidemiologic evidence that heavy coffee drinking is associated with cancer of the ovary, bladder, pancreas, and large bowel (*101*).

Cooking also accelerates the rancidity reaction of cooking oils and fat in meat (*70, 71*), thus increasing consumption of mutagens and carcinogens.

Anticarcinogens

We have many defense mechanisms to protect ourselves against mutagens and carcinogens, including continuous shedding of the surface layer of our skin, stomach, cornea, intestines, and colon (*102*). Understanding these mechanisms should be a major goal of cancer, heart, and aging research. Among the most important defenses may be those against oxygen radicals and lipid peroxidation if, as discussed here, these agents are major contributors to DNA damage (*103*). Major sources of endogenous oxygen radicals are hydrogen peroxide (*83*) and superoxide (*72, 104*) generated as side products of metabolism, and the oxygen radical burst from phagocytosis after viral or bacterial infection or the inflammatory reaction (*105*). A variety of environmental agents could also contribute to the oxygen radical load, as discussed here and in recent reviews (*72, 106*). Many enzymes protect cells from oxidative damage; examples are superoxide dismutase (*104*), DT-diaphorase (*108*), and the glutathione transferases (*109*). In addition, a variety of small molecules in our diet are required for antioxidative mechanisms and appear to be anticarcinogens; some of these are discussed below.

1) *Vitamin E* (tocopherol) is the major radical trap in lipid membranes (*72*) and has been used clinically in a variety

of oxidation-related diseases (*110*). Vitamin E ameliorates both the cardiac damage and carcinogenicity of the quinones adriamycin and daunomycin, which are mutagenic, carcinogenic, cause cardiac damage, and appear to be toxic because of free radical generation (*111*). Protective effects of tocopherols against radiation-induced DNA damage and mutation and dimethylhydrazine-induced carcinogenesis have also been observed (*112*). Vitamin E markedly increases the endurance of rats during heavy exercise, which causes extensive oxygen radical damage to tissues (*113*).

2) *β-Carotene* is another antioxidant in the diet that could be important in protecting body fat and lipid membranes against oxidation. Carotenoids are free-radical traps and remarkably efficient quenchers of singlet oxygen (*114*). Singlet oxygen is a very reactive form of oxygen which is mutagenic and particularly effective at causing lipid peroxidation (*114*). It can be generated by pigment-mediated transfer of the energy of light to oxygen, or by lipid peroxidation, although the latter is somewhat controversial. β-Carotene and similar polyprenes are present in carrots and in all food that contains chlorophyll, and they appear to be the plants' main defense against singlet oxygen generated as a by-product from the interaction of light and chlorophyll (*115*). Carotenoids have been shown to be anticarcinogens in rats and mice (*116*). Carotenoids (in green and yellow vegetables) may be anticarcinogens in humans (*1, 56, 117*). Their protective effects in smokers might be related to the high level of oxidants in both cigarette smoke and tar (*45, 118*). Carotenoids have been used medically in the treatment for some genetic diseases, such as porphyrias, where a marked photosensitivity is presumably due to singlet oxygen formation (*119*).

3) *Selenium* is another important dietary anticarcinogen. Dietary selenium (usually selenite) significantly inhibits the induction of skin, liver, colon, and mammary tumors in experimental animals by a number of different carcinogens, as well as the induction of mammary tumors by viruses (*120*). It also inhibits transformation of mouse mammary cells (*121*). Low selenium concentrations may be a risk factor in human cancer (*122*). A particular type of heart disease in young

people in the Keshan area of China has been traced to a selenium deficiency, and low selenium has been associated with cardiovascular death in Finland (*123*). Selenium is in the active site of glutathione peroxidase, an enzyme essential for destroying lipid hydroperoxides and endogenous hydrogen peroxide and thus helping to prevent oxygen radical–induced lipid peroxidation (*107*), although not all of the effects of selenium may be accounted for by this enzyme (*120*). Several heavy-metal toxins, such as Cd^{2+} (a known carcinogen) and Hg^{2+}, lower glutathione peroxidase activity by interacting with selenium (*107*). Selenite (and vitamin E) has been shown to counter the oxidative toxicity of mercuric salts (*124*).

4) *Glutathione* is present in food and is one of the major antioxidants and antimutagens in the soluble fraction of cells. The glutathione transferases (some of which have peroxidase activity) are major defenses against oxidative and alkylating carcinogens (*109*). The concentration of glutathione may be influenced by dietary sulfur amino acids (*125, 126*). N-Acetyl-cystein, a source of cysteine, raises glutathione concentrations and reduces the oxidative cardiotoxicity of adriamycin and the skin reaction to radiation (*127*). Glutathione concentrations are raised even more efficiently by L-2-oxo-thiazolidine-4-carboxylate, which is an effective antagonist of acetaminophen-caused liver damage (*126*). Acetaminophen is thought to be toxic through radical and quinone oxidizing metabolites (*128*). Dietary glutathione may be an effective anticarcinogen against aflatoxin (*129*).

5) Dietary *ascorbic acid* is also important as an antioxidant. It was shown to be anticarcinogenic in rodents treated with ultraviolet radiation, benzo[*a*]pyrene, and nitrite (forming nitroso carcinogens) (*64, 65, 130*), and it may be inversely associated with human uterine cervical dysplasia (although this is not proof of a cause-effect relationship) (*131*). It was recently hypothesized that ascorbic acid may have been supplemented and perhaps partially replaced in humans by uric acid during primate evolution (*132*).

6) *Uric acid* is a strong antioxidant present in high concentrations in the blood of humans (*132*). The concentration of uric acid in the blood can be increased by dietary purines; however, too much causes gout. Uric acid is also present in

high concentrations in human saliva (*132*) and may play a role in defense there as well, in conjunction with lactoperoxidase. A low uric acid level in blood may possibly be a risk factor in cigarette-caused lung cancer in humans (*133*).

7) Edible plants and a variety of substances in them, such as phenols, have been reported to inhibit (cabbage) or to enhance (beets) carcinogenesis (*11, 55, 134*) or mutagenesis (*3, 66, 92, 135*) in experimental animals. Some of these substances appear to inhibit by inducing cytochrome P-450 and other metabolic enzymes [(*134*); see also (*11*)], although on balance it is not completely clear whether it is generally helpful or harmful for humans to ingest these inducing substances.

The hypothesis that as much as 80 percent of cancer could be due to environmental factors was based on geographic differences in cancer rates and studies of migrants (*136*). These differences in cancer rates were thought to be mainly due to life-style factors, such as smoking and dietary carcinogens and promoters (*136*), but they also may be due in good part [see also (*1*)] to less than optimum amounts of anticarcinogens and protective factors in the diet.

The optimum levels of dietary antioxidants, which may vary among individuals, remain to be determined; however, at least for selenium (*120*), it is important to emphasize the possibility of deleterious side effects at high doses.

Oxygen Radicals and Degenerative Diseases Associated with Aging

Aging. A plausible theory of aging holds that the major cause is damage to DNA (*102, 137*) and other macromolecules and that a major source of this damage is oxygen radicals and lipid peroxidation (*43, 84, 103, 138–141*). Cancer and other degenerative diseases, such as heart disease (*102*), are likely to be due in good part to this same fundamental destructive process. Age pigment (lipofuscin) accumulates aging in all mammalian species and has been associated with lipid peroxidation (*73, 84, 138, 139*). The fluorescent products in age pigment are thought to be formed by malondialdehyde (a mutagen and carcinogen and a major end product of rancidity) cross-linking protein and lipids (138). Metabolic rate is directly correlated with the rate of lipofuscin formation (and inversely correlated with longevity) (139).

Cancer increases with about the fourth power of age, both in short-lived species such as rats and mice (about 30 percent of rodents have cancer by the end of their 2- to 3-year life-span) and in long-lived species such as humans (about 30 percent of people have cancer by the end of their 85-year life-span) (142). Thus, the marked increase in life-span that has occurred in 60 million years of primate evolution has been accompanied by a marked decrease in age-specific cancer rates; that is, in contrast to rodents, 30 percent of humans do not have cancer by the age of 3 (142). One important factor in longevity appears to be basal metabolic rate (139, 141), which is much lower in man than in rodents and could markedly affect the level of endogenous oxygen radicals.

Animals have many antioxidant defenses against oxygen radicals. Increased levels of these antioxidants, as well as new antioxidants, may also be a factor in the evolution of man from short-lived prosimians (143). It has been suggested that an increase in superoxide dismutase is correlated (after the basal metabolic rate is taken into account) with increased longevity during primate evolution, although this has been disputed (141). Ames et al. proposed (132) that as uric acid was an antioxidant and was present in much higher concentrations in the blood of humans than in other mammals, it may have been one of the innovations enabling the marked increase in life span and consequent marked decrease in age-specific cancer rates which occurred during primate evolution. The ability to synthesize ascorbic acid may have been lost at about the same time in primate evolution as uric acid levels began to increase (144).

Cancer and promotion. Both DNA-damaging agents (initiating mutagens) (21, 41, 42) and promoters (145) appear to play an important role in carcinogenesis (21, 146). It has been postulated that certain promoters of carcinogenesis act by generation of oxygen radicals and resultant lipid peroxidation (73, 146–149). Lipid peroxidation cross-links proteins (43, 150) and affects all aspects of cell organization (72), including membrane and surface structure, and the mitotic apparatus. A common property of promoters may be their ability to produce oxygen radicals. Some examples are fat and hydrogen peroxide (which may be among the most important promoters) (67, 68, 81), TCDD (151), lead and cadmium (152), phorbol esters (147, 149, 153), wounding of tissues (154), asbestos (155), peroxides (156), catechol (45) (see quinones above), mezerein and teleocidin B (147), phenobarbital (157), and radiation (72, 158). Inflammatory reactions involve the production of oxygen radicals by phagocytes (105), and this could be the basis of promotion for asbestos (155) or wounding (154). Some of the antioxidant anticarcinogens (discussed above) are also antipromoters (73, 121, 146, 159, 160), and phorbol ester–induced chromosome damage (149) or promotion of transformation (159) is suppressed by superoxide dismutase, as would be expected if promoters were working through oxidative mechanisms. Many "complete" carcinogens cause the production of oxygen radicals (73, 161); examples are nitroso compounds, hydrazines, quinones, polycyclic hydrocarbons (through quinones), cadmium and lead salts, nitro compounds, and radiation. A good part of the toxic effects of ionizing radiation damage to DNA and cells is thought to be due to generation of oxygen radicals (103, 162), although only a tiny part of the oxygen radical load in humans is likely to be from this source.

Recent studies give some clues as to how promoters might act. Promoters disrupt the mitotic apparatus, causing hemizygosity and expression of recessive genes (163). Phorbol esters generate oxygen radicals, which cause chromosome breaks (164) and increase gene copy number (165). Promoters also cause formation of the peroxide hormones of the prostaglandin and leukotriene family by oxidation of arachidonic acid and other C_{20} polyenoic fatty acids, and inhibitors of this process appear to be antipromoters (160). These hormones are intimately involved in cell division, differentiation, and tumor growth (166) and could have arisen in evolution as signal molecules warning the cell of oxidative damage. Effects on the cell membrane have also been suggested as the important factor in promotion, causing inhibition of intercellular communication (167) or protein kinase activation (167a).

Heart disease. It has been postulated that atherosclerotic lesions, which are derived from single cells, are similar to benign tumors and are of somatic mutational origin (*102, 168*). Fat appears to be one major risk factor for heart disease as well as for colon and breast cancer (*69*). In agreement with this, a strong correlation has been observed between the frequency of atherosclerotic lesions and adenomatous polyps of the colon (*69*). Thus, the same oxidative processes involving fat may contribute to both diseases. Oxidized forms of cholesterol have been implicated in heart disease (*169*), and atherosclerotic-like lesions have been produced by injecting rabbits with lipid hydroperoxide or oxidized cholesterol (*169*). The anticarcinogens discussed above could be anti–heart disease agents as well. As pointed out in the preceding section, vitamin E ameliorates both the cardiac damage and carcinogenicity of the free-radical-generating quinones adriamycin and daunomycin; *N*-acetycysteine reduces the cardiotoxicity of adriamycin; and selenium is an antirisk factor for one type of heart disease.

Other diseases. The brain uses 20 percent of the oxygen consumed by man and contains an appreciable amount of unsaturated fat. Lipid peroxidation (with consequent age pigment) is known to occur readily in the brain (*72*), and possible consequences could be senile dementia or other brain abnormalities (*84*). Several inherited progressive diseases of the central nervous system, such as Batten's disease, are associated with lipofuscin accumulation and may be due to a lipid peroxidation caused by a high concentration of unbound iron (*170*). Mental retardation is one consequence of an inherited defective DNA repair system (XP complementation group D) for depurinated sites in DNA (*171*).

Senile cataracts have been associated with light-induced oxidative damage (*172*). The retina and an associated layer of cells, the pigment epithelium, are extremely sensitive to degeneration in vitamin E and selenium deficiency (*173*). The pigment epithelium accumulates massive amounts of lipofuscin in aging and dietary antioxidant deficiency (*173*). The eye is well known to be particularly rich in antioxidants.

The testes are quite prone to lipid peroxidation and to the accumulation of age pigment. A number of agents, such as gossypol, which cause genetic birth defects (dominant lethals) may be active by this mechanism. The various agents known to cause cancer by oxidative mechanisms are prospective mutagenic agents for the germ line. Thus, vitamin E, which was discovered 60 years ago as a fertility factor (72), and other antioxidants such as selenium (174), may help both to engender and to protect the next generation.

Risks

There are large numbers of mutagens and carcinogens in every meal, all perfectly natural and traditional [see also (21, 23)]. Nature is not benign. It should be emphasized that no human diet can be entirely free of mutagens and carcinogens and that the foods mentioned are only representative examples. To identify a substance, whether natural or man-made, as a mutagen or a carcinogen, is just a first step. Beyond this, it is necessary to consider the risks for alternative courses of action and to quantitate the approximate magnitude of the risk, although the quantification of risk poses a major challenge. Carcinogens differ in their potency in rodents by more than a millionfold (175), and the levels of particular carcinogens to which humans are exposed can vary more than a billionfold. Extrapolation of risk from rodents to humans is difficult for many reasons, including the longevity difference, antioxidant factors, and the probable multicausal nature of most human cancer.

Tobacco smoking is, without doubt, a major and well-understood risk, causing about 30 percent of cancer deaths and 25 percent of fatal heart attacks (as well as other degenerative diseases) in the United States (1). These percentages may increase even more in the near future as the health effects of the large increase in women smokers become apparent (1). Diet, which provides both carcinogens and anticarcinogens, is extremely likely to be another major risk factor. Excessive alcohol consumption is another risk, although it does not seem to be of the same general importance as smoking and diet. Certain other high-dose exposures might also turn out to be important for particular groups of people—

for instance, certain drugs, where consumption can reach hundreds of milligrams per day; particular cosmetics; and certain occupational exposures (2), where workers inhale dusts or solvents at high concentration. We must also be prudent about environmental pollution (41, 54). Despite all of these risks, it should be emphasized that the overall trend in life expectancy in the United States is continuing steadily upward (176).

The understanding of cancer and degenerative disease mechanisms is being aided by the rapid progress of science and technology, and this should help to dispel confusion about how important health risks can be identified among the vast number of minor risks. We have many methods of attacking the problem of environmental carcinogens (and anticarcinogens), including human epidemiology (1), short-term tests (41, 42, 177), and animal cancer tests (175). Powerful new methods are being developed [for instance, see (58, 177)] for measuring DNA damage or other pertinent factors with great sensitivity in individuals. These methods, which are often noninvasive as they can be done on blood or urine (even after storage), can be combined with epidemiology to determine whether particular factors are predictive of disease. Thus, more powerful tools will be available for optimizing antioxidants and other dietary anti-risk factors, for identifying human genetic variants at high risk, and for identifying significant health risks.

References and Notes

1. R. Doll and R. Peto, *J. Natl. Cancer Inst.* **66**, 1192 (1981).

2. R. Peto and M. Schneiderman, Eds., *Banbury Report 9. Quantification of Occupational Cancer* (Cold Spring Harbor Laboratory, Cold Spring Harbor, N.Y., 1981).

3. *Cancer Facts and Figures, 1983* (American Cancer Society, New York, 1982).

4. National Research Council, *Diet, Nutrition and Cancer* (National Academy Press, Washington, D.C., 1982).

5. E. C. Miller, J. A. Miller, I. Hirono, T. Sugimura, S. Takayama, Eds., *Naturally Occurring Carcinogens-Mutagens and Modulators of Carcinogenesis* (Japan Scientific Societies Press and University Park Press, Tokyo and Baltimore, 1979); E. C. Miller *et al.*, *Cancer Res.* **43**, 1124 (1983); C. Ioannides, M. Delaforge, D. V. Parke, *Food Cosmet. Toxicol.* **19**, 657 (1981).

6. G. J. Kapadia, Ed., *Oncology Overview on Naturally Occuring Dietary Carcinogens of Plant Origin* (Interna-

tional Cancer Research Data Bank Program, National Cancer Institute, Bethesda, Maryland, 1982).

7. A. M. Clark, in *Environmental Mutagenesis, Carcinogenesis, and Plant Biology*, E. J. Klekowski, Jr., Ed. (Praeger, New York, 1982), vol. 1, pp. 97–132.

8. A. M. Pamukcu, S. Yalciner, J. F. Hatcher, G. T. Bryan, *Cancer Res.* 40, 3468 (1980); J. F. Hatcher, A. M. Pamukcu, E. Erturk, G. T. Bryan, *Fed. Proc. Fed. Am. Soc. Exp. Biol.* 42, 786 (1983).

9. H. F. Stich, M. P. Rosin, C. H. Wu, W. D. Powrie, *Mutat. Res.* 90, 201 (1981); A. A. Aver'yanov, *Biokhimiya* 46, 256 (1981); A. F. Hanham, B. P. Dunn, H. F. Stich, *Mutat. Res.* 116, 333 (1983).

10. K. H. Pegel, *Chem. Eng. News* 59, 4 (20 July 1981).

11. L. K. T. Lam, V. L. Sparnins, L. W. Wattenberg, *Cancer Res.* 42, 1193 (1982).

12. S. J. Jadhav, R. P. Sharma, D. K. Salunkhe, *CRC Crit. Rev. Toxicol.* 9, 21 (1981).

13. R. L. Hall, *Nutr. Cancer* 1 (No. 2), 27 (1979).

14. H. W. Moore and R. Czerniak, *Med. Res. Rev.* 1, 249 (1981).

15. I. Hirono, *CRC Crit. Rev. Toxicol.* 8, 235 (1981).

16. J. P. Brown, *Mutat. Res.* 75, 243 (1980).

17. M. J. Ashwood-Smith and G. A. Poulton, *ibid.* 85, 389 (1981).

18. A. Ya. Potapenko, M. V. Moshnin, A. A. Krasnovsky, Jr., V. L. Sukhorukov, *Z. Naturforsch.* 37, 70 (1982).

19. G. W. Ivie, D. L. Holt, M. C. Ivey, *Science* 213, 909 (1981); R. C. Beier and E. H. Oertli, *Phytochemistry*, in press; R. C. Beier, G. W. Ivie, E. H. Oertli, in "Xenobiotics in Foods and Feeds," *ACS Symp. Ser.*, in press; ——, D. L. Holt, *Food Chem. Toxicol.* 21, 163 (1983).

20. G. Tamura, C. Gold, A. Ferro-Luzzi, B. N. Ames, *Proc. Natl. Acad. Sci. U.S.A.* 77, 4961 (1980).

21. T. Sugimura and S. Sato, *Cancer Res. (Suppl.)* 43, 2415s (1983); T. Sugimura and M. Nagao, in *Mutagenicity: New Horizons in Genetic Toxicology*, J. A. Heddle, Ed. (Academic Press, New York, 1982), pp. 73–88.

22. W. W. Kilgore, D. G. Crosby, A. L. Craigmill, N. K. Poppen, *Calif. Agric.* 35 (No. 11) (November 1981); D. G. Crosby, *Chem. Eng. News* 61, 37 (11 April 1983); C. D. Warren, *ibid.*, p. 3 (13 June 1983).

23. H. F. Stich, M. P. Rosin, C. H. Wu, W. D. Powrie, in *Mutagenicity: New Horizons in Genetic Toxicology*, J. A. Heddle, Ed. (Academic Press, New York, 1982), pp. 117–142; ——, W. D. Powrie, *Cancer Lett.* 14, 251 (1981).

24. N. Katsui, F. Yagihashi, A. Murai, T. Masamune, *Bull. Chem. Soc. Jpn.* 55, 2424 (1982); ——, *ibid.*, p. 2428; R. M. Bostock, R. A. Laine, J. A. Kuc, *Plant Physiol.* 70, 1417 (1982).

25. H. Griesebach and J. Ebel, *Angew. Chem. Int. Ed. Engl.* 17, 635 (1978).

26. J. M. Concon, D. S. Newburg, T. W. Swerczek, *Nutr. Cancer* 1 (No. 3), 22 (1979).

27. H. W. Renner and R. Munzner, *Mutat. Res.* 103, 275 (1982); H. W. Renner, *Experientia* 38, 600 (1982); D. Mourelatos, J. Dozi-Vassiliades, A. Granitsas, *Mutat. Res.* 104, 243 (1982); J. H. Gans, *Toxicol. Appl. Pharmacol.* 63, 312 (1982).

28. B. Toth, in *Naturally Occurring Carcinogens-Mutagens and Modulators of Carcinogenesis*, E. C. Miller, J. A. Miller, I. Hirono, T. Sugimura, S. Takayama, Eds. (Japan Scientific Societies Press and University Park Press, Tokyo and Baltimore, 1979), pp. 57–65; A. E. Ross, D. L. Nagel, B. Toth, *J. Agric. Food Chem.* 30, 521 (1982); B. Toth and K. Patil, *Mycopathologia* 78, 11 (1982); B. Toth, D. Nagel, A. Ross, *Br. J. Cancer* 46, 417 (1982).

29. R. Schoental, *Toxicol. Lett.* 10, 323 (1982); R. J. Huxtable, *Perspect, Biol. Med.* 24, 1 (1980); H. Niwa, H. Ishiwata, K. Yamada, *J. Chromatogr.* 257, 146 (1983).

30. M. Chevion and T. Navok, *Anal. Biochem.* 128, 152 (1983); V. Lattanzio, V. V. Bianco, D. Lafiandra, *Experientia* 38, 789 (1982); V. L. Flohe, G. Niebch, H. Reiber, *Z. Klin. Chem. Klin. Biochem.* 9, 431 (1971); J. Mager, M. Chevion, G. Glaser, in *Toxic Constituents of Plant Foodstuffs*, I. E. Liener, Ed. (Academic Press, New York, 1980), pp. 265–294.

31. J. K. Dunnick *et al.*, *Fundam. Appl. Toxicol.* 2, 114 (1982).

32. L. C. Berardi and L. A. Goldblatt, in *Toxic Constituents of Plant Food-*

stuffs, I. E. Liener, Ed. (Academic Press, ed. 2, New York, 1980), pp. 183–237.

33. S. P. Xue, in *Proceedings, Symposium on Recent Advances in Fertility Regulation* (Beijing, 2 to 5 September, 1980), p. 122.

34. R. K. Haroz and J. Thomasson, *Toxicol. Lett. Suppl.* 6, 72 (1980).

35. M. Coburn, P. Sinsheimer, S. Segal, M. Burgos, W. Troll, *Biol. Bull. (Woods Hole, Mass.)* 159, 468 (1980).

36. C. Campbell, personal communication.

37. G. D. Manners, G. W. Ivie, J. T. MacGregor, *Toxicol. Appl. Pharmacol.* 45, 629 (1978); G. W. Ivie and D. A. Witzel, in *Plant Toxins*, vol. 1, *Encyclopedic Handbook of Natural Toxins*, A. T. Tu and R. F. Keeler, Eds. (Dekker, New York, in press).

38. J. C. M. Van der Hoeven *et al.*, in *Mutagens in Our Environment*, M. Sorsa and H. Vainio, Eds. (Liss, New York, 1982), pp. 327–338; J. C. M. van der Hoeven, W. J. Lagerweij, I. M. Bruggeman, F. G. Voragen, J. H. Koeman, *J. Agric. Food Chem.*, in press.

39. T. Hirayama and Y. Ito, *Prev. Med.* 10, 614 (1981); E. Hecker, *J. Cancer Res. Clin. Oncol.* 99, 103 (1981).

40. M. R. Malinow, E. J. Bardana, Jr., B. Pirofsky, S. Craig, P. McLaughlin, *Science* 216, 415 (1982).

41. B. N. Ames, *ibid.* 204, 587 (1979). "Mutagen" will be used in its broad sense to include clastogens and other DNA-damaging agents.

42. H. F. Stich and R. H. C. San, Eds., *Short-Term Tests for Chemical Carcinogens* (Springer-Verlag, New York, 1981).

43. P. Hochstein and S. K. Jain, *Fed. Proc. Fed. Am. Soc. Exp. Biol.* 40, 183 (1981).

44. D. E. Levin, M. Hollstein, M. F. Christman, E. Schwiers, B. N. Ames, *Proc. Natl. Acad. Sci. U.S.A.* 79, 7455 (1982). Many additional quinones and aldehydes have now been shown to be mutagenic.

45. S. G. Carmella, E. J. LaVoie, S. S. Hecht, *Food Chem. Toxicol.* 20, 587 (1982).

46. K. Morimoto, S. Wolff, A. Koizumi, *Mutat. Res. Lett.* 119, 355 (1983); T. Sawahata and R. A. Neal, *Mol. Pharmacol.* 23, 453 (1983).

47. H. Kappus and H. Sies, *Experientia* 37, 1233 (1981).

48. L. Tikkanen, T. Matsushima, S. Natori, *Mutat. Res.* 116, 297 (1983).

49. P. K. Singal, N. Kapur, K. S. Dhillon, R. E. Beamish, N. S. Dhalla, *Can. J. Physiol. Pharmacol.* 60, 1390 (1982).

50. A. Kasamaki *et al.*, *Mutat. Res.* 105, 387 (1982).

51. J. D. Hendricks, R. O. Sinnhuber, P. M. Loveland, N. E. Pawlowski, J. E. Nixon, *Science* 208, 309 (1980); R. A. Phelps, F. S. Shenstone, A. R. Kemmerer, R. J. Evans, *Poult. Sci.* 44, 358 (1964); N. E. Pawlowski, personal communication.

52. I. Emerit, A. M. Michelson, A. Levy, J. P. Camus, J. Emerit, *Hum. Genet*, 55, 341 (1980).

53. *FDA Compliance Program Report of Findings. FY79 Total Diet Studies—Adult* (No. 7305.002); (available from National Technical Information Service, Springfield, Va.). It is estimated that the daily dietary intake of synthetic organic pesticides and herbicides is about 60 μg, with chlorpropham, malathion, and DDE accounting for about three-fourths of this. An estimate of 150 μg of daily exposure in Finland to pesticide residues has been made by K. Kemmimki, H. Vainio, M. Sorsa, S. Salminen [*J. Environ. Sci. Health* C1 (No. 1), 55 (1983)].

54. N. K. Hooper, B. N. Ames, M. A. Saleh, J. E. Casida, *Science* 205, 591 (1979).

55. L. W. Wattenberg, *Cancer Res. (Suppl.)* 43, 2448s (1983).

56. J. Hoey, C. Montvernay, R. Lambert, *Am. J. Epidemiol.* 113, 668 (1981); A. J. Tuyns, G. Pequignot, M. Gignoux, A. Valla, *Int. J. Cancer* 30, 9 (1982); A. Tuyns, in *Cancer Epidemiology and Prevention*, D. Schottenfeld and J. F. Fraumeni, Jr., Eds. (Saunders, Philadelphia, 1982), pp. 293–303; R. G. Ziegler *et al.*, *J. Natl. Cancer Inst.* 67, 1199 (1981); W. D. Flanders and K. J. Rothman, *Am. J. Epidemiol.* 115, 371 (1982).

57. E. L. Abel, *Hum. Biol.* 54, 421 (1982); H. L. Rosset, L. Weiner, A. Lee, B. Zuckerman, E. Dooling, E. Oppenheimer, *Obstet. Gynecol.* 61, 539 (1983).

57a. R. A. Anderson, Jr., B. R. Willis, C. Oswald, L. J. D. Zaneveld, *J. Pharmacol. Exp. Ther.* 225, 479 (1983).

58. H. F. Stich and M. P. Rosin, *Int. J. Cancer* **31**, 305 (1983).

59. R. P. Bird, H. H. Draper, P. K. Basrur, *Mutat. Res.* **101**, 237 (1982); M. A. Campbell and A. G. Fantel, *Life Sci.* **32**, 2641 (1983).

60. V. J. Feron, A. Kruysse, R. A. Woutersen, *Eur. J. Cancer Clin. Oncol.* **18**, 13 (1982).

61. T. Suematsu *et al.*, *Alcoholism: Clin. Exp. Res.* **5**, 427 (1981); G. W. Winston and A. I. Cederbaum, *Biochem. Pharmacol.* **31**, 2301 (1982); L. A. Videla, V. Fernandez, A. de Marinis, N. Fernandez, A. Valenzuela, *Biochem. Biophys. Res. Commun.* **104**, 965 (1982); T. E. Stege, *Res. Commun. Chem. Pathol. Pharmacol,* **36**, 287 (1982).

62. M. G. Cutler and R. Schneider, *Food Cosmet. Toxicol.* **12**, 451 (1974).

63. Y. Tazima, in *Environmental Mutagenesis, Carcinogenesis and Plant Biology,* E. J. Klekowski, Jr., Ed. (Praeger, New York, 1982), vol. 1, pp. 68–95.

64. P. N. Magee, Ed., *Banbury Report 12, Nitrosamines and Human Cancer* (Cold Spring Harbor Laboratory, Cold Spring Harbor, N.Y., 1982); P. E. Hartman, in *Chemical Mutagens,* F. J. de Serres and A. Hollaender, Eds. (Plenum, New York, 1982), vol. 7, pp. 211–294; P. E. Hartman, *Environ. Mutagen.* **5**, 111 (1983).

65. Committee on Nitrite and Alternative Curing Agents in Food, Assembly of Life Sciences, National Academy of Sciences, *The Health Effects of Nitrate, Nitrite, and N-Nitroso Compounds* (National Academy Press, Washington, D.C. 1981).

66. H. F. Stich, P. K. L. Chan, M. P. Rosin, *Int. J. Cancer* **30**, 719 (1982); H. F. Stich and M. P. Rosin, in *Nutritional and Metabolic Aspects of Food Safety,* M. Friedman, Ed. (Plenum, New York, in press).

67. L. J. Kinlen, *Br. Med. J.* **286**, 1081 (1983); D. J. Fink and D. Kritchevsky, *Cancer Res.* **41**, 3677 (1981).

68. C. W. Welsch and C. F. Aylsworth, *J. Natl. Cancer Inst.* **70**, 215 (1983).

69. P. Correa, J. P. Strong, W. D. Johnson, P. Pizzolato, W. Haenszel, *J. Chronic Dis.* **35**, 313 (1982).

70. F. B. Shorland *et al.*, *J. Agric. Food Chem.* **29**, 863 (1981).

71. M. G. Simic and M. Karel, Eds., *Autoxidation in Food and Biological Systems* (Plenum, New York, 1980).

72. W. A. Pryor, Ed., *Free Radicals in Biology* (Academic Press, New York, 1976 to 1982), vols. 1 to 5.

73. H. B. Demopoulos, D. D. Pietronigro, E. S. Flamm, M. L. Seligman, *J. Environ. Pathol. Toxicol.* **3**, 273 (1980).

74. F. Bischoff, *Adv. Lipid Res.* **7**, 165 (1969).

75. N. L. Petrakis, L. D. Gruenke, J. C. Craig, *Cancer Res.* **41**, 2563 (1981).

76. H. S. Black and D. R. Douglas, *ibid.* **32**, 2630 (1972).

77. H. Imai, N. T. Werthessen, V. Subramanyam, P. W. LeQuesne, A. H. Soloway, M. Kanisawa, *Science* **207**, 651 (1980).

78. M. Ferrali, R. Fulceri, A. Benedetti, M. Comporti, *Res. Commun. Chem. Pathol. Pharmacol.* **30**, 99 (1980).

79. N. R. Artman, *Adv. Lipid Res.* **7**, 245 (1969).

80. J. K. Reddy, J. R. Warren, M. K. Reddy, N. D. Lalwani, *Ann. N.Y. Acad. Sci.* **386**, 81 (1982); J. K. Reddy and N. D. Lalwani, *CRC Crit. Rev. Toxicol.,* in press.

81. H. L. Plaine, *Genetics* **40**, 268 (1955); A. Ito, M. Naito, Y. Naito, H. Watanabe, *Gann* **73**, 315 (1982); G. Speit, W. Vogel, M. Wolf, *Environ. Mutagen.* **4**, 135 (1982); H. Tsuda, *Jpn. J. Genet.* **56**, 1 (1981); N. Hirota and T. Yokoyama, *Gann* **72**, 811 (1981).

82. S. Horie, H. Ishii, T. Suga, *J. Biochem. (Tokyo)* **90**, 1691 (1981); D. P. Jones, L. Eklow, H. Thor, S. Orrenius, *Arch. Biochem. Biophys.* **210**, 505 (1981).

83. B. Chance, H. Sies, A. Boveris, *Physiol. Rev.* **59**, 527 (1979).

84. D. Harman, *Proc. Natl. Acad. Sci. U.S.A.* **78**, 7124 (1981); in *Free Radicals in Biology,* W. A. Pryor, Ed. (Academic Press, New York, 1982), vol. 5, pp. 255–275.

85. I. Emerit, M. Keck, A. Levy, J. Feingold, A. M. Michelson, *Mutat. Res.* **103**, 165 (1982).

86. C. E. Neat, M. S. Thomassen, H. Osmundsen, *Biochem. J.* **196**, 149 (1981); J. Bremer and K. R. Norum, *J. Lipid Res.* **23**, 243 (1982); M. S. Thomassen, E. N. Christiansen, K. R. Norum, *Biochem. J.* **206**, 195 (1982); H. Osmundsen, *Int. J.*

Biochem. **14,** 905 (1982); J. Norseth and M. S. Thomassen, *Biochim, Biophys. Acta,* in press.

87. M. G. Enig, R. J. Munn, M. Keeney, *Fed. Proc. Fed. Am. Soc. Exp. Biol.* **37,** 2215 (1978); J. E. Hunter, *J. Natl. Cancer Inst.* **69,** 319 (1982); A. B. Awad, *ibid.,* p. 320; H. Ruttenberg, L. M. Davidson, N. A. Little, D. M. Klurfeld, D. Kritchevsky, *J. Nutr.* **113,** 835 (1983).

88. R. Wood, *Lipids* **14,** 975 (1979).

89. E. N. Christiansen, T. Flatmark, H. Kryvi, *Eur. J. Cell Biol.* **26,** 11 (1981).

90. Council for Agricultural Science and Technology, *Diet, Nutrition, and Cancer: A Critique* (Special Publication 13, Council for Agricultural Science and Technology, Ames, Iowa, 1982).

91. L. F. Bjeldanes *et al., Food Chem. Toxicol.* **20,** 357 (1982); M. W. Pariza, L. J. Loretz, J. M. Storkson, N. C. Holland, *Cancer Res. (Suppl.)* **43,** 2444s (1983).

92. H. F. Stich, W. Stich, M. P. Rosin, W. D. Powrie, *Mutat. Res.* **91,** 129 (1981); M. P. Rosin, H. F. Stich, W. D. Powrie, C. H. Wu, *ibid.* **101,** 189 (1982); C.-I. Wei, K. Kitamura, T. Shibamoto, *Food Cosmet. Toxicol.* **19,** 749 (1981).

93. E. Yamasaki and B. N. Ames, *Proc. Natl. Acad. Sci. U.S.A.* **74,** 3555 (1977).

94. R. Baker, A. Arlauskas, A. Bonin, D. Angus, *Cancer Lett.* **16,** 81 (1982).

95. D. Schuetzle, D. Cronn, A. L. Crittenden, R. J. Charlson, *Environ. Sci. Technol.* **9,** 838 (1975); G. Gartrell and S. K. Friedlander, *Atmos. Environ.* **9,** 279 (1975); L. D. Kier, E. Yamasaki, B. N. Ames, *Proc. Natl. Acad. Sci. U.S.A.* **71,** 4159 (1974); J. N. Pitts, Jr., *Environ. Health Perspect.* **47,** 115 (1983).

96. J. E. Vena, *Am J. Epidemiol.* **116,** 42 (1982); R. Cederlof, R. Doll, B. Fowler, *Environ. Health Perspect.* **22,** 1 (1978); F. E. Speizer, *ibid.* **47,** 33 (1983).

97. B. Brunekreef and J. S. M. Boleij, *Int. Arch. Occup. Environ. Health* **50,** 299 (1982).

98. H. Kasai *et al., Gann* **73,** 681 (1982).

99. V. Armuth and I. Berenblum, *Carcinogenesis* **2,** 977 (1981).

100. S. Fabro, *Reprod. Toxicol.* **1,** 2 (1982).

101. D. Trichopoulos, M. Papapostolou, A. Polychronopoulou, *Int. J. Cancer* **28,** 691 (1981); P. Hartge, L. P. Lesher, L. McGowan, R. Hoover, *ibid.* **30,** 531 (1982); B. MacMahon, *Cancer (Brussels)* **50,** 2676 (1982); H. S. Cuckle and L. J. Kinlen, *Br. J. Cancer* **44,** 760 (1981); R. L. Phillips and D. A. Snowdon, *Cancer Res. (Suppl.)* **43,** 2403s (1983); L. D. Marrett, S. D. Walter, J. W. Meigs, *Am J. Epidemiol.* **117,** 113 (1983); D. M. Weinberg, R. K. Ross, T. M. Mack, A. Paganini-Hill, B. E. Henderson, *Cancer (Brussels)* **51,** 675 (1983).

102. P. E. Hartman, *Environ. Mutagen.,* in press.

103. J. R. Totter, *Proc. Natl. Acad. Sci. U.S.A.* **77,** 1763 (1980).

104. I. Fridovich, in *Pathology of Oxygen,* A. Autor, Ed. (Academic Press, New York, 1982), pp. 1–19; L. W. Oberley, T. D. Oberley, G. R. Buettner, *Med. Hypotheses* **6,** 249 (1880).

105. B. Halliwell, *Cell Biol. Int. Rep.* **6,** 529 (1982); A. I. Tauber, *Trends Biochem. Sic.* **7,** 411 (1982); A. B. Weitberg, S. A. Weitzman, M. Destrempes, S. A. Latt, T. P. Stossel, *N. Engl. J. Med.* **308,** 26 (1983). Neutrophils also produce HOCl, which is both a chlorinating and oxidizing agent.

106. M. A. Trush, E. G. Mimnaugh, T. E. Gram, *Biochem. Pharmacol.* **31,** 3335 (1982).

107. L. Flohe, in *Free Radicals in Biology,* W. A. Pryor, Ed. (Academic Press, New York, 1982), vol. 5, pp. 223–254.

108. C. Lind, P. Hochstein, L. Ernster, *Arch. Biochem. Biophys.* **216,** 178 (1982).

109. M. Warholm, C. Guthenberg, B. Mannervik, C. von Bahr, *Biochem. Biophys. Res. Commun.* **98,** 512 (1981).

110. J. G. Bieri, L. Corash, V. S. Hubbard, *N. Engl. J. Med.* **308,** 1063 (1983).

111. Y. M. Wang *et al.,* in *Molecular Interrelations of Nutrition and Cancer,* M. S. Arnott, J. van Eys, Y.-M. Wang, Eds. (Raven, New York, 1982), pp. 369–379.

112. C. Beckman, R. M. Roy, A. Sproule, *Mutat. Res.* **105,** 73 (1982); M. G. Cook and P. McNamara, *Cancer Res.* **40,** 1329 (1980).

113. K. J. A. Davies, A. T. Quintanilha, G. A. Brooks, L. Packer, *Biochem. Biophys. Res. Commun.* **107,** 1198 (1982).

114. C. S. Foote, in *Pathology of Oxy-*

gen, A. Autor, Ed. (Academic Press, New York, 1982), pp. 21–44; J. E. Packer, J. S. Mahood, V. O. Mora-Arellano, T. F. Slater, R. L. Willson, B. S. Wolfenden, *Biochem. Biophys. Res. Commun.* 98, 901 (1981); W. Bors, C. Michel, M. Saran, *Bull. Eur. Physiopathol. Resp.* 17 (Suppl.), 13 (1981).

115. N. I. Krinsky and S. M. Deneke, *J. Natl. Cancer Inst.* 69, 205 (1982); J. A. Turner and J. N. Prebble, *J. Gen. Microbiol.* 119, 133 (1980); K. L. Simpson and C. O. Chichester, *Annu. Rev. Nutr.* 1, 351 (1981).

116. G. Rettura, C. Dattagupta, P. Listowsky, S. M. Levenson, E. Seifter, *Fed. Proc. Fed. Am. Soc. Exp. Biol.* 42, 786 (1983); M. M. Mathews-Roth, *Oncology* 39, 33 (1982).

117. R. Peto, R. Doll, J. D. Buckley, M. B. Sporn, *Nature (London)* 290, 201 (1981); R. B. Shekelle *et al.*, *Lancet* 1981-II, 1185 (1981); T. Hirayama, *Nutr. Cancer* 1, 67 (1979); G. Kvale, E. Bjelke, J. J. Gart, *Int. J. Cancer* 31, 397 (1983).

118. W. A. Pryor, M. Tamura, M. M. Dooley, P. I. Premovic, D. F. Church, in *Oxy-Radicals and Their Scavenger Systems: Cellular and Medical Aspects*, G. Cohen and R. Greenwald, Eds. (Elsevier, Amsterdam, 1983), vol. 2, pp. 185–192; W. A. Pryor, B. J. Hales, P. I. Premovic, D. F. Church, *Science* 220, 425 (1983).

119. M. M. Mathews-Roth, *J. Natl. Cancer Inst.* 69, 279 (1982).

120. A. C. Griffin, in *Molecular Interrelations of Nutrition and Cancer*, M. S. Arnott, J. Vaneys, Y. M. Wang, Eds. (Raven, New York, 1982), pp. 401–408; D. Medina, H. W. Lane, C. M. Tracey, *Cancer Res. (Suppl.)* 43, 2460s (1983); M. M. Jacobs, *Cancer Res.* 43, 1646 (1983); H. J. Thompson, L. D. Meeker, P. J. Becci, S. Kokoska, *ibid.* 42, 4954 (1982); D. F. Birt, T. A. Lawson, A. D. Julius, C. E. Runice, S. Salmasi, *ibid.*, p. 4455; C. Witting, U. Witting, V. Krieg, *J. Cancer Res. Clin. Oncol.* 104, 109 (1982).

121. M. Chatterjee and M. R. Banerjee, *Cancer Lett.* 17, 187 (1982).

122. W. C. Willett *et al.*, *Lancet*, in press.

123. J. T. Salonen, G. Alfthan, J. Pikkarainen, J. K. Huttunen, P. Puska, *ibid.* 1982-II, 175 (1982).

124. M. Yonaha, E. Itoh, Y. Ohbayashi, M. Uchiyama, *Res. Commun. Chem. Pathol. Pharmacol.* 28, 105 (1980); L. J. Kling and J. H. Soares, Jr., *Nutr. Rep. Int.* 24, 39 (1981).

125. N. Tateishi, T. Higashi, A. Naruse, K. Hikita, Y. Sakamoto, *J. Biochem. (Tokyo)* 90, 1603 (1981).

126. J. M. Williamson, B. Boettcher, A. Meister, *Proc. Natl. Acad. Sci. U.S.A.* 79, 6246 (1982).

127. CME Symposium on "*N-Acetylcysteine* (NAC): A Significant Chemoprotective Adjunct," *Sem. Oncol.* 10 (Suppl. 1), 1 (1983).

128. J. A. Hinson, L. R. Pohl, T. J. Monks, J. R. Gillette, *Life Sci.* 29, 107 (1981).

129. A. M. Novi, *Science* 212, 541 (1981).

130. W. B. Dunham *et al.*, *Proc. Natl. Acad. Sci. U.S.A.* 79, 7532 (1982); G. Kallistratos and E. Fasske, *J. Cancer Res. Clin. Oncol.* 97, 91 (1980).

131. S. Wassertheil-Smoller *et al.*, *Am. J. Epidemiol.* 114, 714 (1981).

132. B. N. Ames, R. Cathcart, E. Schwiers, P. Hochstein, *Proc. Natl. Acad. Sci. U.S.A.* 78, 6858 (1981).

133. A. Nomura, L. K. Heilbrun, G. N. Stemmermann, in preparation.

134. J. N. Boyd, J. G. Babish, G. S. Stoewsand, *Food Chem. Toxicol.* 20, 47 (1982).

135. A. W. Wood, *et al.*, *Proc. Natl. Acad. Sci. U.S.A.* 79, 5513 (1982).

136. T. H. Maugh II, *Science* 205, 1363 (1979) (interview with John Higginson).

137. H. L. Gensler and H. Bernstein, *Q. Rev. Biol.* 6, 279 (1981).

138. A. L. Tappel, in *Free Radicals in Biology*, W. A. Pryor, Ed. (Academic Press, New York, 1980), vol. 4, pp. 1–47.

139. R. S. Sohal, in *Age Pigments*, R. S. Sohal, Ed. (Elsevier/North-Holland, Amsterdam, 1981), pp. 303–316.

140. J. E. Fleming, J. Miquel, S. F. Cottrell, L. S. Yengoyan, A. C. Economos, *Gerontology* 28, 44 (1982).

141. J. M. Tolmasoff, T. Ono, R. G. Cutler, *Proc. Natl. Acad. Sci. U.S.A.* 77, 2777 (1980); R. G. Cutler, *Gerontology*, in press; J. L. Sullivan, *ibid.* 28, 242 (1982).

142. R. Peto, *Proc. R. Soc. London Ser.*

B **205**, 111 (1979); D. Dix, P. Cohen, J. Flannery, *J. Theor. Biol.* **83**, 163 (1980).
143. R. G. Cutler, in *Testing the Theories of Aging,* R. Adelman and G. Roth, Eds. (CRC Press, Boca Raton, Fla., in press).
144. D. Hersh, R. G. Cutler, B. N. Ames, in preparation.
145. E. Boyland, in *Health Risk Analysis* (Franklin Institute Press, Philadelphia, 1980), pp. 181–193; E. Boyland, in *Cancer Campaign,* vol. 6, *Cancer Epidemiology,* E. Grundmann, Ed. (Fischer, Stuttgart, 1982), pp. 125–128.
146. J. L. Marx, *Science* **219**, 158 (1983).
147. B. D. Goldstein, G. Witz, M. Amoruso, D. S. Stone, W. Troll, *Cancer Lett.* **11**, 257 (1981); W. Troll, in *Environmental Mutagens and Carcinogens,* T. Sugimura, S. Kondo, H. Takebe, Eds. (Univ. of Tokyo Press, Tokyo, and Liss, New York, 1982), pp. 217–222.
148. B. N. Ames, M. C. Hollstein, R. Cathcart, in *Lipid Peroxide in Biology and Medicine,* K. Yagi, Ed. (Academic Press, New York, 1982), pp. 339–351.
149. I. Emerit and P. A. Cerutti, *Proc. Natl. Acad. Sci. U.S.A.* **79**, 7509 (1982); *Nature (London)* **293**, 144 (1981); P. A. Cerutti, I. Emerit, P. Amstad, in *Genes and Proteins in Oncogenesis,* I. B. Weinstein and H. Vogel, Eds. (Academic Press, New York, in press); I. Emerit, A. Levy, P. Cerutti, *Mutat. Res.* **110**, 327 (1983).
150. J. Funes and M. Karel, *Lipids* **16**, 347 (1981).
151. S. J. Stohs, M. Q. Hassan, W. J. Murray, *Biochem. Biophys. Res. Commun.* **111**, 854 (1983).
152. C. C. Reddy, R. W. Scholz, E. J. Massaro, *Toxicol. Appl. Pharmacol.* **61**, 460 (1981).
153. H. Nagasawa and J. B. Little, *Carcinogenesis* **2**, 601 (1981); V. Solanki, R. S. Rana, T. J. Slaga, *ibid.,* p. 1141; T. W. Kensler and M. A. Trush, *Cancer Res.* **41**, 216 (1981).
154. R. H. Simon, C. H. Scoggin, D. Patterson, *J. Biol. Chem.* **256**, 7181 (1981); T. S. Argyris and T. J. Slaga, *Cancer Res.* **41**, 5193 (1981).
155. G. E. Hatch, D. E. Garder, D. B. Menzel, *Environ. Res.* **23**, 121 (1980).
156. A. J. P. Klein-Szanto and T. J. Slaga, *J. Invest. Dermatol.* **79**, 30 (1982).

157. C. C. Weddle, K. R. Hornbrook, P. B. McCay, *J. Biol. Chem.* **251**, 4973 (1976).
158. A. G. Lurie and L. S. Cutler, *J. Natl. Cancer Inst.* **63**, 147 (1979).
159. C. Borek and W. Troll, *Proc. Natl. Acad. Sci. U.S.A.* **80**, 1304 (1983); C. Borek, in *Molecular Interrelations of Nutrition and Cancer,* M. S. Arnott, J. van Eys, Y.-M. Wang, Eds. (Raven, New York, 1982), pp. 337–350.
160. T. J. Slaga *et al.,* in *Carcinogenesis: A Comprehensive Treatise* (Raven, New York, 1982), vol. 7, pp. 19–34; K. Ohuchi and L. Levine, *Biochim. Biophys. Acta* **619**, 11 (1980); S. M. Fischer, G. D. Mills, T. J. Slaga, *Carcinogenesis* **3**, 1243 (1982).
161. R. P. Mason, in *Free Radicals in Biology,* W. A. Pryor, Ed. (Academic Press, New York, 1982), vol. 5, pp. 161–222.
162. G. McLennan, L. W. Oberley, A. P. Autor, *Radiat. Res.* **84**, 122 (1980).
163. J. M. Parry, E. M. Parry, J. C. Barrett, *Nature (London)* **294**, 263 (1981); A. R. Kinsella, *Carcinogenesis* **3**, 499 (1982).
164. H. C. Birnboim, *Can. J. Physiol. Pharmacol,* **60**, 1359 (1982).
165. A. Varshavsky, *Cell* **25**, 561 (1981).
166. T. J. Powles *et al.,* Eds. *Prostaglandins and Cancer; First International Conference* (Liss, New York, 1982).
167. J. E. Trosko, C.-C. Chang, A. Medcalf, *Cancer Invest.,* in press.
167a. I. B. Weinstein, *Nature (London)* **302**, 750 (1983).
168. J. A. Bond, A. M. Gown, H. L. Yang, E. P. Benditt, M. R. Juchau, *J. Toxicol. Environ. Health* **7**, 327 (1981).
169. Editorial, *Lancet* **1980-I**, 964, (1980); K. Yagi, H. Ohkawa, N. Ohishi, M. Yamashita, T. Nakashima, *J. Appl. Biochem.* **3**, 58 (1981).
170. J. M. C. Gutteridge, B. Halliwell, D. A. Rowley, T. Westermarck, *Lancet* **1982-II**, 459 (1982).
171. J. E. Cleaver, in *Metabolic Basis of Inherited Disease,* J. B. Stanbury, J. B. Wyngaarden, D. S. Fredrickson, J. L. Goldstein, Eds. (McGraw-Hill, ed. 5, New York, 1983), pp. 1227–1250.
172. K. C. Bhuyan, D. K. Bhuyan, S. M. Podos, *IRCS Med. Sci.* **9**, 126 (1981); A. Spector, R. Scotto, H. Weissbach, N.

Brot, *Biochem. Biophys. Res. Commun.* **108**, 429 (1982); S. D. Varma, N. A. Beachy, R. D. Richards, *Photochem. Photobiol.* **36**, 623 (1982).

173. M. L. Katz, K. R. Parker, G. J. Handelman, T. L. Bramel, E. A. Dratz, *Exp. Eye Res.* **34**, 339 (1982).

174. D. Behne, T. Hofer, R. von Berswordt-Wallrabe, W. Elger, *J. Nutr.* **112**, 1682 (1982).

175. B. N. Ames, L. S. Gold, C. B. Sawyer, W. Havender, in *Environmental Mutagens and Carcinogens*, T. Sugimura, S. Kondo, H. Takebe, Eds. (Univ. of Tokyo Press, Tokyo, and Liss, New York, 1982), pp. 663–670.

176. National Center for Health Statistics, Advance Report, Final Mortality Statistics, 1979, *Monthly Vital Statistics Report* **31**, No. 6, suppl. [DHHS publication (PHS) 82–1120, (Public Health Service, Hyattsville, Md., 1982]; Metropolitan Life Insurance Company Actuarial Tables, April 1983.

177. B. A. Bridges, B. E. Butterworth, I. B. Weinstein, Eds., *Banbury Report 13. Indicators of Genotoxic Exposure* (Cold Spring Harbor Laboratory, Cold Spring Harbor, N.Y., 1982); R. Montesano, M. F. Rajewsky, A. E. Pegg, E. Miller, *Cancer Res.* **42**, 5236 (1982); H. F. Stich, R. H. C. San, M. P. Rosin, *Ann. N.Y. Acad. Sci.*, in press; I. B. Weinstein, *Annu. Rev. Public Health* **4**, 409 (1983).

178. I am indebted to G. Ferro-Luzzi Ames, A. Blum, L. Gold, P. Hartman, W. Havender, N. K. Hooper, G. W. Ivie, J. McCann, J. Mead, R. Olson, R. Peto, A. Tappel, and numerous other colleagues for their criticisms. This work was supported by DOE contract DE-AT03-76EV70156 to B.N.A. and by National Institute of Environmental Health Sciences Center Grant ES01896. This article has been expanded from a talk presented at the 12th European Environmental Mutagen Society Conference, Espoo, Finland, June 1982 [in *Mutagens in Our Environment*, M. Sorsa and H. Vainio, Eds. (Liss, New York, 1982)]. I wish to dedicate this article to the memory of Philip Handler, pioneer in the field of oxygen radicals.

Some Original Scientific Literature

JOURNAL OF THE AMERICAN GERIATRICS SOCIETY
Copyright © 1976 by the American Geriatrics Society

Vol. XXIV, No. 7
Printed in U.S.A.

Free Radical Theory of Aging: Effect of Dietary Fat on Central Nervous System Function*

DENHAM HARMAN, MD, PhD**, SHELTON HENDRICKS, PhD†, DENNIS E. EDDY, PhD‡
and JON SEIBOLD, MA‖

University of Nebraska, Omaha, Nebraska

ABSTRACT: Free radical reactions have been implicated in aging. A rise in the level of random free radical reactions in a biologic system might have a greater effect on the central nervous system (CNS) than elsewhere, partly because of the presence of glial cells and the unique connections between neurons. To evaluate this possibility, some animal experiments were conducted. The initial experiment involved old male Sprague-Dawley rats fed (since shortly after weaning) with semisynthetic diets characterized by fat differing in amount or degree of unsaturation. The number of errors made in a Hebb-Williams maze was determined and found to be higher as the amount or degree of unsaturation of the fat was increased. Likewise rats aged 6 and 9 months, fed semisynthetic diets containing 20 percent by weight of lard, oleinate, or safflower oil+α-tocopherol performed significantly better in a discrimination learning situation (Skinner box) than did rats fed a diet containing 20 percent by weight of safflower oil. The diets employed in these studies did not have a significant effect on the mortality rates. These results are compatible with the possibility that enhancing the level of lipid peroxidation has an adverse effect on the CNS, out of proportion to the effect on the body as a whole, as measured by the mortality rate.

Chronic organic brain syndrome (COBS) is a major health problem (1, 2). In this disease the central nervous system (CNS), at least that part involved in higher functions, can be regarded as aging faster than the body as a whole, becoming "old" to the point where the individual is deprived of intellectual and emotional life for a significant period before death. The incidence of COBS rises rapidly with advancing age, beginning at about age 70 (1). Since the median age of the 65+ group is increasing (3), marked increases can be expected in the number of persons with COBS.

COBS patients can be divided into three large groups on the basis of the major brain lesions: a) senile plaques 47 percent; b) vascular disease 30 percent; and c) mixed "a" and "b" 23 percent (4). Recent work indicates that degenerative changes in aging dendrites (5) may also be involved in COBS.

The etiology of COBS is unknown. Free radical reactions may be involved in the pathogenesis. This class of chemical reaction (6, 7), ubiquitous in biologic systems (8, 9), has been implicated in the degradation of such systems. On this basis, one possible means of decreasing the rate of degradation in the central nervous system and elsewhere, would be to decrease the ingestion of dietary components that might reasonably be expected to participate significantly in more-or-less random free radical reactions in vivo. Fat is such a dietary factor (10), and it is a major component of most human diets. The fatty-acid moieties present in dietary fat differ markedly

* This investigation was supported in part by grants from the NIH (HE-06979) and the U.S. Department of Agriculture.
** Departments of Biochemistry and Medicine, University of Nebraska Medical Center.
Address for correspondence: Denham Harman, MD, Department of Biochemistry, University of Nebraska Medical Center, 42nd and Dewey Ave., Omaha, NB 68105.
† Department of Psychology, University of Nebraska at Omaha.
‡ Departments of Biochemistry and Medicine, University of Nebraska Medical Center.
‖ St. Paul, Minnesota.

in the ease with which they are peroxidized (11), i.e., react with molecular oxygen; peroxidation of a polyunsaturated fatty acid such as linolenic acid proceeds much more rapidly than that of stearic acid, a saturated fatty acid. Thus, decreasing the amount or degree of unsaturation of dietary fat might be expected to result in a decreased rate of biologic degradation.

In general, dietary fat might be expected to have an effect on the CNS similar to that on the body as a whole. However, the CNS response may be greater than elsewhere in the organism because the neurons are fixed postmitotic cells with unique connections with other neurons (12), while exchange with the capillaries, in contrast with parenchymal cells elsewhere, is modified by the presence of glial cells. The foregoing characteristics could conceivably make the CNS more susceptible than the rest of the body to accumulative deleterious changes which in turn could be reflected in CNS degradation becoming clinically evident for varying periods before death, the duration of disability being different for each individual.

To evaluate this possibility – that increases in the level of more-or-less random free radical reactions secondary to increased lipid peroxidation might have a selective adverse effect on the CNS – two experiments were conducted in which the relative efficiency in a learning situation was used as a measure of CNS deterioration. In the first study the effect of the amount or degree of unsaturation of dietary fat on the mortality rate for rats was determined, as well as the maze-learning abilities of the animals when old. The second experiment was designed to assess the influence of dietary fats and of one antioxidant, vitamin E, on the learning behavior of relatively young rats, aged 3, 6 and 9 months; operative behavior was evaluated using a discrimination learning paradigm.

EXPERIMENT 1

Method

Four hundred Sprague-Dawley male rats were obtained from Charles River Breeding Laboratories, Wilmington, Massachusetts shortly after weaning and caged, 4 per cage (stainless steel, $11^{1}/_{2} \times 18^{1}/_{4} \times 6^{1}/_{2}$ inches). The rats were maintained in an air-conditioned room at 76–78°F at a humidity of 50–60 percent. Cages were cleaned 2–3 times per week. The bedding consisted of sterilized shredded corn cobs (San-i-Cel, Paxton

Processing Company, Paxton, Illinois). At age 2 months the rats were divided at random into groups and given semisynthetic diets (13) containing 5, 10 or 20%w (percent by weight) of lard, olive oil, corn oil, safflower oil or distilled triglycerides of menhaden oil (Technological Laboratory, Bureau of Commercial Fisheries, Fish and Wildlife Service, U. S. Department of the Interior, Seattle, Washington). There were. 28 rats in each of the 5 percent and 10 percent groups and 24 rats in each of the 20 percent groups. The lard (antioxidant-free), olive oil, corn oil and safflower oil were all edible grade, marketed for human consumption.

The composition of the 5%w lipid diet has been published (14); 10 and 20%w lipid diets were prepared at the expense of glucose monohydrate. These diets meet the nutritional requirements of rats (15). Although the amount and type of dietary fat are the only significant variables in these diets, they are not the only variables. Thus, the thiamine requirement of a diet increases with the percentage of carbohydrate. α-Tocopherol acetate was added in the proportion of 20 mg per 100 gm of finished diet, to obviate the possibility of vitamin-E deficiency.

The 5%w, 10%w and 20%w fat diets contained 408, 433 and 483 calories, respectively, per 100 gm. The diets were fed isocalorically; for each gram of diet fed the 20 percent groups, the 10 percent groups received 1.12 gm, and the 5 percent group 1.19 gm. Food consumption was determined once a month for a period of one week; the average amount of food eaten per rat per day in the dietary groups eating the least during the week period was fed to all the groups during the ensuing month. Despite the foregoing, the body weights tended to increase with the level of dietary fat. Judging from the animals' appetites, all the diets were about equally palatable.

The diets were made up once a week and stored in glass jars prior to use; the safflower and menhaden oil diets were kept in a deep-freeze, while the other diets were stored in a cold-room at refrigerator temperature. Samples of the diets were analyzed several times for peroxides by the iodiometric method (AOCS Official Method Cd 8–53), but no peroxides were found.

The rats, ear-coded, were weighed and counted each month. No adjustments were made when deaths decreased the number (originally 4) in a cage.

Learning behavior was assessed at age 32–35 months, with use of an adaptation (16) of the Hebbs-Williams closed field maze (17). In this maze the positions of the start and goal boxes remain constant while the pathway to the goal box is determined by the positions of adjustable barriers. The field is divided into 36 alternate black and white 5-inch squares. Entrances to any squares which were not in the direct path between the start and goal boxes were counted as errors. The rats were tested under 23-hour food deprivation; reinforcement was accomplished with 45-mg Noyes pellets (P. J. Noyes Co., Lancaster, New Hampshire). The maze floor was covered by a ⁵⁄₈-inch layer of water which served as an additional motivating factor. This supplementary aversive stimulus was found to be necessary for the elicitation of maze-running behavior in these old rats. The animals were given 8 trials in each specific maze configuration. Six practice mazes were run by each rat, to adapt him to the apparatus and handling and to establish the habit of eating in the goal box. The rats were habituated to the test situation between 29 and 31 months of age. Testing in the maze occurred between 32 and 35 months of age.

Results

The percentage surviving, and average weight for each of the 15 dietary fat groups are shown in Table 1 as a function of age in months. The amount or degree of unsaturation did not have a significant effect on the mortality rate (13). However, the mortality rates for the 20 percent groups were somewhat higher than those for the corresponding 5 percent and 10 percent groups. The mortality rates for the 20 percent groups tended to increase, except for the menhaden oil rats, with increasing unsaturation of the dietary fat. The mortality rates for the menhaden oil groups were lower than had been expected from the degree of unsaturation of the oil; this same effect was also noted in studies at the same time with C3H and Swiss mice (13). The unexpectedly relatively low mortality rates for the menhaden oil groups possibly may have been a result of the less ready enzymatic hydrolysis of the 20:5 and 22:6 fatty acids present in menhaden oil (18) (so that the lipid actually absorbed from the intestinal tract may have been more saturated than that ingested), and of a preferential utilization of highly unsaturated fatty acids for energy production (19).

The maze data are presented in Table 2. The maze study was conducted at a time when the mortality rates for the 15 dietary groups were high, so many rats did not live to complete all the mazes. For this reason the data are divided into three parts; the top third of the table show data for rats that completed mazes 1–4, the

TABLE 1
Effect of Dietary Fat on Mortality Rate (Sprague-Dawley Male Rats)

Fat in Diet, % by Weight	Age of Rats (mos.)	Lard		Olive Oil		Corn Oil		Safflower Oil		Menhaden Oil	
		W[1]	S[2]	W	S	W	S	W	S	W	S
5% w groups		N = 28[3]		N = 28		N = 28		N = 28		N = 28	
	28	625	71.4	633	64.3	613	64.3	633	67.9	644	57.4
	30	566	50.0	600	50.0	556	60.7	569	46.4	664	39.3
	32	512	42.9	557	35.7	535	53.6	535	42.9	550	28.6
	34	508	21.4	508	25.0	510	35.7	479	39.3	509	21.4
	36	515	14.3	502	14.3	497	21.4	467	21.4	522	10.7
	38	650	3.6	–	0.0	590	7.2	518	14.3	373	3.6
10% w groups		N = 28		N = 29		N = 28		N = 28		N = 28	
	28	610	53.6	581	72.4	634	60.7	612	64.3	664	67.9
	30	602	32.1	606	55.2	636	53.5	612	50.0	614	57.1
	32	541	28.6	545	44.8	607	39.3	551	39.3	582	50.0
	34	543	17.9	549	31.0	550	32.1	614	39.3	561	39.3
	36	556	3.6	544	13.8	475	17.9	581	17.9	574	10.7
	38	–	0.0	554	3.5	599	3.6	540	7.2	–	0.0
20% w groups		N = 24		N = 24		N = 23		N = 24		N = 24	
	28	662	70.8	704	58.3	762	47.8	678	29.2	679	62.5
	30	626	45.8	659	37.5	689	13.0	731	12.5	718	54.2
	32	612	33.7	575	25.0	646	10.5	668	12.5	638	29.2
	34	582	25.0	546	12.5	574	10.5	561	12.5	673	20.8
	36	504	12.5	–	0.0	715	5.3	662	4.2	735	12.5
	38	532	4.2	–	0.0	–	0.0	–	0.0	540	4.2

[1] = Weight in grams.
[2] = Percentage of original group still alive.
[3] = Initial number of rats.

D. HARMAN ET AL. *Vol. XXIV*

TABLE 2

Effect of Dietary Fat on Average Number of Errors in a Modified Version of the Hebb-Williams Closed-Field Intelligence Test (Sprague-Dawley Male Rats)

% Fat (by Weight) in Diet	Dietary Fat				
	Lard	Olive	Corn	Safflower	Menhaden
	Mazes 1–4: (Age 32–33 months)				
5%w	17.8±5.2[1] [12]	20.1±5.6 [10]	23.2±8.4 [13]	21.8±6.4 [11]	25.5±9.8 [7]
10%w	19.5±7.2 [6]	20.6±6.0 [11]	22.6±6.3 [10]	22.9±6.4 [9]	23.1±7.9 [12]
20%w	21.3±6.6 [8]	21.3±6.5 [6]	17.5±7.0 [2]	22.3±7.2 [3]	24.2±5.7 [5]
	Mazes 1–8: (Age 32–34 months)				
5%w	17.0±6.6 [7]	19.5±4.6 [5]	21.8±7.1 [10]	20.0±7.2 [9]	24.8±10.3 [5]
10%w	17.9±7.3 [6]	21.0±6.0 [7]	21.1±7.6 [8]	22.1±7.7 [6]	24.3±7.5 [9]
20%w	21.3±6.5 [7]	19.5±7.2 [3]	19.4±7.0 [2]	23.7±8.0 [2]	23.6±5.3 [3]
	Mazes 1–12:(Age 32–35 months)				
5%w	18.6±7.1 [5]	21.8±6.0 [4]	22.9±7.0 [7]	19.1±7.3 [6]	26.7±10.3 [4]
10%w	20.5±9.8 [4]	24.9±8.7 [6]	24.1±8.8 [6]	25.0±7.4 [4]	25.8±7.4 [8]
20%w	22.0±7.8 [5]	21.7±6.9 [2]	24.8±8.2 [1]	28.4±10.4 [2]	27.0±7.5 [3]

[1] = Standard deviation.
[2] = Number of rats.

middle third for those finishing mazes 1–8, and the bottom third for those completing all 12 of the standardized mazes. Each figure in the table is the average number of errors per maze ± the standard deviation made by each rat completing the maze series; thus, each of the 12 rats in the 5%w lard group that completed mazes 1–4 made an average of 17.8 ± 5.2 errors (i.e. the total number of errors made in running a given maze 8 times) for each of the four mazes.

In general the number of maze errors increased both with an increase in the amount of dietary fat and an increase in unsaturation of the dietary fat. Statistical analysis (variance) of the data for the animals that completed all 12 mazes — combining the data of the 10 percent and 20 percent groups because of the small number of rats in the latter — showed that this conclusion was valid at $P < 0.05$.

EXPERIMENT 2

Six-Month-Old Rats

Method

Male and female Sprague-Dawley rats were obtained at weaning and caged and maintained as in the initial study. At the age of 1 month the females were given semisynthetic diets (13) containing either 5 or 20%w (percent by weight) of lard, oleinate, safflower oil, or safflower oil plus 20 mg of α-tocopherol acetate per 100 gm of finished diet; the lipids were of edible grade. The fatty acid composition of the three dietary lipids is shown in Table 3. When the rats were 3 months old, one male of the same age as the females and

TABLE 3

Dietary Lipids: Fatty Acid Analysis

Carbon Number	Safflower (%)	Lard[d] (%)	Safflower-Olive (%)
10			0.1[a]±0.1[c]
12			0.2±0.1
14	0.5[a]±0.3[c]	1.7[b]±0.1[c]	0.4±0.3
16	6.7±0.6	26.5±0.2	5.8±0.6
16:1ω7		2.1±0.4	0.1±0.05
18	1.6±0.3	12.1±0.7	1.2±0.1
18:1ω9	11.1±0.05	49.8±1.7	75.5±0
18:2ω6	79.7±0.1	10.3±0.2	15.8±0.9
20 or 22 acids	0.1±0.05	2.4±1.4	

[a] The average of two samples taken at a 6-month interval from the dietary oil.
[b] The average of three samples taken at intervals within a year.
[c] Standard error of the mean.
[d] The lard contained a trace amount of 22:6ω3 as the free acid.

fed prior to mating on a commercial pelleted diet (Rockland, Teklad, Inc., Monmouth, Ill.), was placed in a cage with 4 females for a period of 7 days and then removed. The offspring at 23 days of age, were weaned, sexed, caged 4 per cage, and maintained on the same diet as their mothers.

At 6 months of age, 4 male rats from each of the groups — 20%w lard, 5%w lard, 20%w safflower oil + vitamin E, and 20%w safflower oil — were drawn randomly for behavior testing. The operator did not know the composition of the diets; the dietary groups were simply labeled A, B, C, and D: A represented lard 20%w; B, lard 5%w; C, safflower oil 20% + vitamin E; and D, safflower oil 20%w.

The rats were maintained at approximately 80 percent of their free-feeding body weights and tested under conditions of 48-hour food deprivation. Testing was conducted in a Skinner box

(Lehigh Valley operant chamber; Lehigh Valley Electronics, Lehigh Valley, Pa.). This device was provided with two manipulanda (bars) which operated a food delivery magazine placed midway between the bars. Noyes reinforcement pellets (40 mg) were delivered when appropriate responses were emitted. Contingencies between responses (bar depression), cue lights (on or off) and the delivery of reinforcements were automatically controlled. A cue light was available over each bar. Animals were first placed in the testing chamber for 30 minutes with both bars set to deliver a food pellet after one press. This procedure was continued for 5 sessions conducted every other day. Animals which had not by that time begun to bar-press spontaneously were shaped by hand. After that time the reinforcement contingency was switched to FR-4 (the rat received a reinforcement consequent to emitting a total of 4 bar presses on one or both of the bars). These tests lasted 15 minutes and were conducted every other day. Three such test sessions were conducted for each animal. There were no differences between the groups under FR-4 testing.

After FR-4 training, a discrimination procedure was introduced in which only responses on the bar over which a cue light was lighted would result in reinforcement. After every correct response there was a 50:50 probability that the light would switch to the other bar. The tests were also of 15 minutes' duration and conducted every other day. Three such tests were conducted.

Results

The average number of correct responses ± standard deviation per rat for the 3 tests conducted under FR-4 discrimination for the 4 groups are tabulated in Table 4. Group D (safflower 20%w) exhibited significantly fewer correct responses (P < 0.01, Mann-Whitney U test). There were no significant differences among the other groups. Group D (safflower oil) exhibited a significantly lower percentage of correct responses (P < 0.05) on tests 2 and 3 but not on test 1 (Table 4); there were no significant differences among the other groups.

To confirm these data, two additional groups of 4 rats each, labelled A and B, were given to the operator for evaluation. These rats were females, aged 9 months, and they had been given the semisynthetic diets since age 2 months. As in the case of the 6-month-old rats, there were no differences among groups under FR-4 testing.

The number and the percentages of correct responses under FR-4 discrimination are shown in Table 5. Group B (20%w safflower) exhibited significantly fewer correct responses than Group A (20%w lard) (P < 0.01). The percentage of correct responses by Group B was significantly lower on the first test (P < 0.01) but the differences were not significant for tests 2 and 3.

Three-Month-Old Rats

Method

This study employed 3-month-old male rats. The rats, born of mothers from the groups re-

TABLE 4
Effect of Dietary Fat on Discrimination Learning at Age 6 Months (Sprague-Dawley Male Rats*)

Number of Correct Responses			
	No. of Correct Responses ± S.D.		
Diet†	Test 1	Test 2	Test 3
A. Lard, 20%w	359±283	463±152	350±350
B. Lard, 5%w	291±171	409±103	398±102
C. Saff., 20%w + 20 mg vit.E	314±179	519±177	705±292
D. Saff., 20%w	90±49‡	118±80‡	104±76‡

Percent Correct Responses			
	% Correct Responses ± S.D.		
	Test 1	Test 2	Test 3
A. Lard, 20%w	56±24	53±5	65±16
B. Lard, 5%w	59±12	55±8	60±5
C. Saff., 20%w + 20 mg vit.E	50±4	53±7	65±6
D. Saff., 20%w	49±7	46±5‡	43±17‡

* Born of mothers receiving the same diets.
† Four rats in each group.
‡ Significantly smaller, P < 0.01, than the value for the other three groups.

TABLE 5
Effect of Dietary Fat on Discrimination Learning at Age 9 Months (Sprague-Dawley Female Rats*)

Number of Correct Responses			
	No. of Correct Responses ± S.D.		
Diet†	Test 1	Test 2	Test 3
A. Lard, 20%w	166±144	190±88	400±78
B. Safflower, 20%w	16±16‡	145±64‡	162±76‡

Percent Correct Responses			
	% Correct Responses ± S.D.		
	Test 1	Test 2	Test 3
A. Lard, 20%w	59±28	50±20	80±27
B. Safflower, 20%w	26±16‡	61±19	73±25

* Diets started at age 2 months.
† Four rats in each group.
‡ Significantly less, P < 0.01, than the value for Group A.

ceiving 20%w lard, 20% safflower oil+vitamin E, or 20%w safflower oil, as well as from mothers fed standard laboratory chow pellets (Rockland), were maintained with the same diet as their mothers. As before, except for the Rockland group, the operator did not know the composition of the diet. The diets were labeled A, B, C, D: Group A, Rockland; Group B, 20%w lard; Group C, 20%w safflower oil+vitamin E; and Group D, 20%w safflower oil.

The animals were tested in the operant chamber in the same manner as in Experiment 2A.

Results

Only in one aspect of the operant behavior testing was there a reliable effect of diet. This influence was on the percentage of rats spontaneously shaping; the values for the Rockland, 20%w lard, 20%w safflower oil+vitamin E, and 20%w safflower oil groups were, 76, 78, 95 and 25 percent, respectively. The 20%w safflower oil group was significantly poorer in this respect than the other three groups (P < 0.01). Responding under FR-4, or FR-4–discrimination, did not differentiate among the groups.

The earlier discrimination studies demonstrated that rats aged 6 months and 9 months in the safflower oil group, without the vitamin E supplement, had a severely depressed capacity to deal with the operant situation. With 3-month-old rats this suppression was evident only when the free shaping situation was considered.

DISCUSSION

Dietary fat did not significantly alter the lifespan of rats employed in the initial experiment with the Hebb-Williams maze or of those employed in the second experiment (20) with a Skinner box. However, in both studies, dietary fat modified learning behavior and, by implication, the functioning of the CNS. The results of both experiments are compatible with the possibility that enhancing the level of lipid peroxidation has an adverse effect on the CNS out of proportion to its effect on the body as a whole, as measured by mortality rate. Thus variation in the amount or degree of unsaturation of dietary fat and of factors (e.g., vitamin E) that can modify lipid peroxidation rates, may contribute to the variability in age of onset of evident degradative CNS changes such as senility, above and beyond the variations expected from differences in mortality rates.

The manner in which increases in the amount or degree of unsaturation of dietary fat modifies CNS function is unknown. Several mechanisms may be operating. Neuronal dysfunction may be mediated in part through deleterious effects of dietary fat on the glial cells. The rate of peroxidation of serum and vessel-wall constituents may be increased, leading to a more rapid development of arteriocapillary fibrosis (21). Increased lipid peroxidation in the synaptic areas, areas rich in polyunsaturated fatty acids (22) such as $22:5\omega6$ and $22:6\omega3$, could cause damage in a manner similar to that caused by β-hydroxy dopamine (23), or by the anesthetic, halothane (24, 25).

REFERENCES

1. Kay DWK: Epidemiological aspects of organic brain disease in the aged, *in* Aging and the Brain, ed. by CM Gaitz. New York, Plenum Press, 1972, pp 15–27.
2. Redick RW, Kramer M and Taube CA: Epidemiology of mental illness and utilization of psychiatric facilities among older persons, *in* Mental illness in Later Life, ed. by EW Busse and E Pfeiffer. Washington, DC, American Psychiatric Association, 1973, pp 201–230.
3. Brotman HB: Who are the aging? *Ibid*, pp 19–39.
4. Malamud N: Neuropathology of organic brain syndromes associated with aging, *in* Aging and the Brain, ed. by CM Gaitz. New York, Plenum Press, 1972, pp 63–87.
5. Feldman ML: Degenerative changes in aging dendrites, Gerontologist 14(No. 5, part II): 36, 1974.
6. Pryor WA: Free Radicals. New York, McGraw-Hill, 1966.
7. Nonhebel DC and Walton JC: Free-Radical Chemistry. Cambridge, Mass., University Press, 1974.
8. Isenberg I: Free radicals in tissue, Physiol Rev 44: 487, 1964.
9. Swartz HM, Bolton JR and Borg DC (Eds.): Biological Applications of Electron Spin Resonance. New York, Wiley-Interscience, 1972.
10. Lea CH: The oxidative deterioration of food lipids, *in* Symposium on Foods: Lipids and Their Oxidation, ed. by HW Schultz, EA Day and RO Sinnhuber. Westport, Conn., Avi Publ Co, 1962, pp 3–28.
11. Lundberg WO: Mechanisms, *Ibid*, pp 31–50.
12. Peters A, Palay SL, and Webster H: The Fine Structure of the Nervous System. New York, Harper & Row, 1970.
13. Harman D: Free radical theory of aging: effect of the amount and degree of unsaturation of dietary fat on mortality rate, J Gerontol 26: 451, 1971.
14. Harman D: Free radical theory of aging: effect of free radical reaction inhibitors on the mortality rate of male LAF₁ mice, J Gerontol 23: 476, 1968.
15. Committee on Animal Nutrition: Nutrient Requirements of Domestic Animals (No. 10). Publication 990, Natl Acad Sci, Natl Res Council, Washington, DC, 1962.
16. Rabinovitch MS, and Rosvold HE: A closed-field intelligence test for rats, Canad J Psych 5: 122, 1951.
17. Hebb DO and Williams K: A method of rating animal intelligence, J Genetic Psych 34: 59, 1946.
18. Botting NR, Vandenburg GA and Riser R: Resistance of certain long-chain polyunsaturated fatty acids of marine oils to pancreatic lipase hydrolysis, Lipids 2: 489, 1967.
19. Dupont J and Mathias MM: Bio-oxidation of linoleic

acid via methylmalonyl CoA, Lipids 4: 478, 1969.

20. Harman D and Eddy DE: Free radical theory of aging: effect of dietary fat on body weight and mortality rate, (in preparation).

21. Harman D: Prolongation of life: role of free radical reactions in aging, J Am Geriatrics Soc 17: 721, 1969.

22. Galli C and Przegalinski E: Dietary-induced long lasting accumulation of 22:6ω3 fatty acid in rat brain synaptosomal phospholipids, Pharmacol Res Comm 5: 239, 1973.

23. Heikkila RE and Cohen G: β-Hydroxydopamine: evidence for superoxide radical as an oxidative intermediate, Science 181: 456, 1973.

24. Quimby KL, Aschkenase LJ and Bowman RE: Enduring learning deficits and cerebral synaptic malformation from exposure to 10 parts of halothane per million, Science 185: 625, 1974.

25. Van Dyke RA and Wood CL: *In vitro* studies on irreversible binding of halothane metabolite to microsomes, Drug Metab & Dispos, 3: 51, 1975.

Appendix:
A Few More
Life Extension Suppliers

These vendors are listed for informational purposes only, and no endorsement of the effectiveness or safety of the products sold is intended. Moreover, we have no control over their order fulfillment process.

CAUTION: Before using these products, you should familiarize yourself with the precautions we have detailed in *Life Extension A Practical Scientific Approach.* Check the index for specific substances for their cautions and warnings. For example, do *not* use RNA if you have gout, or unneutralized acidic products if you have ulcers, or tyrosine/phenylalanine if you have cardiac arrhythmias, or cysteine if you have kidney stones, or folic acid if you are receiving the widely used cancer treatment drug methotrexate. We have also repeatedly cautioned, and do so again, that you should be under a doctor's supervision, with regular laboratory tests, if you use these materials. For example, only your doctor can tell you if you have diabetes mellitus (a possible reason not to use cysteine) or whether you have a cardiac arrhythmia.

Dajean Gerontological Laboratories
Division of Dajean Foods Corp.
Box #4119
Huntington Station, NY 11746

This firm offers many products which are very similar to some of our own personal nutrient supplements. Many of our friends and research subjects use these products. A catalog is available upon request.

Some of the products offered by this firm include: L-tryptophan, L-tyrosine, L-phenylalanine, L-arginine, L-arginine powder, L-ornithine, L-cysteine, L-cysteine plus vitamin C, L-glutathione (reduced), 55% phosphatidyl choline (5x standard strength lecithin), Oxy-Scavengers™ (a high potency antioxidant formula), ascorbyl palmitate (lipid soluble vitamin C), sodium selenite (yeast-free selenium), Na-PCA lotion, Na-PCA with Aloe Vera lotion, polysorbate 80, polysorbate 80 with biotin and niacin, BHT, beta carotene, choline chloride with B-5, RNA, Micro-sublingual B-12, Hair Vitamin formula (L-cysteine, vitamin C, biotin, PABA, inositol), chapparal herb extract (contains NDGA, an extremely potent natural antioxidant), powdered cooked velvet beans (richest food source of L-Dopa, see special cautions in our *Life Extension*), D, L-phenylalanine, glycine, L-arginine and L-ornithine combination, niacinamide ascorbate and inositol capsules, PABA ester sunscreen, pure powdered and crystalline vitamins, minerals, and amino acids, calcium ascorbate, canthaxanthin, GABA with Niacinamide and Inositol, GTF (glucose tolerance factor) chromium yeast, Nutrimix™ (A pure powder mix which is based on a formula we originated for our own use and have described in *Life Extension*. It differs primarily in that the lower niacin dose is more readily tolerated without very strong flushing, and it does not contain two synthetic food antioxidants, dilauryl thiodipropionate and thiodipropionic acid, two secondary antioxidants which destroy organic peroxides.)

This firm ships UPS COD, and will be obtaining a toll free 800 number for phone orders. Ask for their catalog; they have nearly everything.

This firm will donate 3% of their gross receipts to an outstanding non-profit aging mechanism and intervention research foundation from which we have not and will not be receiving funds. Three percent of the gross is a very large contribution for this type of business.

Health Maintenance Programs, Inc.
Orders: PO Box 252, Valhalla, NY 10595
Business Office: 24 Sycamore Rd., Scarsdale, NY 10583
  Customer Service and Inquiries: (914)592-3155

This firm offers high quality antioxidants, vitamins, and other micronutrient food supplements. Their products contain no lubricants, binders, fillers, gums, starches, sugars, sodium salts, flavorings, artificial colorings, oil bases, additives or excipients of any kind. Health Maintenance Programs is run by a health professional whose highly respected scientific work involves extensive study of free radicals and lipid peroxidation. For this reason, this firm is particularly careful to keep their supplements free of peroxides. A well informed, conservative professional biomedical consultation service is available to customers and potential customers without cost, and is a truly unique feature. This service is not intended to replace your personal physician, but rather to help you to obtain sound professional advice in areas where few physicians have extensive experience. In addition, the firm offers special, professionally designed formulations for children 2-12 years old (chewable tablets), teenagers, pregnant and lactating women, and the elderly, who often have difficulty taking pills or capsules. There is a professionally written newsletter, *Nutrient News*, available.

This firm ships UPS COD. Ask for their catalog.

This firm was created to supply funds for life extension research. We receive none of these funds.

Life Extension Products
2835 Hollywood Blvd.
Hollywood, FL 33020
  to order, phone (305)925-2500 in
Florida, or (800)327-6110 outside Florida

Life Extension Products features nutrient formulas designed to improve health, decrease the risk of degenerative diseases, and retard premature aging. Among the nutritional products currently offered by this firm are the following: Cognitex-1® (a combination of choline, pantothenic acid, and

RNA/DNA), which is designed to help improve memory; the nutrient amino acid cysteine; Ca-X-1® (a combination of 8 antioxidants including beta-carotene, cysteine, and selenium), which is designed to help lower the risk of cancer and premature aging; and a new anti-aging cosmetic cream that includes NaPCA.

Life Extension Products also offers books such as *Life Extension* by Durk Pearson & Sandy Shaw; *Maximum Lifespan* by Roy Walford, M.D., and *The Life-Extension Revolution* by Saul Kent; *Anti-Aging News*—a monthly newsletter that includes a column by Durk Pearson & Sandy Shaw; audio tapes featuring authorities on life extension; and even life extension T-shirts.

The Life Extension Foundation maintains a current list of life extension doctors, whose names may be obtained by telephone: outside of Florida (toll free), 1-800-327-6110; in Florida, 305-925-2500.

Life Extension Products is owned by individuals dedicated to the extension of the human life span. As a result, the firm donates 10% of its gross revenues to The Life Extension Foundation—a non-profit, tax-exempt organization for the support of basic scientific research. The firm also spends at least 75% of its profits on research designed to develop new and better life extension products. We receive none of these funds.

A catalog is available upon request.

Advanced Research Health Products Corp.
Box R
Summit, NJ 07901
(212)977-9579

Products offered include AN83 (an encapsulated very high potency antioxidant nutrient mix which is based on a formula we originated for our own personal experimental mixture), Phylan 100 (100 milligram tablets of phenylalanine), and AR19 (a tabletted high potency nutrient formulation). This firm has a policy of donating a substantial portion of the profits of the business to legitimate non-profit charitable research foundations for research on biological aging mechanisms and means of intervention. We have no control over these foundations and have never received grants from them, nor will we ever do so, thereby avoiding a potential conflict of interest.

Multinational Nutrient Trading Company
P.O. Box 5344
Austin, TX, 78763 (512)346-9318

This firm deals in the kinds of nutrients discussed in our books on a world-wide basis and is in contact with numerous vitamin and nutrient companies throughout the world. They are particularly interested in supplying the more difficult-to-obtain nutrients. They state that, on most items, they have the lowest prices in this new industry. People who order from outside Texas, where their operation is located, do not have to pay sales tax. If you send your name and address to this firm, along with the names of the particular nutrients that you seek, the firm will see that you receive the names and addresses of companies, if any, near you that handle those vitamins or nutrients. This service is offered whether you live in the United States or elsewhere in the world. Their products include an encapsulated formula similar to that which we use ourselves, amino acids, ascorbyl palmitate, beta carotene, BHT and BHA (for preservative use only), canthaxanthin (for food coloring use only), niacinamide ascorbate, NaPCA lotion, and many others. They also offer capsules and capsule filling equipment.

This firm will donate 3% of the gross receipts of their products to a non-profit research foundation from which we have not and will not be receiving funds.

Longevity Products, Inc.™
2210 Wilshire Blvd., #711
Santa Monica, CA 90403
Nationwide 1-(800)227-3900 and (213)306-6939
California (800)632-2122

Longevity Products, Inc. is a new firm which offers Velvet Bean Protein Plus™ (in capsules or tablets), which is powdered cooked velvet beans, a food that contains about 3% by weight of the amino acid L-Dopa (specific lot analysis will appear on the label), about which we wrote extensively in *Life Extension A Practical Scientific Approach.* Be sure to read our special L-Dopa precautions in *Life Extension* before use! They also offer a NaPCA moisturizing lotion under the name of Silky PCA Moisturizer™ (this lotion contains the principal natural antibacterial found in human mother's milk as a hypoallergenic antimicrobial preservative). Other products include reduced glutathione, ascorbyl palmitate, GTF chromium, L-arginine & vitamin C mix, L-arginine & L-ornithine mix, B-1-C-cysteine mix, polysorbate 80, DL-phenylalanine, BHT, and L-tryptophan, plus urine test strips for glucose and for vitamin C, and very desirable but hard to find reusable humidity indicators to detect unwanted moisture in your stored bulk vitamins. It is easy to be sure that your supplements are stored in a cool dark place, but without these inexpensive humidity indicators, what may seem dry to you may really be destructively moist. Protect your investment and your health.

This firm will donate 3% of the gross receipts of their products to a non-profit research foundation from which we have not and will not be receiving funds.

Vitamin Research Products
2044-A Old Middlefield Way
Mountain View, CA 94043
(800)541-8536 Toll free inside California
(800)541-1623 Toll free outside California
(415)967-7770

Vitamin Research Products is a mail order supplier of a very wide array of bulk nutrients, encapsulations, preservatives, antioxidants, sweeteners, and skin care formulations both to researchers and the general public. They offer virtually all of the products mentioned in this book in powder form or in excipient-free capsules.

The company offers a wide selection of ingredients for a multitude of nutritional applications, with particular focus on life extension and hypoallergenic formulations. A partial list from the Vitamin Research Products catalog includes: ascorbyl palmitate; beta carotene; BHT and BHA; NaPCA in ready-to-use cosmetics and concentrate; polysorbate 80;

GABA; vitamin C in acid and buffered forms; the sweetener aspartame (two amino acids strung together, with no bitter aftertaste, metabolized as food), all B vitamins; over twenty forms of amino acids; naturally and synthetically derived vitamin E; and supplies necessary for home encapsulation. A complete listing may be obtained on request by domestic or international customers.

This firm will donate 3% of the gross receipts of their products to a non-profit research foundation from which we have not and will not be receiving funds.

Bronson Pharmaceuticals
4526 Rinetti Lane
La Canada, CA 91011

intravenous ascorbate solution

Creative Health Products
5148 Saddle Ridge Road
Plymouth, MI 48170
(313)453-5309 or 455-0177

Slim Guide skinfold caliper, $19.95 (with instructions for measuring % body fat)

Edmund Scientific
101 E. Gloucester Pike
Barrington, NJ 08007
(609)547-3488

Fat-O-Meter (catalog no. E33,033, $10.95) is a skinfold caliper for measuring % body fat. Comes with instruction booklet. Windmill spirometer (catalog no. E31,649, $89.95) measures lung air capacity, elasticity, and strength

Wholesale Nutrition Club
Box 3345, Dept. Z
Saratoga, CA 95070

a wide range of low priced nutrients and antioxidants, vitamin C crystals, Drug Rehabilitation kit (relatively comfortable withdrawal from opiates with vitamin C), C-Strips (measure vitamin C in your urine with these test

papers); "Every 2nd Child"
by A. Kalokerinos, M.D.
(tells how the author-M.D.
prevented infant crib
death with vitamin C)

This firm is generously donating about 5 to 6% of all gross business, including re-orders, from "Dept. Z" to a non-profit aging research foundation (from which we do not receive and have never received funding). Be sure to mention "Dept. Z"!

Pure Planet Products
1025 N. 48th St., Dept. AGE
Phoenix, AZ 85008
(602)267-1000

empty gelatin capsules,
"00" and "000"; The
Capsule Machine, a "00"
filling device, $9.95 plus
$1.50 shipping; catalog, $.25

This firm will donate 3% of the gross receipts on orders coming from this book to a non-profit life extension research foundation from which we do not receive and have never received funding, if you will *mention AGE on your order*!

CARTOONIST SERVICES

Many of the hilarious cartoons and comics in *Life Extension A Practical Scientific Approach* and in this book were contributed by the following artists. We invite other artists to write to us at PO Box 758, Redondo Beach, CA 90277 concerning art for upcoming books and for our large personal art collection. Please do *not* send letters about medical matters to this address! (All such letters will be forwarded to the Life Extension Foundation in Hollywood, Florida, usually after a substantial delay.) We are *not* physicians!

Aaron Bacall
204 Arlene Street
Staten Island, NY 10314

Aaron Bacall has contributed numerous hilarious cartoons to this book and to *Life Extension*. He is a member of the Cartoonist's Association and the Cartoonist's Guild. A good example of his work follows:

Sidney Harris
8 Polo Road
Great Neck, NY 11023

Sidney Harris has three books of scientific cartoons in print. His cartoons were prominently featured in *Life Extension* and more appear in this book. His cartoons have appeared regularly in *American Scientist* since January 1970.

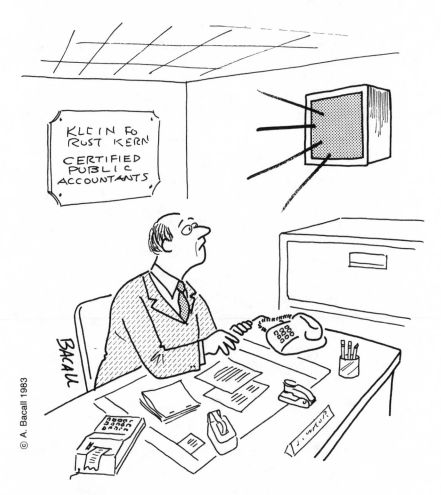

"Attention, attention! This is a tax shelter alert. Everyone to the tax shelter."

Sandy Dean
742 N. Citrus
Pensacola, FL 32505

Several of Sandy Dean's cartoons can be seen in *Life Extension* and in this book. Ms. Dean's favorite of her cartoons is reproduced below:

NON-PROFIT RESEARCH FOUNDATIONS

The following institutions support aging research which is, in our opinions, of excellent quality. Donations to the American organizations are generally tax-deductible. Write them for information concerning their activities; very informative newsletters are often available. Listing these institu-

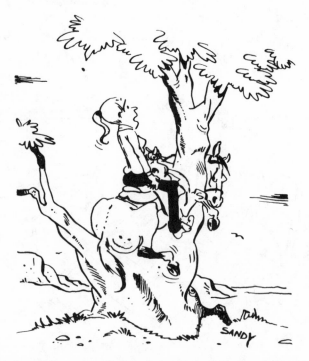

Cartoon by Sandy Dean

"Mom wanted me to be a nurse; Dad wanted me to be a teacher; Auntie wanted me to be a stewardess—but, no, *I* wanted to be a horse trainer!"

tions here does not imply their approval of our ideas. We do not receive funds from these foundations.

The American Aging Association, Inc. (AGE)
Attn.: Denham Harman, M.D.
University of Nebraska Medical Center
Omaha, Nebr. 68105

AGE publishes *AGE News*, a newsletter on aging research, written for scientists and interested laymen. Membership is $20 per year. Dr. Harman is the originator of the free radical theory of aging. **Patients seeking a physician may write AGE for the office addresses and phone numbers of physicians in their area with a professional interest in the treatment of aging and the aged.** AGE may be reached by telephone at 1-(402) 559-4416. For a toll-free 800 number, call 1-(800) 555-1212 and ask for the number of the American Aging Association.

Fund for Integrative Biomedical Research (FIBER)
1000 Connecticut Ave., N.W., Suite 803
Washington, D.C. 20036
(202)293-7660

Contributors of $20 or more to FIBER become Sustaining Members and receive quarterly reports on the latest biomedical advances in extending human life.

The Linus Pauling Institute of Science and Medicine
440 Page Mill Road
Palo Alto, CA 94306

The Pauling Institute publishes a very informative Newsletter, with emphasis on research with vitamin C.

The Life Extension Foundation
PO Box 1067
Hollywood, FL 33022
(305)925-2500 in Florida; (800)327-6110 outside Florida

The Life Extension Foundation publishes *Anti-Aging News*, an excellent publication about aging research. Subscriptions are $27 per year, $50 per two years. A column by Durk and Sandy is usually included. **Referrals to physicians in your area with a professional interest in life extension can be obtained without charge by calling the toll-free 800 number.**

Foundation for Experimental Ageing Research
Felix Platter-Spital
4055 Basel, Switzerland
061/440031
Attn.: Dr. Marco Ermini

Glossary:
A Layman's Guide
to Word Usage

Note: These are generally not full technical definitions.

acetaldehyde—an aldehyde found in cigarette smoke, auto exhaust, smog, and created in the liver from alcohol. Acetaldehyde autoxidizes (spontaneously oxidizes in the presence of air) to produce the organic peroxide peracetic acid (an eye irritant in smog) and damaging free radicals, and is a mutagen, carcinogen, and cross-linker.

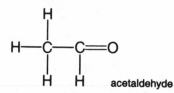

acetaldehyde

acetylcholine—ACh, a natural chemical which is used as a neurotransmitter in the brain (especially for memory and the control of sensory input signals and muscular output signals), and as a neuromuscular transmitter (ACh released by muscle nerves makes muscles contract). It is made by the brain from the precursor nutrient choline.

adrenergic—of or pertaining to nervous activities controlled by adrenaline (epinephrine) or noradrenaline (norepinephrine).

aerobic—oxygen-requiring metabolic processes and organisms.

aging—the decline of physiological functions which occurs with time, accompanied by a falling probability of survival.

aging clocks—biological clocks which turn physiological processes on or off at specific genetically programmed times. Examples are menopause and male pattern balding.

agonists—substances that increase responsiveness of specific nerve receptors.

aldehydes—a class of organic compounds which have an end group with a carbon and oxygen double bonded to each other and with a hydrogen bonded to the same carbon. These compounds, related to formaldehyde, are cross-linkers, mutagens, and carcinogens. Malonaldehyde, created in the breakdown of peroxidized fats is also carcinogenic and an extremely potent cross-linker. Acetaldehyde is made from alcohol in the liver (the acetaldehyde is a major reason alcoholics have such heavily wrinkled skin) and is found in cigarette smoke and smog. Most aldehydes autoxidize, producing damaging free radicals.

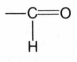

aldehyde group

amino acid—an organic acid containing an amine (ammonia-like) chemical group. Amino acids are connected together in specific ways in small numbers to form polypeptides and in large numbers to form proteins. The simplest amino acid is glycine; its structure is shown under that entry in the glossary.

anaerobic—metabolic processes and organisms that do not require oxygen. Also means "without oxygen."

androgens—male sex hormones.

anecdotal evidence—observations of treatment effects in individual cases or in informal clinical studies, without controls, not blind. These observations cannot prove anything in themselves but sometimes provide leads for useful research.

anoxia—the absence of oxygen.

antibody—a large Y-shaped protein molecule made by B-cells of the immune system which very selectively binds to other specific protein molecules called antigens. Specific antibodies combine with and inactivate specific viruses, while other specific antibodies mark invading bacteria and cancer cells for destruction by other cells of the immune system.

antigen—a protein which is recognized by antibodies and other parts of the immune system. Different antigens distinguish enemies (such as bacteria, cancer cells, viruses, and foreign tissue) from your own normal cells.

antioxidant—a chemical which combines with free radicals and/or other chemicals that release free radicals that would otherwise attack molecules in the body, and abnormally oxidize them. Susceptible molecules include such vital entities as DNA, RNA, lipids (fats), and proteins. The antioxidant, by reacting with the oxidant, protects these important molecules from being damaged. Examples of antioxidants include vitamins A, C, E, B-1, B-5, B-6, beta carotene, the amino acid cysteine, reduced glutathione, the synthetic food antioxidants BHT and BHA, and certain enzymes containing the minerals selenium and zinc.

arginine—an amino acid which is an immune system stimulant and causes the pituitary gland to release growth hormone.

arrhythmias—irregular heart beat.

atherogenic—causes atherosclerosis.

atherosclerosis—a common degenerative disease of the arteries, often caused by free radical damage. Atherosclerotic plaques are tumors which grow into and damage the artery lining. Cholesterol and other fats deposited into the injured area become oxidized, further increasing free radical activity and resulting in adherence of platelets (blood clot-making particles) to plaques. The platelets attract red blood cells which burst (hemolyze), leaking iron and copper, which are powerful free radical autoxidation catalysts. Eventually atherosclerotic arteries narrow and may become blocked by a blood clot, causing a heart attack, stroke, or other circulatory insufficiency. Herpes viruses have also been implicated as another cause of some plaques.

ATP—adenosine triphosphate, the universal energy storage molecule. Energy released during the oxidation of foodstuffs to carbon dioxide and water are stored in the high energy phosphate bonds of ATP.

autoantibodies—antibodies which attack other molecules or cells of their own body.

autoimmune—a state in which a person's immune system erroneously attacks some of his or her own cells, damaging them. Rheumatoid arthritis and multiple sclerosis are examples of conditions thought to be autoimmune diseases. As people age, autoimmunity becomes more and more prevalent.

autoxidation—a spontaneous oxidation reaction in which a molecule reacts with oxygen via a free radical, self-catalyzed route. The development of rancidity in fatty foods, the formation of gum in old gasoline, and the spontaneous combustion of rags soaked with oil-base paint are examples of autoxidation.

B-cells—white blood cells which make antibodies, usually under instructions from the white blood cells called T-cells. B-cells are made in your bone marrow, either directly or by division of cells originally made there, and so the name "B-cells."

benzoalphapyrene—a type of polynuclear aromatic hydrocarbon, carcinogenic substances produced during combustion of fuels.

benzodiazepine—a class of compounds that includes Valium® and Librium® which stimulate certain anti-anxiety brain receptors.

beta adrenergic—certain nerve receptors responsive to adrenalin and noradrenalin (norepinephrine).

BHA—butylated hydroxyanisole, a synthetic antioxidant frequently added to foods to prevent fat rancidity (peroxidation).

BHT—butylated hydroxytoluene, a synthetic antioxidant often added to foods to prevent fat rancidity (peroxidation).

bioavailability—the amount of ingested nutrients that are actually absorbed by the body.

biological clocks—long-term clocks involving DNA that keep track of time, and which turn on and off various genetic programs which are "set" for various times. Menopause, male pattern balding, and the spawning of salmon are examples of biological aging clocks. A major theory of aging proposes that an aging clock may drastically alter production and use of certain hypothalamic and pituitary gland hormones, thereby causing death. Sleeping and waking take place as a result of a circadian (daily) biological clock, which probably involves somewhat different mechanisms.

carcinogenesis—the process of causing cancer, usually by altering DNA.

carcinogens—cancer causing agents.

carotenoid—a class of very important antioxidants produced by plants which protects them from damage caused by singlet and triplet oxygen and free radicals produced during photosynthesis. Carotenoids also provide protection from ultraviolet damage and can prevent the development of cancer in experimental animals. They are usually colored bright yellow, orange, or red. Carotenoids make carrots orange and fall leaves a beautiful array of colors. Recent findings suggest that they are very effective in preventing certain cancers, especially lung cancer due to cigarette smoking.

catalase—an enzyme which catalyzes the breakdown of hydrogen peroxide in the body. Catalase is found in all organisms which require oxygen or can survive in its presence.

catalyst—a chemical which acts to stimulate a particular chemical reaction, usually without itself being permanently chemically changed in the process. Enzymes are a form of biological catalyst. Iron and copper are powerful free radical autoxidation catalysts. The products of free radical autoxidation of lipids (oils and fats) catalyze further autoxidation, hence the process is called autocatalytic. The spontaneous combustion of oil-based paint-soaked rags is autocatalytic autoxidation.

catecholamines—a class of brain neurotransmitters (chemicals which serve to carry communications between nerves) which includes norepinephrine and dopamine. Both of these decline with age, particularly dopamine, with consequent decline of functions dependent on these catecholamines. The autoxidation of dopamine results in 6-OH-dopamine, hydrogen peroxide, and free radicals which damage the receptors for dopamine. 6-OH-dopamine autoxidation is suspected as being responsible for the pathetic "burnt out" schizophrenic and may be involved in producing Parkinsonism.

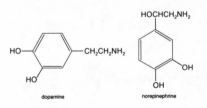

dopamine   norepinephrine

CCK—cholecystokinin, a polypeptide hormone found in the brain and gastrointestinal tract which, among other functions, causes you to feel full after eating.

central nervous system—the brain, spinal cord, optic nerves, retinas, auditory nerves, pituitary and pineal glands, hypothalamus, and other structures enclosed within the special membranes surrounding the brain and spinal cord.

chelation—the process of forming a closely associated complex with a metal in which the metal is surrounded by and multiply bound to part of an organic structure, thereby usually altering both the chemical reactivity and transport properties of the metal.

cholinergic—those parts of the nervous system, both peripheral and in the brain, using acetylcholine as a neurotransmitter. Acetylcholine released at the synapse (junction) between a motor nerve and a muscle fiber causes the muscle fiber to contract. Acetylcholine is an important brain neurotransmitter, too, being involved in memory, long-term planning, control of mental focus, sexual activity, and other functions. It is made in the body from choline in reactions requiring the availability of adequate vitamin B-5 (as part of the enzyme acetyl co-enzyme A).

chromosomes—double stranded DNA helixes which contain the basic blueprints for physiological activities, including some of their associated control and regulation proteins. The DNA from a human cell would be about 1 meter long if stretched out; it is normally stored in compact supercoiled (coiled coils) packages, the microscopic chromosomes.

Citric Acid Cycle (also called the Kreb's Cycle and the Tricarboxylic Acid Cycle)—this cycle stores energy, released by the oxidation of fats, proteins, and carbohydrates in foodstuffs, in high energy phosphate bonds of ATP. About 90% of the energy released from food occurs in this Citric Acid Cycle. In the process, a series of acids are oxidized to release the energy used in forming high-energy ATP phosphate bonds, plus carbon dioxide and water. ATP is life's universal energy supply.

clone—an identical twin of another cell or animal, with the same genetic instructions (DNA). Nowadays, this term is sometimes also used to refer to mass-produced copies of a DNA strand, as in cloned DNA, or of a particular antibody, such as monoclonal antibodies.

collagen—a connective tissue protein, the most abundant protein in the human body, about 30% of total body protein.

complement—a system of protein molecules produced by the immune system which kills antibody-tagged foreign cells by making holes in their cell membranes.

controls—a technique used to evaluate experimental treatments by having two groups of experimental subjects, one to receive treatment, and one subjected to the same conditions but not given the treatment. This way, scientists can find out whether effects they are seeing are due to treatment or some other experimental condition. Non-controlled experiments are considered very difficult to evaluate because of the absence of controls with which to compare treated subjects.

cross-linking—an oxidation reaction in which undesirable bonds form between nucleic acids (RNA and DNA, the genetic blueprint material) or between proteins, often as links between sulfur atoms called disulfide bonds, or between lipids or any combination thereof. The links may be between different proteins or nucleic acids or lipids or between parts of the same protein or nucleic acid or lipid. The result is that the molecule cannot assume the correct shape for proper functioning. Some cross-links are required in proteins for rigidity and structural strength. However, cross-links of an inappropriate, undesired nature form throughout life, resulting in such conditions as artery rigidity, skin wrinkling, and loss of eye focus accommodation due to aging. The hardening and fluid loss ("weeping") of an old gelatin dessert and the deterioration of your automobile's windshield wiper blades and rubber hoses is caused by cross-linking. Free radicals, aldehydes, ozone, ultraviolet light, and x-rays are powerful cross-linkers. The vulcanization which converts soft latex gum into a hard rubber comb involves disulfide bond cross-linking.

dehydroascorbic acid—toxic oxidized form of vitamin C (ascorbic acid); it is a pro-oxidant rather than antioxidant.

diastolic—the part of the heartbeat cycle during which blood pressure is lowest, when the heart is relaxed; if you have a blood pressure of 115/70, 70 is your diastolic blood pressure.

dimethylbenzanthracene—a type of polynuclear aromatic hydrocarbon, a tarry carcinogenic substance produced during the combustion of fuels.

disulfide bond—a sulfur to sulfur bond found in both normal and abnormal cross-linked proteins, bonding a protein to parts of the same molecule or to other molecules. These bonds provide the three dimensional structure of molecules containing them. Latex is vulcanized to form rubber by the controlled formation of disulfide bonds.

disulfide bond

DMSO—dimethyl sulfoxide, a hydroxyl radical-scavenging solvent that rapidly penetrates the skin.

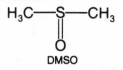

DMSO

DNA—deoxyribonucleic acid, the genetic material, encoding full plans for how living organisms are constructed and how they function. Damage to DNA is believed to be a central feature of both aging and cancer.

L-Dopa—precursor to dopamine.

dopamine—an important brain neurotransmitter (chemical which enables nerve cells to communicate with each other) which plays a role in body movement, motivation, primitive drives and emotions including sexual behavior, and immune system function. See molecular structure under "catecholamines."

dopaminergic—those parts of the nervous system in the brain which use dopamine as neurotransmitter.

double blind—a technique used in modern scientific research to separate facts from the hopes and wishes of both scientists and experimental subjects. A treatment which is to be tested is administered by scientists who do not know whether they are using the active treatment or the inactive placebo. The experimental subjects don't know which is which, either. The test results are evaluated by scientists who also do not know which group received the active treatment and which the placebo. At the end of the experiment, the secret code is broken, and the responses of the subjects to the real experimental treatment are compared with their responses to the placebo.

EEG—electroencephalogram, the brain's electrical output as measured on the scalp.

EGF—epidermal growth factor, a hormone which causes epithelial tissues, such as skin and the cells lining the gastrointestinal tract and lungs, to grow and heal.

EKG—electrocardiogram, the heart's electrical output as measured by electrodes placed on the skin of the torso.

enzyme—a protein which acts as a catalyst in certain metabolic reactions, usually specifically acting on a particular substance or class of substances. Enzymes are generally not themselves destroyed in these reactions. Proper enzyme function depends on the three dimensional configuration of the enzyme molecule, and often requires that the enzyme be properly integrated into a cell membrane.

epidemiology—study of the possible causes and frequency of occurrence of diseases in natural human or animal populations outside the laboratory.

epistemology—the study of the sources of knowledge; that is, the principles by which one may distinguish what is true from what is not true.

epithelial—referring to rapidly dividing tissues such as skin, the lining of the gastrointestinal tract, and the lining of the lung.

epoxide—a very reactive oxidized form of organic compound, in which two carbon atoms are bonded both to each other and to a single oxygen atom in an organic molecule (see figure). For example, polynuclear aromatic hydrocarbon epoxides and cholesterol epoxides are carcinogenic and mutagenic. Epoxides are excellent cross-linkers, and this reaction is catalyzed by free radicals; this is what happens when you mix epoxy resin and catalyst—the pastes or liquids cross-link to form a hard solid.

epoxide group

esters—the class of organic compounds formed in the reaction of an alcohol and an acid, by the elimination of water. Amyl acetate, the principal aroma note in bananas, is an ester, as are many fruity and floral scents.

estrogens—female sex hormones.

fibroblasts—connective tissue cells.

free radical—an atom or molecule with an unpaired electron. These chemically reactive entities are produced in the course of normal metabolism, in the breakdown of peroxidized fats in the body, by radiation (radiation sickness is a free radical disease), in ozone interactions with lipids, in the attack of oxidizing agents on fatty acids, particularly those that are unsaturated, and so on. Free radicals are major sources of damage that cause aging, cardiovascular disease, and cancer. Free radical scavengers, molecules which can block free radical chain reactions, have extended experimental animals' life spans and reduced cardiovascular disease and cancer incidence.

GABA—gamma aminobutyric acid. GABA is an amino acid which functions as an inhibitory neurotransmitter in the central nervous system.

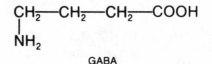

GABA

gene—the basic unit of DNA in chromosomes which codes for a protein or affects the expression of genetic information.

GH—see growth hormone.

glutamate or **glutamic acid**—an excitatory amino acid neurotransmitter in the central nervous system.

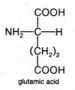

glutamic acid

glutathione peroxidase—selenium - and - cysteine - containing enzyme which, with the required help of reduced glutathione, catalyzes the breakdown of peroxides, while controlling the potentially dangerous free radicals. It also directly scavenges free radicals.

glycine—aminoacetic acid, the simplest amino acid. It is an inhibitory neurotransmitter in the central nervous system.

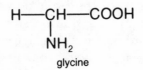

glycine

glycoprotein—a molecule containing both carbohydrate and protein parts. Many antigens are glycoproteins.

growth hormone (GH)—a polypeptide hormone secreted by the anterior lobe of the pituitary gland in the brain. Growth hormone (GH) plays a crucial role in growth and repair, as well as stimulating the immune system. The GH peaks during sleep which are typical of young people are frequently absent or small in older people, and in those who are obese.

HDL—high density lipoproteins, a fat-transporting fraction of blood higher levels of which are believed to be associated with a reduced risk of heart disease.

hemolysis—bursting (lysis) of red blood cells. One way of measuring vitamin E deficiency is by finding out how easily the red blood cells burst when subjected to lysing agents such as hydrogen peroxide. Higher serum levels of vitamin E protect the red blood cells against hemolysis, unless they are then exposed to even higher concentrations of the oxidant hydrogen peroxide.

5-HIAA—5-hydroxyindoleacetic acid, a breakdown product of the neurotransmitter serotonin.

histamine—an amine which is released during traumas and under stressful conditions. Histamine is necessary for growth and healing, is a capillary dilator (widens these small blood vessels), stimulates stomach acid secretion, and is required for orgasm. Excess histamine release can be toxic. Vitamin C can help detoxify histamine in the body.

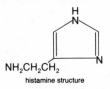

histamine structure

hormone—a chemical messenger that is transported (often by the bloodstream) a relatively long distance from its source to the cells it affects. Insulin, vasopressin, testosterone, and cortisone are all examples.

hydroperoxide—a type of organic peroxide.

hydroxyl radicals—a particularly reactive, damaging type of free radical, formed when superoxide radicals react with hydrogen peroxide. Hydroxyl radicals are thought to be the principal damaging agent to joint membranes in arthritis. X-rays do most of their damage via hydroxyl radicals. Hydroxyl radicals can attack and damage any molecule in your body.

hypercholesterolemia—a class of conditions, often hereditary, in which the cholesterol levels in the blood are extremely high.

hypothalamus—the master gland of neuroendocrine (hormone) control in the brain. It controls the pituitary's production and release of its own hormones. Appetite and body temperature control centers are located in the hypothalamus. It releases many hormones including LHRH, a natural aphrodisiac. An aging clock or clocks may be located in the hypothalamus.

hypoxia—a condition of oxygen deficiency (but not total absence) in part or all of the body. Under conditions of hypoxia, free radical production is often greatly stimulated.

immune system—specialized cells, organs, glycoproteins, and polypeptides which protect the body by locating, killing, and eating foreign invaders (bacteria, parasites, viruses), atherosclerotic plaques, and cancer cells. Includes white blood cells, thymus gland, lymphatic system, spleen, bone marrow, antibodies, complement, and interferon.

infarct—tissue which has died due to lack of oxygen resulting from a blood clot blocking an artery.

inhibitory neurotransmitter—decreases the activity of neurons; examples are GABA (gamma aminobutyric acid), serotonin, and glycine.

interferon—a class of protective proteins produced by the white cells and fibroblasts which prevent viruses from penetrating body cells and which may also help to regulate cell development.

involution—atrophy, shrinking in volume and mass.

LDL—low density lipoproteins, a fraction of blood associated with an increased risk of heart disease and, possibly, cancer.

leukocyte—scientific term for white blood cell. There are several types of leukocytes.

lipids—fats and oils. Fats are solid at body temperature, while oils are liquid at that temperature. Especially important are lipids found in the cellular membranes. Lipids, especially polyunsaturated, are sensitive to damage by oxidants and free radicals.

lipid soluble—dissolves in fats or oils.

lipoproteins—substances found in the bloodstream that are composed of proteins and lipids (fats); two types of lipoproteins are HDL and LDL.

lymphocyte—type of white blood cell which arises in lymph glands, spleen, thymus, or marrow.

macrophage—a type of white blood cell, which kills and eats bacteria, viruses, and cancer cells.

malonaldehyde—an aldehyde formed as a breakdown product of peroxidized polyunsaturated lipids in the body. Malonaldehyde is a mutagen, carcinogen, and cross-linker.

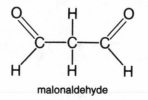

malonaldehyde

melanoma—a type of often deadly skin cancer.

membrane stabilizers—compounds which can protect cellular membranes from damage. Some examples are vitamin E, PABA, inositol, and hydrocortisone.

mitochondria—structures in cells that act as power plants. Mitochondria oxidize food to water, carbon dioxide, and energy. This energy is used by the mitochondria to convert low energy ADP (adenosine diphosphate) to high energy ATP (adenosine triphosphate), the cell's universal energy molecule. Free radicals are a normal and essential part of mitochondrial oxidation, but dangerous if they escape from the protective control systems in the mitochondria.

monamine oxidase (MAO)—an enzyme which, in the brain, degrades certain neurotransmitters (such as serotonin, dopamine, and norepinephrine). In aging brains, these neurotransmitters may decline in concentration or receptors may be lost or develop insensitivity to them. Monamine oxidase inhibitors are sometimes used as anti-depressants. By reducing the degradation of neurotransmitters, their concentrations can be increased. Examples of monamine oxidase (MAO) inhibitors are isocarboxazid, phenelzine, and tranylcypromine.

monounsaturated fat—a fat which contains a single carbon to carbon double bond. This double bond can react more readily with oxygen in a free radical reaction than the single bonds. Most monounsaturated fats are more similar to saturated fats than polyunsaturated fats in their ease of free radical autoxidation (the process that causes rancidity.)

mutagen—a chemical which causes alterations in DNA structure, usually resulting in faulty cell function and sometimes in cancer.

NaPCA—the sodium salt of pyrollidone carboxylic acid, the primary natural moisturizer found in human skin.

NE—see norepinephrine.

neurites—thin tendrils growing from each neuron in the brain in large numbers, through which the neurons communicate with each other. There may be over 100,000 neurites growing from a single neuron. The natural hormone nerve growth factor (NGF) stimulates growth of neurites (required for learning). Hydergine® (Sandoz) may also stimulate neurite growth via the same mechanism as nerve growth factor.

neurochemical—a chemical found in and active in the nervous system.

neuromodulators—substances that modify nerve function.

neurons—nerve cells.

neurotransmitter—a chemical which serves to carry messages between neurons in the brain. Dopamine, norepinephrine, acetylcholine, serotonin, and GABA are several important known neurotransmitters; there are many others under investigation.

NGF—nerve growth factor, a hormone important in the growth of nerves.

niacin—a form of vitamin B-3, also called nicotinic acid.

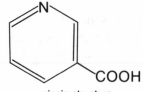

niacin structure

noradrenaline—see norepinephrine.

norepinephrine—an important brain neurotransmitter (chemical which enables brain cells to communicate with each other) which plays a role in primitive drives and emotions such as motivation, aggression, and acquisition of food and sex, and body movement. It is sometimes called noradrenaline and is, in fact, the brain's version of adrenaline.

normobaric—normal oxygen pressure.

nucleases—enzymes that take strings of nucleic acids apart.

oxidants—substances that cause oxidation.

oxidation—a type of chemical reaction in which an electron is attracted away from the oxidized entity. Oxygen is the most familiar oxidizer.

ozone—an excited, highly oxidized form of oxygen; its formula is O_3. It attacks a wide variety of organic molecules, particularly lipids, often producing free radicals in the process.

perfuse—to pour over or through.

peroxidase—an enzyme which catalyzes the breakdown of peroxides in the body.

peroxides—highly oxidized compounds like hydrogen peroxide (H-O-O-H), which not only oxidize lipids directly but in so doing create free radicals which spread in a chain reaction until stopped (quenched) by enzymes like peroxidases, catalases, and superoxide dismutase or by antioxidants like vitamin E and BHT.

peroxidized—a chemical which has been oxidized, so that a peroxide (relative of hydrogen peroxide, H-O-O-H) forms. Unsaturated fats (lipids) in the body are particularly susceptible to peroxidation.

PGI$_2$—see prostacyclin.

pituitary gland—a gland in the brain which produces and releases several hormones, including growth hormone, LH, FSH, TSH, vasopressin, ACTH, and others. An aging clock may be located in the pituitary.

placebo—a non-active substance used in an experiment to find out the purely psychological effects of the experimental design, and distinguish these from physiological drug effects. When pain patients are given a placebo which they are told is morphine, for example, about 40% of these patients obtain pain relief, though this percentage rapidly drops with repeated doses of placebo.

plaques—tumors which form in arteries, damaging the lining and resulting in deposition of platelets, red blood cells, cholesterol and other lipids which are subsequently autoxidized, swelling the wall and subsequently narrowing the artery.

plasma—the watery part of the blood, from which corpuscles have been removed.

platelet—structures found in the bloodstream which aggregate in the formation of blood clots. They are tiny fragments of cells derived from the bone marrow. Lipid peroxides stimulate platelets to make thromboxane A_2, which in turn causes platelets to adhere and aggregate, as in the formation of atherosclerotic plaques and clotting.

polycyclic aromatic hydrocarbons (PAH)—compounds found in combustion tars, created in the burning of nearly all fuels, which are metabolically activated (especially in the liver) to a mutagenic and carcinogenic form. These are probably the most important human chemical carcinogens and are suspected of being responsible for many of human cancers other than solar ultraviolet induced skin cancers. Tobacco smoke is by far the most important source for humans. They are also found in relatively large quantities on charcoal broiled meats.

polynuclear aromatic hydrocarbons—PAH, same as polycyclic aromatic hydrocarbons.

polypeptides—small proteins, such as hormones. The bond between adjacent amino acids in a protein is called a peptide bond.

polyunsaturated fats—fats containing two or more sets of double bonds between some of their carbon atoms; these bonds are susceptible to autoxidation attack by oxygen and free radicals, which converts polyunsaturated fats to carcinogenic, immune suppressive, clot promoting, cross-linking peroxidized fats. Antioxidants can protect these polyunsaturated fats from such chemical attacks. The more unsaturated (the more double bonds), the more readily autoxidized.

precursor—a chemical which can be converted to another is a precursor of the latter.

prolactin—a hormone released by the pituitary gland which has several functions, including stimulating milk production.

prophylactic—as a preventive.

prostacyclin—the prostaglandin hormone PGI_2, a natural hormone made by normal artery wall lining cells (intima) to inhibit the formation of abnormal blood clots. Peroxidized lipids can block prostacyclin manufacture, thus fostering the development of blood clots.

proteases—enzymes which break down proteins. An example is bromelain, found in raw pineapple. Some proteases have been found to stimulate the immune system.

psychobiochemistry—the biochemistry of mental processes.

psychopharmacology—the effects of drugs on mental processes.

quench—to terminate a chemical reaction, as in quenching a fire, or to return an excited energetic reactive molecule to its most stable lowest energy state.

receptors—special biological structures found on cells where active molecules such as hormones, enzymes, and neurotransmitters are attached to the cell surface. The cell then responds to the presence of the chemical in the receptors. Loss of and/or damage to receptors is one important event in aging.

reduction—a chemical reaction in which an electron is donated to the reduced entity.

refereed journals—scientific journals in which a committee of scientists review papers before they are published, checking for adequate experimental design and whether the experimental results support the conclusions reached.

retinoid—a substance closely related chemically to vitamin A. (Vitamin A is retinoic acid and its esters, or retinyl alcohol.) Retinoids regulate growth of epithelial cells (skin, lung, and gut) and are often powerful antioxidants and cancer preventing agents. The early stages of some epithelial cancers can be converted back into normal tissue by some retinoids. Retinoids are also chemically closely related to and made from carotenoids.

RNA—ribonucleic acid, which carries instructions from DNA (deoxyribonucleic acid) in the nucleus to cell polyribosomes, where proteins are made according to the RNA instructions copied from the DNA master version of the cell's blueprints.

saturated fats—fats containing no carbon-to-carbon double bonds; these fats are less susceptible to autoxidation (conversion to a peroxidized, immune-suppressive, clot promoting, carcinogenic form) than are polyunsaturated fats.

serotonin—an inhibitory neurotransmitter required for sleep; its natural precursor is the essential amino acid tryptophan, found in relatively large quantities in bananas and milk.

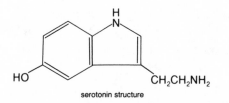

serotonin structure

singlet oxygen—an activated, energetic, reactive form of oxygen, which is produced by the reaction of ultraviolet light with oxygen in the skin, as well as in other chemical reactions.

Singlet oxygen can damage important macromolecules such as DNA. Singlet oxygen quenchers include beta-carotene (gives carrots their yellow color), which is pro-vitamin A, converted in the body to vitamin A on demand.

stimulatory neurotransmitter—increases activity of neurons; examples are norepinephrine and glutamate.

stimulus barrier—a mental state or drug state in which a person's brain can more readily filter out unwanted sensory stimuli. Examples include some of the most commonly used drugs: nicotine, alcohol, tranquilizers, caffeine. After regular use of these chemical stimulus barriers, discontinuing their use can result in the opposite effect, an increased sensitivity to sensory stimuli (as in withdrawal from cigarettes or alcohol).

sulfhydryl—a sulfur atom bonded to a hydrogen atom is a sulfhydryl group. A sulfhdryl compound contains one or more sulfhydryl groups. Examples include vitamin B-1, the amino acid cysteine, and the triple amino acid reduced glutathione.

superoxide dismutase (SOD)—a zinc and copper or manganese containing enzyme which reacts with superoxide radicals to convert them to less dangerous chemical entities. It is the fifth most common protein in the human body. All organisms not killed by air contain SOD. Intracellular cytoplasmic SOD generally contains zinc and copper, while mitochondrial SOD contains manganese.

superoxide radical—a free radical thought to play a central role in arthritis, cancer promotion, and cataract formation. Our major intracellular (inside of cells) defense against them is the enzyme superoxide dismutase.

synapse—the gap between nerve cells. One nerve cell stimulates another one to fire an electric pulse by secreting special chemicals called neurotransmitters into the synapse between the cells.

synergy—when chemicals or drugs are used together, they may show negative or positive synergy. Positive synergy occurs when the sum of the effects of chemicals acting together is greater than the additive effects of the individual chemicals. Negative synergy occurs when the sum of effects of the mixture is less than that of the individual components of the mix. Antioxidant mixtures commonly exhibit positive synergy, although negative synergy can also occur.

systemic—throughout the body.

systolic—the maximum blood pressure which occurs when the ventricle of the heart contracts; if your blood pressure is 115/70, 115 is your systolic blood pressure.

T-cells—thymus-derived white blood cells which kill and eat foreign invaders (bacteria, viruses, and cancer cells), or control the production or attack of other T-cells or the antibody-making B-cells.

thiol—a sulfhydryl compound. An example is vitamin B-1 (thiamine).

thrombogenic—causes blood clots to form.

thrombosis—blood clot blocking a blood vessel.

thromboxane A₂—a hormone that causes blood to clot.

thymocyte—white blood cell arising in or processed in the thymus.

thymotropic—causes enlargement of the thymus gland.

thymus—the master gland of the immune system, located behind the breastbone. The thymus "instructs" T-cells when to mature or reproduce, and what targets to go after. This gland shrinks in young adulthood, and immune system decline follows. The shrinkage and decline can be prevented or reversed by several methods and materials.

tissue culture—the growth of cells as tissue in a special medium. While the properties of tissue in culture differs in some ways from tissues in the body, particularly in lacking many of the protective mechanisms of the whole animal, tissue culture research can provide valuable data at relatively low cost.

topical—applied externally.

toxic—poisonous. Toxic effects of a substance are dependent on the dose. At sufficiently high doses, air, water, anything, even the inert gas helium, is toxic. (High pressure helium causes lethal convulsions even when adequate oxygen is present.)

Tricarboxylic Acid Cycle—see Citric Acid Cycle.

triglycerides—a class of fats found in the bloodstream.

tumorigenesis—the process of initiating a tumor.

uric acid—a chemical formed in the body during the metabolic breakdown of RNA, caffeine, and related substances by the enzyme xanthine oxidase. Uric acid or sodium hydrogen urate crystals precipitating into joints and kidneys can cause gout, with severe pain and possibly even permanent damage.

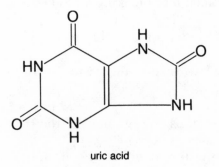

uric acid

water soluble—dissolves in water.

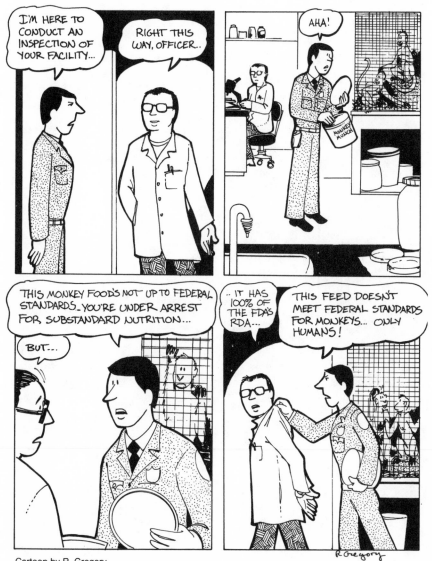

Cartoon by R. Gregory
© 1982 Durk Pearson and Sandy Shaw

BIMODAL DISTRIBUTION

INDEX OF INDEXES

Index of Indexes
Safety Index for *The Life Extension Companion*
Safety Index for *Life Extension, A Practical Scientific Approach*
Substance Index for *The Life Extension Companion*
Substance Index for *Life Extension, A Practical Scientific Approach*
General Index for *The Life Extension Companion*
General Index for *Life Extension, A Practical Scientific Approach*
Name Index for *The Life Extension Companion*
Name Index for *Life Extension, A Practical Scientific Approach*
Index Generation, Word Processing, and Personal Computers: A Colophon for the Late Twentieth Century

The indexes have been arranged in this order to facilitate the concurrent use of our two books. We believe that you can gain both greater benefits and safety by referring to both books, rather than just one or the other. Check both Safety Indexes before taking any actions based on what you have read in these books. Even essential nutrients can be dangerous under certain circumstances.

The Safety Indexes often have the same information presented under different headings to lessen the chance that you will miss some vital information. Before taking or doing anything, check the relevant entries in both Safety Indexes, reading the WARNINGs and CAUTIONs first, then the other relevant material.

The Substance Indexes, General Indexes, and Name Indexes usually *do not* list the items in the Safety Indexes. They also contain far less redundancy. When you look something up, especially in the Substance Indexes, you may find that the index entry has some additional relevant terms in parentheses—look up these, too!

Word Processing, Personal Computers, and Software

A COLOPHON FROM THE LATE TWENTIETH CENTURY

The traditional colophon tells the reader about the production of the book, describing type styles, paper, end boards, and sometimes even the printing press. Colophons have not changed much since Gutenberg, about 500 years ago.

Personal computers have been essential in producing both of our books, and our colophon will describe a bit of this process.

If you write as little as a page or two per week, but do not already use a word processor, you should seriously consider getting a personal computer and *quality* word processing software. First, see pages 722 to 724 in *Life Extension, A Practical Scientific Approach.* If that attracts your interest, purchase the most recent edition of *The Word Processing Book* by Peter A. McWilliams. Don't bother looking for a copy in a used book store; the buyers guide part of an old copy would be useless, and that is where you will need the most help.

We wrote most of this book in our trusty old Northstar Horizon® computer system, which was described in "A very special thank you" on pages 722 to 724 of our first book. When this system was occupied with other tasks, parts of *The Companion* were written on our Morrow Design Co. Micro-decision®, and on our two transportable computers, an old Osborne-1® and a new Kaypro 4®.

The Northstar Horizon® is still one of the fastest personal computers, but we purchased a much faster machine with over 1,000,000 bytes of RAM memory and 16,000,000 bytes of very fast hard disk memory for the indexing task. (Thank you very much for buying over a million copies of our first book!) This super personal computer is an Ithaca Intersystems Encore®, with their cache memory CP/M® operating system. (This is not a computer for a beginner.) Durk loves it, and Sandy now has full time use of our Northstar Horizon®, which she prefers.

We write with Micropro's Wordstar®, using the newest version #3.3 toward the end of the process. If you have an older version, it is worth getting an update; the earlier versions will crash if your text file exceeds about 500 kilobytes. There is an average of 2 kilobytes of information per printed page in our first book. (*The Life Extension Companion* text, exclusive of indexes, is 476 kilobytes, and *Life Extension, A Practical Scientific Approach,* exclusive of index, is 1,652 kilobytes.)

The new version can handle the 1,652,000 bytes of our first book without losing a single bit. This #3.3 version has other new goodies too, such as improved column and table editing facilities. We sure could have used those! Although the choice of word processing software certainly involves personal style and taste, all the professional writers we know use Wordstar®. We would like to specially thank Mr. Peter Schakow of Micropro® for his help in getting the ultra long file crash bug exterminated. Normally, we write using a separate file for each chapter, but the indexing process that Durk used required that the entire text be in one piece.

How did Durk produce these indexes?

First, Durk had to generate lists of words to be indexed. It soon became obvious that a *comprehensive* index required more than our memories; we already needed computer assistance. We use a splendid spelling checking program called Word+® from Oasis Systems. This spelling checker allows you to view the questionable word in context, and to assign it to any one of a number of special dictionaries if it is correct, or to correct it automatically. We rapidly realized that the large dictionary supplied with Word+® contained words that should be indexed, so he couldn't just use our special technical dictionaries that he had created using this program.

One of the best features of Word+® is that is is modular. Normally, it runs as a truly user friendly menu driven (just pick what you want to do from a menu and it does it) spelling checker. This program is constructed from several modules which can be used independently and this capability was essential for Durk's task. One of the modules is Dictsort, a program which sorts a list of words alphabetically so that they can be used as a special dictionary for the spelling checker. Chapter, by chapter, Dictsort sorted both books, pass by pass, into a list of about 13,000 words. A quick look at that list gave us a real shock: half of the words were technical.

To make a long story short (all the unneeded ordinary words had to be edited out by hand), by the time phrases were included in the lists of things to be indexed, the lists contained 14,153 words.

We also discovered that we had cited the work of approximately 1,000 scientists!

Clearly, one index for each book would be difficult to use; for example, important safety warnings would be buried. After Durk separated the lists of words and phrases by index type (safety, substance, general, and name), he was ready to index.

There are two types of indexing programs. Nearly all of them, including Micropro's StarIndex®, require marking the beginning and end of words and phrases in the text with special non-printing control characters. That is very distracting while writing, and a great deal of work.

Durk was rescued from this ghastly manual task by a module called Phrase from an Oasis Systems® software package called Punctuation+Style®. (This is in effect a considerable part of the Bell Telephone Laboratories Writers Workbench® which costs $4,000 and runs on maxicomputers. The Oasis Systems® software package costs $125, and it runs nearly as fast on your personal computer as the $4,000 software does on a million dollar computer. Wayne Holder of Oasis Systems is a fine programmer, and we would like to thank him for his help in making his software modules do things that he never had in mind when he wrote them. How many writers need to process unusual "words" like 6-ethoxy-1-2-dihydro-2-2-4-trimethylquinoline?)

The Phrase module accepts a list of words and phrases and marks them in the text with any characters that you specify. It is usually used as part of the Punctuation+Style® software package for improving writing style, a task it performs amazingly well.

If you use an indexing program like StarIndex® which requires marked text, you will definitely want Punctuation-+Style® to automate the text marking, and Word+® to help you generate the list of words and phrases to be indexed. Durk had already started indexing with another program when we got StarIndex®, but he did have a chance to try it out on a few chapters. It works with the WordStar® Mail-Merge® form letter printing option to index the book a chapter at a time. It has a very flexible output format so that you can specify exactly how you want the index to look, and it produces a very attractive output. It has one sometimes unfortunate feature; it also produces a reformatted output file of the extire text whether you want it or not. If you like the regular WordStar® print formatting (which is already exceptionally good), and if your disk space is limited, this feature can be inconvenient. Hopefuly the next version will allow you to turn it off.

Durk generated these indexes using the second type of indexing program, one which reads an input file of words and phrases to be indexed, reads an input text file of any length, and generates an index file as output. He used a not-quite-ready for sale developmental version of Phrase Index® from Oasis Systems.

With plenty of Wayne Holder's help, Durk modified this program to handle our odd "words." In its present incomplete pre-release form, it does not do a fancy job of formatting the index, so he had to do that by hand. He is certainly looking forward to avoiding that task on our next book.

The Punctuation+Style® software package has a program called Cleanup, which does precisely that; it cleans up text for phototypesetting directly from your disk. That is how

The Life Extension Companion is being produced. Cleanup found nearly 1,000 punctuation errors, most of them being an absence of two, rather than one, spaces after each period. It also found several unpaired parentheses and quotation marks and a few run together words. We missed these flaws and so did the professionals hired by Warner. Now we understand why manual typesetting costs so much and is so time consuming. What attention to minute detail! With Cleanup, Durk found and fixed all these errors in one day.

Another thunder storm is brewing—it really does rain in Los Angeles—the one yesterday killed the power twice, and we do not yet have uninterruptable power supplies for our computers. A power failure while the computer is modifying the disk directory scrambles everything abysmally, so Durk is going to stop writing right now, edit the text with WordStar®, check the spelling with Word+®, and clean it up with Cleanup from Punctuation+Style®, and send these indexes to our publisher.

Live Long and Prosper,
Durk & Sandy

PS: The Word+® found and corrected 13 spelling errors in this colophon, and Cleanup from Punctuation+Style® found 42 errors of spacing, and 3 repeated words (as in this this example.)

SUPPLIERS:

Ithaca Intersystems
P.O. Box 91
Ithaca, New York, 14850

Northstar® Computer
    Company
P.O. Box 947
Pinellas Park, Florida, 34209

MicroPro International
33 San Pablo Ave.
San Rafael, California, 94903

Oasis Systems
2765 Reynard Way
San Diego, California, 92103

The Word Processing Book is $10 postpaid from:
Prelude Press
P.O. Box 19937
Los Angeles, California, 90019
(If you have Visa® or MasterCard®, call 1-800-421-1809 toll free, or 1-213-733-1111 in California.)

INDEX TO:
GENERAL TOPICS

IMPORTANT NOTICE:

Do not use any information from our *Life Extension Companion* or our *Life Extension. A Practical Scientific Approach* without first checking the Safety Indexes for both books for the supplement, drug, or action that you plan to take. Also check the Safety Indexes for any illness that you might have and for any drugs that you are now using, since this may influence the safety of your intended actions. It is important that you heed these warnings.

Live Long and Prosper,

Durk Pearson & Sandy Shaw

abilities verbal and visual 39, 40
abortion 158
abstinence 124
abstract reasoning 38, 41
abstracts of scientific papers 182, 231, 242–43, 250, 251
accelerated hazard test 168
accidents 10
acclimation to time zone changes 10, 108
acne 127
acromegaly 334
adaptation 5, 10, 102, 108, 113, 114
additives 55, 63, 96, 178, 202–03, 205–06, 301, 333
adenohypophyseal growth hormone 328
adipokinesis 254
adrenal cortex 6
adrenergic 21, 43, 103, 311, 315
advertising 64, 69, 126, 165, 176, 192, 240
aerobic 312
aftertaste 305
aggression 25, 30, 33, 36, 43, 140, 143, 327
aggressiveness 25, 30, 33, 35, 36, 43, 121, 140, 143, 327
aging 24, 28, 41, 46, 49, 59, 76, 79, 83, 84, 86, 89, 91, 92, 97, 122, 125, 127, 131, 142, 149, 152, 161, 175, 178, 186, 196, 198, 201, 202, 208, 218, 219, 220, 223, 225, 226, 227, 228, 230, 231, 232, 233, 234,

235, 236, 238, 239, 300, 301–02, 306,309, 310, 312, 315, 318, 319, 322, 326,331
aging clocks 76, 145, 312, 315, 324, 328
aging mechanisms 41, 84, 302
air cleaners 57
air pollution 29, 49, 91–92, 94, 172
airtight containers, for vitamins and foods 187, 204
alcoholism 29, 82, 83, 312
alertness 110, 113, 117
allergies 176, 239
alpha receptors 21
alternative health care 62, 254
alveolar macrophages 60, 61, 83, 198, 203–04, 207
Alzheimer's disease 67, 134
amendment, Kefauver 66, 170, 171, 237
American Aging Association (AGE) 208, 226, 227, 228, 229, 309
amnesia 39, 124
amphetamine abuse 48, 111, 122–23
amphibians 139
anaerobic 312
analogs 151
anecdotal evidence 213, 313
anemia 67, 133, 134, 135
anger 35–37
angina pectoris 40, 146
angiology 199

animal studies 19–20, 29, 32, 50, 51, 55, 56, 66, 70, 72, 74, 75, 80, 81, 97, 98, 118, 121, 128, 134, 142, 143, 148, 152, 168, 169, 170, 171, 175–76, 182, 183, 189, 194, 198–99, 202, 205, 206, 207, 216–17, 232, 235, 250, 253, 254, 316, 318, 321, 334
anorexia nervosa 66
anoxia 313
anterior lobe 323
anterior pituitary 249
Anti-Aging News 234, 302, 309
anti-anxiety 26, 37, 38, 315
anticancer agents 207, 208, 236
antiinflammatory 100
antiviral agents 157
anxiety 26, 32, 37–38, 103–04, 315
aortic 199
appetite 51, 324
approval, drugs 62, 63, 66–68, 85, 107, 134–35, 154–55, 166, 167, 237, 309
approved uses, drugs 66–68, 165–66
aqueous solutions 85
aroma 321
arousal 44, 115
arrhythmias 66, 107, 299, 313
art 306
arteries 19, 21, 80, 84, 159, 196, 314, 318, 324, 329, 330
arteriosclerosis 29
arthritis 45, 49, 63, 86, 92, 98, 99, 126, 127, 128, 131, 195, 239, 314, 324, 332
artists 306
ascites 61, 73
assays 119, 142, 184, 189
assertiveness 32, 33
asthma 103
astronauts 232
atherogenic 50, 120, 142, 195, 313
atherosclerosis 29, 50, 51, 98, 100, 122, 142, 188, 195, 199, 313, 314
atherosclerotic plaques 6, 45, 72, 112, 314, 324, 329
athletics 248, 251
atmosphere 24, 171
atoms 16, 71, 77–78, 92, 127, 194, 318, 321, 329, 332
atrophy 7, 159, 325
attitudes xi
auditory nerves 317
autocatalytic process 316
autoimmunity 314
automobiles 15, 21, 25, 40, 80, 111, 149, 157, 224
autoxidation 16, 18, 24, 60, 74, 77, 81, 85, 187, 189, 194, 196, 199, 201, 202, 311, 312, 314, 316, 326, 329, 330, 331
average life span 80, 216
awake state 117, 122–23

B-cells 7, 46, 51, 313, 314–15, 333
babies. See Infants
bacteria 6, 39, 45, 50, 51, 60, 72, 80, 112, 122, 197, 203, 207, 238, 313, 324, 325, 333
baldness 76, 77, 312, 315
balloon and catheter xvii
ban on artificial sweeteners 170
baseline laboratory studies xiv, 155, 255

bedridden patients, deep vein clotting in 159
benzodiazepine receptors 37, 38, 43, 115
beta receptors 21, 103
bibliography 114, 215, 233, 234, 238
binding 37, 38, 84, 85, 96, 97, 99, 119, 313
bioactivity 184
bioavailability 82, 176, 177, 178, 315
biochemistry 6, 25, 27, 32, 36, 38, 41, 79, 84, 92, 97, 108, 110, 117, 118, 135, 139, 143, 183, 185, 194, 330
biofeedback 21, 22
biogenic 124, 149, 250
biological clocks 11, 312, 315
biological rhythms vii, 10–11, 108, 114
biologist 47
biology 30, 60, 115, 131, 149, 199
biomedicine iii, xvi, xvii, 22, 74, 161, 218, 219, 220, 223, 228, 240, 243, 244, 248, 301, 309
biophysics 91, 183
biopotency 184
biorhythms. See biological rhythms
birds 10
birth 41, 91, 158, 159, 160, 175
bitter 305
black market 168
blacks 135
bladder 9, 13–14, 24, 27, 54, 78, 100
blindness 151, 171
blockers 19, 21, 35, 43, 53, 75, 78, 79, 103, 104, 107, 127, 133, 159, 174, 202, 314, 322, 324, 330, 334
blood pressure 7, 11, 21, 22, 28, 33–34, 48, 66, 103, 107, 111, 140, 238, 319, 333
blood pressure gauge 21–22
blood-brain barrier 18, 33, 109, 152, 197, 237, 253
bloodstream 6, 8, 25, 119, 164, 237, 313, 323, 325, 329, 334
blood vessels xii, 19, 129, 321, 334
body fat 49, 305
bonds, chemical 18, 24, 75, 81, 146, 151, 194, 314, 317, 318, 319, 321, 326, 329, 332
bones 7, 18, 25, 45, 121, 314, 324, 329. See also marrow
brain 6, 7, 9, 11, 16, 18, 19, 20, 25, 26, 30, 33, 35, 35–36, 37, 39, 40, 41, 43, 45, 48, 54, 84, 86, 89, 98, 102, 103, 107, 108, 109, 110, 111, 114, 115, 116, 117, 118–19, 121, 122–23, 124, 125, 131, 133, 134, 135, 139, 140, 141, 143, 149, 151, 168, 196–97, 205, 209, 236, 239, 311, 315, 316–17, 320, 323, 324, 326, 327, 328, 332
brain waves 22
brand names 119, 142, 179, 180
breakfast 51, 114, 190
breast cancer 53, 55, 60, 150, 159
breastbone 45, 80, 121, 334
breathing 25, 40, 72, 92, 171, 175, 197, 202
Brevispina 98, 100
bristlecone pines 207
brittleness 80
broiled foods, carcinogens and 329
bronchodilating drugs 103
browning 96, 97, 129
bruises 92, 96, 97, 127, 196, 258
buffered 305

Burkitt's lymphoma 55, 150
bush 103, 161
businessmen 22, 101, 104
bypass. *See* cardiac bypass surgery
byproduct 77, 128

C-Strips® 305
cadavers 24
caliper, skinfold thickness 305
calories 114, 199, 263
cancer xiii, xiv, xvi, 6, 7, 10, 14, 22–23, 25, 30,
    45, 47–48, 49, 50, 51, 53, 54, 55, 56, 58,
    59, 60, 70, 72, 73, 78, 79, 80, 83, 85–86,
    87, 91, 92, 94, 95, 97, 101, 112, 120, 122,
    127, 131, 142, 150, 151, 159, 160, 169,
    170, 172, 173, 194, 195, 198, 199, 201,
    202, 204, 205–6, 207, 219, 231, 235–36,
    238, 239, 240, 241, 299, 302, 313, 315,
    316, 319, 322, 324, 325, 326, 329, 331,
    332, 333
cancer incidence 91–92, 322
cancer causing agents 71, 85
cans 170
capillaries 18, 33, 97, 98, 133, 197, 323
capsules xiii, 66, 180, 188, 189, 190, 191, 300,
    301, 303, 304, 305, 306
carcinogens 13, 50, 55, 56, 71, 120, 142, 151,
    168, 169, 170, 195, 205, 311, 312, 315,
    319, 321, 325, 329, 330, 331
carcinogenesis 73, 87, 95, 313
carcinoma. *See* cancer
cardiac arrythmias. *See* arrythmias
cardiac bypass surgery xvii
cardiovascular conditioning 232
cardiovascular disease 49, 54, 58, 70, 79, 86,
    92, 112, 127, 160, 175, 195, 202, 219,
    238, 322
Cartoonist services 306
cartoons 5, 8, 14, 15, 23, 34, 37, 40, 42, 46,
    47, 51, 64, 65, 68, 71, 72, 76, 77, 79, 87,
    88, 102, 112, 120, 123, 129, 153, 154,
    155, 251, 306–07, 308
case histories viii, 63, 76, 213, 218
catalogs 300–06
catalysis 56, 62, 96, 97, 131, 316, 321, 322,
    328
cataracts 54, 70, 128, 195, 332
catnaps 122
cats 16, 97, 131
cavities 40
cells vii, 6, 18–19, 22, 25, 30, 47–48, 50, 51,
    59, 60, 67, 71, 78, 80, 81, 89, 96, 97, 103,
    124, 127, 129, 133, 134, 135, 139, 175,
    197, 205, 242, 253, 317, 318, 320, 325,
    326, 327, 330, 331, 332, 333, 334
central nervous system ix, 31, 132, 171, 198,
    199, 208, 237, 317, 322
cerebral cortex 102
cerebrospinal fluid (CSF) 6
cervical carcinoma 150
chain reaction, free radical 18, 81, 92, 97,
    322, 328
characterization, systems 183
charitable antiaging research foundations
    xviii, 237, 302
charts 115, 158, 232
chelation vi, 8, 9, 27, 51, 54, 78, 88, 96,
    97–98, 99, 100. 120, 190. 317

chemicals 13, 17, 24, 25, 33, 38, 41, 48, 50,
    63, 80, 84, 94, 97, 109, 112, 117, 119,
    122, 131, 139, 142, 143, 149, 174, 175,
    179, 181, 182, 184, 185, 186, 187, 188,
    193, 194, 195, 201, 253, 311, 312, 313,
    316, 317, 320, 323, 327, 328, 329, 330,
    331, 332, 333, 334
chemistry 75, 122, 208
chemists 91
chemotactic 59
chemotherapy 241
chest 3, 34, 173
chickens 51, 157
children 41, 46, 134, 135, 301, 305
cholinergic 115, 119, 142, 317
chromatography 119, 142, 207
chromosomes 56, 205, 317, 322
chronobiology 114
circadian rhythms 10, 108, 114, 125, 315
circulation 16, 236, 314
citations 114, 231, 249
claims 64, 66, 188, 190
clinical gerontologists 226
clincal laboratory tests, personal 218, 219,
    220
clinical research 69
clocks 117, 125, 235, 315, 325
clones 318
clotting 19, 50, 72, 92, 120, 142, 159, 188–89,
    195, 196–97, 314, 324, 329, 330, 331, 334
coal burning power plants 172
codes 222, 223, 226, 229, 320, 322
cognitive abilities 44, 102, 104, 115, 121
coils, DNA 317
cold sores 150
cold water stress 148
colds 45, 46, 59, 235
collapse, respiratory, drug interactions and
    156
colon 53, 55, 150
combustion 10, 25, 55, 56, 172, 205, 314, 316,
    319, 329
common cold 59, 235
commuting 22, 24
competition xvii
complete blood count (CBC) 155
computers ix, xvi, 219, 231, 240, 242
computer system xvi
concentration, mental 39, 111, 121, 141
conception 218
concussion 131
conditioning 232
condom 158
confusion, mental 228
congestion 25
connective tissue 17, 24, 51, 80, 235, 318, 321
consciousness xi, 117, 121
consultation, physician xiv, 7, 24, 81, 103,
    129, 131
consultation service 301
consumers 64–65, 66, 119, 142, 178, 189, 192
containers 80, 187, 203–04
contraceptives 158, 159, 160
contractions 48, 144
contraindications xvi, 209
control systems 92, 99, 326
controlled experiments xii, 66, 135–36, 142,
    213–14, 313, 318, 320, 324

convulsions 123, 171, 334
cooking 199, 202, 203, 208, 300, 303
coping xiv, 7, 12, 13, 26
cornea 128
coronary 19, 209
corpuscles 329
correlation 95
cortex 6, 29, 149
cosmetics 85, 165, 180, 302, 304
cosmetic formulations 85
cosmetics industry 85
cost-effectiveness 178
coughs 14
cracked lips, vitamin A overdose symptom 8,
    51, 87
cramps 40, 148
creativity 40, 121, 305
creosote bush 207
crippling 103
crises 133, 134, 135–36
cross-linkers 85, 312, 319, 321
cross-linking 75–76, 80, 81, 83, 84, 85, 89, 91,
    312, 318, 319, 321, 330
cruciform vegetables 206–07
crushing injury 20, 97–98, 129–30, 131
crystalline 300
crystals 75, 76, 113, 305, 334
CT (CAT scan, computerized tomography)
    243
cycles 10, 17, 109, 114, 117, 122, 123, 146,
    175, 251, 317, 319, 334
cystine stone formation 9, 13, 24, 27, 54, 78,
    100
cystitis 63, 126
cytologist 152
cytoplasmic 332

dam, relative hazard 172, 173, 174
dandruff 78, 92, 127, 196
DATA ix, 218, 219, 220–221, 222, 225, 226,
    227, 228, 229
data bank of geriatrics and clinical
    gerontology physicians. See DATA
data base xvi, 218–19, 231
DATA physicians' register. See DATA
deerhounds 55
deficiencies 17, 54, 72, 74, 76, 85, 86–87, 121,
    147, 171, 324
degenerative diseases 151, 301, 314
Delaney amendment 170, 171
delusions, safety, 122, 231
depletion 6, 7, 18, 19, 20, 21, 35, 48, 111,
    122, 197
depression 6, 7, 32, 33, 34, 35, 36, 43, 48, 50,
    87, 108, 111, 115, 139, 141, 143, 199, 221
desensitization 102
detoxification 19, 56, 152, 176, 323
diabetes insipidus 67
diabetes mellitus 81–82, 103, 239, 255, 299
diagnoses, need for professional xii
diaphragm 158
diarrhea 148
diastolic blood pressure 319
diet 3, 21, 30, 55, 59, 62, 71, 73, 76, 80, 86,
    115–16, 117, 147, 178, 194, 196, 199,
    205, 206, 208, 235, 238, 239
dietary restriction, 235
diffusion barriers 189, 191

dilator 323
discontinue phenylalanine and tyrosine if
    overstimulated 33–34
discontinue vitamin A supplements if
    overdose symptoms develop 51
discontinuing stimutus barrier substances 332
disease 3, 9, 14, 26, 45, 46, 49, 50, 54, 58, 67,
    70, 74, 79, 86, 92, 101, 112–13, 116, 127.
    133, 134, 135, 150, 157, 175, 195, 196,
    202, 209, 219, 238, 239, 314, 321, 322
distillation 181
dizziness 103
DNA synthesis 151, 253
doctors xvi, 3, 21, 28, 107, 134–35, 153, 155,
    213, 221, 226, 227, 232–33, 299, 302
Doctors' Registry for the Treatment of the
    Aging (DATA) 218, 226, 227
dogs 20, 55, 60
donations xviii, 300, 302, 303, 304, 305, 306,
    308
dopaminergic stimulation 144, 253
Dorland's Illustrated Medical Dictionary 5
doses 6, 8, 9, 13, 16, 20, 24, 25–26, 27, 28, 30,
    33, 35, 36, 37, 38, 39, 41, 42, 48, 51, 53,
    54, 55, 56, 57, 58, 59, 62, 66, 70, 72–73,
    81, 82, 88–89, 104, 107, 109, 110, 111,
    118, 119, 124, 128, 134, 139–40, 141,
    143, 144, 148, 152, 154, 157, 160,
    168–70, 171, 175, 186, 189, 196, 198,
    210, 219, 223–24, 226, 232, 238, 300,
    329, 334
double blind experimental method. See
    controlled experiment
dreams 41, 117, 121, 124, 125
drinking 11, 12, 13, 15–16, 18, 24, 56, 57, 70,
    75, 80, 87, 89, 170
driving 15–16, 25, 40, 111
drug approval 63, 66, 166, 237
drug interactions 232
drug regulation 66, 236–37
drugstores 6, 21, 26, 38, 63, 75, 99, 113

E deficiency 323
earplugs 11
economics 149, 232
edema 131, 171
EEG. See electroencephalogram
efficacy 135, 237
Ehrlich ascites tumor 61, 73
EKG. See electrocardiogram
elasticity of skin 24
elderly 67, 125, 141, 228, 250, 301
electrocardiogram (EKG) 320
electroencephalogram (EEG) 22, 320
electromyography 22
electron spin resonance (ESR) spectrometer
    131
electrons, unpaired 16, 49, 71, 77, 92, 97,
    127, 195, 321
electronic precipitator 91
embalming 24, 56
embryo 175
emergency medicine and dmso use 131
EMG. See electromyography
emmissions 172
emotions 33, 39, 102, 109, 110, 121, 173, 185,
    186, 205, 234, 320, 327
emphysema 81, 127

346

encapsulation 179, 180, 189
encapsulators 180, 189
endometrial carcinoma 160
energy 16, 17, 20, 22, 35, 92, 110, 128, 146,
    171, 173, 187, 197, 202, 236, 314, 317,
    326, 330
enhancers 39
environment 110, 121, 170, 213, 238
enzymatic 16, 80, 195, 196, 197
epidemics 53, 64, 150, 203
epidemiology xiii, 15, 54, 58, 70, 91, 221, 321
epideremal 86, 91, 320
epilepsies 127
epistemology 321
epithelial 51, 86–87, 126, 160, 212, 320, 321,
    331
equipment 21, 111, 157, 207, 213, 303
ergometer 251
erythropoietic protoporphyria 89
esterification 187, 188
estrogenic 159, 160, 181
ethics 192, 221
excitation 25–26, 27–28, 35, 36, 42, 110, 118,
    143, 323, 328, 330
executive lifestyle 4
executives vii, 3, 6, 10, 11, 17, 22, 26, 108,
    227, 228
exercise 55, 122, 232, 248, 251, 252
exhaustion 6, 17, 147
experimental subjects 8, 218, 219, 221, 223,
    225, 318, 320
experimental treatment 37, 161, 219, 320
experts 103, 114, 151, 184
eyebrows 8, 87
eyes xii, 23, 41, 94, 121, 128, 171, 237, 311,
    318

face 24, 202
fads vii, 107, 163, 230
fallacies vii, 66, 107, 163, 168, 180
family 160, 182–83, 254
fantasy 177
farms 23, 74, 105, 253
fasting 55, 114, 122, 169
Fat-O-Meter®, skinfold caliper 305
fatalities 103
fatigue 108
fats. See unsaturated fats
FDA label regulations 182
fears 11, 102–03, 104–06, 107
feasting 114
feelings. See emotions
feet 63, 122
females 40, 80, 145, 148, 159–60, 175, 250,
    254–55, 321
fermentation 178
fertility control 158, 160
fetal 89
fiber 39, 309, 317
fibrillation 20
fibrocystic breast disease 53, 60
fight or flight reaction 5–6, 102, 106, 107,
    150
fillers, 188, 189, 190, 191, 301
filters 11, 39, 56–57, 332
fingers 103
fires 330, 332
fishy odor 39

fitness 232
flatworms 254
flavors 205, 208
flexible 133
flies 104, 172
flu 45, 49, 235–36
flush, niacin 143–44, 300
flush, niacin (similar to Masters and Johnson
    sex flush) 144
flying 10, 11, 101, 104–05, 108, 109, 111
followup 155
food ages, just as living organisms do 201
Food Chemicals Codex 181
foundations 302–03, 308–09
free radical damage 18–19, 77–78, 86, 92, 97,
    129, 196, 205, 314
free radical disease 49, 92, 127, 195, 196,
    321–22
free radical pathology ix, 31, 132, 133, 231,
    236
free radical theory of aging ix, xiii, 83, 92,
    127, 131, 152, 196, 198, 208, 226, 227,
    309
frogs 17, 148
frying 190
fuels 10, 70, 315, 319, 329
funding xviii, 134, 161, 170, 221, 223, 249,
    300, 301, 302, 303, 304, 305, 306, 309
future 3, 32, 38, 65, 131, 135, 234

galvanic skin response (GSR) 22
garlic breath, urine, and sweat, selenium
    warning 73
gas chromatography/mass spectrometry 131
gas-liquid chromatography 119, 142
gastric cancer 60
gastrointestinal tract 19, 40, 51, 148, 317,
    320, 321. See also gut
genes 134, 135, 322
genetics 32, 101, 150, 175, 315, 318, 319, 322
genetic defects 89, 91
genetic disease 133
genetic engineering 135
genital herpes 150, 152, 153
genitalia 150
geriatrics ix, 83, 226, 227, 228, 229, 233
germs 175–76, 181, 182
gerontologists 226, 235
gerontology xi, 43, 115, 125, 226, 227, 228,
    229, 234, 236, 250, 300
gestation 183
GH. See growth hormone
giants xii
glands 7, 8, 39, 45, 48, 49, 53, 54, 80, 121,
    171, 313, 315, 317, 323, 324, 325, 328,
    330, 334
gout 20–21, 299, 334
grants xviii, 55, 303
greenness 96
grief 7
groggy, jet lag 108
growth 41, 45, 48, 49, 53, 54–55, 61, 75,
    76–77, 78, 82, 86, 91, 100, 112–13, 115,
    121, 122, 124, 125, 143, 219, 249, 250,
    251, 252–53, 254–55, 256, 313, 320, 322,
    323, 327, 328, 331, 334
growth hormone (GH) release 121, 122, 249,
    253, 254

347

growth hormone (GH) secretion viii, 59, 248, 250, 251, 255, 256
GSR. *See* galvanic skin response
guinea pigs 18, 19–20, 80, 82, 220, 232
gum 76, 314, 319
gut 15, 39, 66, 86, 109, 148, 152, 188, 331
gynecologists 152

habits 113
hair vii, 8, 51, 62, 63, 75, 76, 77–78, 87, 88, 205, 300
hair follicles 78
hair loss 51
hallucinations 122, 124
hallucinogenics 117
hands xii, 5, 11, 66, 104
hangovers 15–16, 57, 81
hard disc xvi
hardware 35, 126
hard work 3
hardback 231, 232, 236
hardening of the arteries 80, 84
Hawthorne effect 213. *See also* placebo effect
head 11, 63, 78, 122, 168, 214–16, 232
headaches 36, 39, 42, 51, 87, 141, 143, 210
healing 17–18, 49, 86, 97, 127, 143, 236, 238, 251, 320, 323
health food 6, 26, 38, 62, 63, 75, 99, 126, 179
health food stores 62, 63, 64, 66, 112, 117, 119, 142, 168, 176, 182, 203
hearing 21
hearsay 231
heart xiii, 19, 20, 21, 25, 28, 30, 34, 48, 66, 111, 194, 197, 199, 228, 232, 238, 313, 319, 333
heart attacks 3, 19, 20, 103, 159, 194, 197, 238, 239, 314
heart disease xiv, 30, 49, 50, 209, 323, 325
heartbeat 319
heat 129
heavy metals poisoning 98
height 223
helixes 317
hemolysis 98, 129, 314, 323
HEPA filter 56
herpes viii, 53, 55, 63–64, 150, 151, 152, 153, 154, 156, 203, 238, 314
heterozygote 134
high blood pressure 7, 11, 21, 22, 28, 33–34, 48, 66, 103, 107, 111, 140, 209, 238
high pressure liquid chromatography 207
homeostasis 199, 237
homozygote 134
hormesis 95
hospitals 16, 18, 55, 131, 151, 157, 159, 221
humidity indicators 304
humoral 30, 59
hydroelectric power 171
hydrolysis 191
hydrophobic 157
hypercholesterolemia 199, 324
hyperglycemia 255
hypersensitivity to sunlight 89
hypersexuality 143
hypertension. *See* high blood pressure
hypervitaminosis A 58, 87
hypoallergenic 304
hypoglycemia 75, 81, 239

hyponatremia 171
hypophyseal 249
hypopituitarism 254–55
hypotension 7, 34, 157
hypothalamus 65, 254, 255, 315, 317, 324
hypoxia 19, 41, 133, 134, 209, 324

ice 180
identical twin 318
ideology, 230
illegal 63, 134
illegally 126
illness xi, 26, 34, 99, 150, 219
immune system vii, 6, 7, 8, 45, 46, 47, 48, 49, 50, 52, 53, 54, 72, 75, 80, 92, 101, 112, 120, 121, 124, 142, 150, 151, 188, 195, 198, 203, 207, 248, 251, 313, 314, 318, 320, 323, 324, 330, 334
immune system decline 334
immune system stimulant 8, 53, 313
immunity 10, 29, 30, 46, 47–48, 59, 80, 92, 198, 330
immunization 46
immunocompetence 29, 61
immunological theory of aging 235
immunology 30, 59, 73, 125
immunosuppression 195
immunotherapy xvi
impotence 194
indicators 83
individualization, use and 28, 33, 109, 111
inducible, protective enzymes 93, 94
industry 65, 85, 126, 179, 180, 189, 190, 192, 303
infants 46, 171, 306
infarction 30, 199, 324
infections 9, 14, 24, 27, 30, 53, 54, 60, 63, 78, 100, 150, 151, 152, 157, 159, 203, 238, 239
inflammation 31
infrared 126
infusions xii, 251, 253
inhibitory 25, 37, 61, 73, 117, 143, 207, 253, 322
injections 20, 53, 97, 128, 131, 159
injuries 6, 7, 16, 20, 49, 50, 60, 97, 126, 127, 129–30, 131, 197, 207, 314
inoculations 53, 61, 73
insects 176
insomnia 25, 27, 36, 42, 110, 118, 140, 143
insulin hypoglycemia 251–52
intelligence 32, 38, 39, 41, 67, 69, 121, 145, 230, 231
intensification, of orgasms 39
interactions, drug 84, 92, 103, 322
intercourse 159
intermediary metabolism 115
internal radiation 92, 127, 196
international unit 180, 191, 192
interstitial cystitis 63, 126
Intersystems Encore® computer xvi
intervention in the aging process 161
intestinal. *See* gastrointestinal tract
intestines 19
intima 330
intoxication 15–16, 98
intranasally 145
intravenous 3, 18

348

intravenous ascorbate (vitamin C) 305
in vitro studies 61, 82, 136, 152, 183, 210
in vivo studies 146, 183, 253
involution 7, 325
ionizing radiation, 92, 95
irritability 51, 87, 140
irritants 78, 94, 311
ischemia 30–31
itching 51, 143–44, 150
itchy scalp 78
IUDs 158

jelly 189
jet   10–11, 108, 109, 111, 113, 114,

jitters 41
jogging 232
joints 98, 128, 324, 334
journals xvi, 134, 230, 231, 234, 237, 240,
    243, 248, 331

Kefauver amendments 237
kidneys 9, 13, 24, 27, 54, 78, 81, 82, 100, 299,
    334
Krebs cycle 17, 146, 317–18

labels 64, 66, 165, 166, 180, 182, 190, 199,
    304
lamb 51
larynx, spasm and vasopressin (Diapid®) 40
learning 38, 39, 41, 43, 67, 103, 106, 110,
    121, 124, 141, 145, 149, 196, 232, 237,
    327
legs 17, 20, 96
lens 128
lesions 50
leukocyte 19, 30, 59, 199, 324
libido 39, 140, 145, 148, 175–76
life extenders do it longer 149
life extension i–xviii, 19, 35, 59, 69, 73, 82,
    90, 96, 100, 107, 114, 122, 124, 149, 152,
    160, 178, 181, 190, 198, 207, 211, 216,
    217, 218, 222, 223, 225, 230, 232, 233,
    234, 235, 236, 248, 251, 299, 300,
    301–02, 304, 306, 307, 308, 309–10
*Life Extension, A Practical Scientific
    Approach* xi–xviii, 7, 8, 12, 14, 28, 35, 38,
    42, 49, 57, 63, 76–77, 112–13, 119, 134,
    149, 179, 181, 183, 186–87, 203, 231,
    236, 248, 251, 299, 304, 306
lifespan 55, 207, 208
lifestyle xiii, xiv, 4
ligands 43, 115
lightheadedness 103, 157
lighting 213
lipid antioxidant 199
lipid coat 151, 157
lipid soluble 300, 325
lipid-coated viruses 151, 152
lipid-containing viruses 60
lips 8, 51, 87
liver 16, 41, 51, 54, 55, 56, 80, 81, 88, 150,
    152, 153, 154, 155–56, 176, 311, 312,
    329
lobe 323
long-lived species 128
long-term study conducted on middle aged
    men in San Mateo 18

longevity 94, 140, 303
lunch 12, 51, 114, 119
lungs 13, 14, 15, 25, 30, 40, 50, 51, 56, 58, 59,
    60, 81, 86, 94, 173, 198, 207, 305, 316,
    320, 321, 331
lymph glands 45, 325
lymphatic system 324
lymphocytes 29, 50, 51, 325
lymphoma 55, 150
lysis 323

macrophages 50, 60, 61, 80, 83, 198, 203–04,
    207, 325
male pattern baldness 76
males 35, 80, 83, 125, 144–45, 148, 175, 250,
    251, 254–55, 312, 315
malignant melanoma. *See* melanoma
malpractice 155, 241
mammals 55, 93, 139, 146
mammary tumors 55
manic-depression 139
marrow 7, 45, 121, 314, 324, 325, 329
maturation 60, 124
maximum life span 93, 235, 302
mazes 196, 205
meals 8–9, 13, 26, 66, 114, 118, 124. *See also*
    diet
measles 151
mechanisms 5, 19, 41, 60, 71, 76, 79, 84, 89,
    97, 101, 108, 123, 127, 133, 144, 157,
    231, 254, 300, 302, 315, 327
media 64, 92, 172, 222, 223
median 253
Medical Hotline® 30, 69
Medlars (National Library of Medicine
    computer literature search service) ix,
    xvi, xvii, 231, 237, 240, 241–42, 243, 248,
    251
Medline (National Library of Medicine
    computer literature search service) ix,
    240, 249
megadoses xiv, 176
melanocytes 78
melanoma 34, 48, 100, 111, 326
membranes 6, 71, 97, 98, 127–28, 130, 175,
    197, 237, 316, 318, 320, 324, 325, 326
memory xvi, 33, 35, 38, 39, 41, 43, 44, 67,
    106, 110, 111, 115, 121, 124, 125, 141,
    142, 145, 149, 232, 237, 302, 311, 317
menopause 145, 159, 160, 312, 315
menstruation 145
Merck Index 181
metabolism 6, 16, 49, 60, 62, 77, 81, 92, 93,
    95, 99, 115, 127–28, 149, 170, 183,
    186–87, 197, 199, 202, 253, 305, 312,
    313, 320, 321, 329, 334
metastases 100
methylate 184, 193
methylation 184
mice 30, 53, 55, 59, 61, 73, 80, 82, 83, 100,
    171, 173, 205, 207, 208, 216, 217
microbes 175, 176
microcirculation 31
microscopy 23, 98, 317
middle-aged men 14
misinformation 202, 230, 235
mitochondrial 187, 326, 332
moisturizers 84, 85, 90, 91, 304, 326

349

molecules 16, 17, 18, 24, 45, 71, 75, 77, 81, 92, 127, 133, 135, 146, 151, 174, 175, 185, 186, 195, 253, 311, 313, 314, 318, 319, 320, 321, 322, 323, 324, 326, 328, 330
Moloney sarcoma virus 53
monitor, blood pressure 21–22
monitored, your health by your personal physician 228
monitoring, your health xiv, 21–22, 28, 33–34, 218, 228
monkeys 148, 152, 157
monoclonal antibodies 66, 318
moods 48, 110, 141
mortality 20, 60, 83, 160, 161, 196
motivation 35, 110, 320, 327
multiple sclerosis 151, 314
muscle tone 141
muscles 17, 19, 39, 49, 55, 63, 102, 103, 110, 148, 253, 311, 317
muscular output 311
mutagenic substances 50, 52–53, 71, 120, 142, 195, 321, 329
mutations 13, 18, 71, 78, 83, 92, 151, 198, 201, 207
myocardial infarction 30, 199

nails 35
nasopharyngeal cancer 150
National Library of Medicine's data base (see Medline and Medlars)
natural substances xii, xiii, xiv, 26, 37, 39, 41, 63, 65, 67, 79–80, 85, 86, 87, 91, 99, 108, 111, 120, 122, 144, 170, 174, 175, 176, 177–78, 179, 180, 181, 182, 183, 184, 185, 186, 187, 188, 189, 190, 191, 192, 193, 206, 209, 304, 311, 320, 324, 327, 330, 331
natural antioxidant 128, 143, 188, 190, 300
natural form 180, 186, 188
natural source 185, 188, 193
natural vitamins 174, 176, 177–8, 179
naturalness 193
nature 25, 29, 36, 43, 59, 83, 91, 115, 131, 170, 172, 178, 182, 183, 187, 193, 256, 318
nausea 41–42, 210
navy 36
neck 307
negative synergy 332–33
neoplasia 29, 61
nerves 18, 19, 25, 33, 35, 36, 41, 48, 59, 89, 109, 110, 117, 119, 123, 139, 197, 236, 256, 311, 312, 315, 316, 317, 320, 327, 332
nervousness ix, 20, 31, 116, 123, 132, 143, 171, 198, 199, 208, 237, 255, 311, 316, 317, 320, 322, 325, 327, 331
neurites 41, 327
neurochemistry 11, 48, 327
neuroendocrinology 255, 324
neuromuscular 311
neurons 327. See also nerves
neurotransmitters 25, 33, 36, 39, 48, 54, 109, 110, 112, 115, 117, 119, 123, 140, 143, 148, 311, 317, 320, 322, 323, 325, 327, 331, 332

newsletters 234, 301, 302, 308, 309
niacin flush (similar to Masters and Johnson sex flush 144
noise 56, 217
non-FDA-approved uses 11
nonsmokers 29
normalizing 7, 34, 111, 140
normobaric, oxygen pressure 173, 327
nose 3, 67, 86, 143, 198
nuclear power plants 172
nucleus 331
nursing 228, 229
nutrients vii, 6, 8, 12, 13, 24, 26, 32–33, 35, 37–38, 48, 53, 63, 64, 70, 75, 81, 99, 109, 110, 112–13, 117, 127, 174, 191, 218, 219, 232, 236, 238, 300, 301–02, 303, 311
nutrient mix 302
nutrition xi, xiv, 3, 4, 6, 10, 28, 70, 74, 82, 99, 115, 117, 125, 131, 182, 186, 192, 199, 208, 218, 219, 221, 223, 225, 226, 239, 301, 304, 305

obesity 254–55, 323
odors 39, 78, 119, 142, 189, 198, 205
organisms 46, 92, 97, 98, 127, 175, 197, 201–02, 312, 316, 319, 332
organs 55, 84, 85, 157, 205, 324
orgasms 33, 41, 143–44, 146, 323
orgy 155
Oroville dam 172
ovaries 159, 160
over-the-counter (non-prescription drugs) 62, 131, 142, 239
overdose 8, 41–42, 51, 72–73
overdose, vitamin A 8, 51
overdose, selenium 72–73
overstimulation 43
overweight 50, 198
overwork 3, 6, 11
oxidation 8, 16, 17, 54, 56, 77–78, 81, 85, 88, 96, 127, 159, 174, 175, 178, 191, 196, 201, 202, 236, 253, 314, 317, 318, 326, 328
oxidized xiii, 9, 24, 27, 54, 78, 100, 128, 146, 175, 187, 188, 195, 201, 203–04, 205, 311, 313, 314, 317, 319, 321, 326, 328
Oxygen Free Radicals and Tissue Damage 100

pacemaker 19
pain 3, 127, 128, 133, 135, 159, 213, 329, 334
paint 314
paralysis 46, 171
paramedics 131
paranoid 122
paraplegia 97, 131
parasites 324
parenteral 254
parents 46, 228
Parkinson's disease 9, 26, 316
patents 107, 127, 154
pathology viii, 31, 77, 79, 86, 117, 132, 133, 189, 231, 236
pathways 17, 20, 79, 115
perception 35, 144
perfusing 17, 148, 328
peristalsis 148

permeability 19
peroxidation xiii, 49, 50, 60, 61, 66, 71, 73, 85–86, 92, 119, 120, 127–28, 135, 142, 180, 183, 188, 189, 195, 198, 199, 210, 310, 312, 315, 321, 325, 328, 330, 331
personal physician, importance of 218, 220, 221, 224, 301
pesticides 126
pharmaceuticals vii, 11, 62, 63, 65, 66, 68, 158, 160, 237, 305
pharmacology xii, xiv, 43–44, 69, 115, 157, 210, 251
phobias vii, 11, 21, 32, 35, 43, 66, 101–02, 103, 104, 105–07
photosynthesis 316
Physician's Desk Reference® 63, 68, 209, 232
physician-patient relationship 10
physicians xi, xiv, xvii, 7, 11, 21, 24, 33, 68, 69, 73, 82, 98, 99, 103, 107, 129, 131, 134, 165–66, 209, 213, 218, 225, 226, 227, 228, 229, 231, 233–34, 240, 241, 242, 243, 301, 306, 309, 310. *See also* personal physician
physiology 5, 6, 7, 11, 13, 26, 85, 125, 232, 251, 312, 317, 329
pigment 23
pigs 14, 18, 19–20, 80, 82, 220, 231, 253
pills 21, 38, 63, 158, 159, 160, 175, 301
pilots 171
pimples 127
pituitary gland 39, 45, 48, 49, 53, 55, 111, 121, 144, 145, 249, 251, 252, 253, 254, 255, 313, 315, 317, 323, 328, 330
placebo effect. *See* Hawthorne effect
placebos 66, 213, 320, 328–29
plants 23, 97, 172, 174, 175, 176, 187, 193, 202, 205, 207, 316, 326
plaques 6, 45, 72, 112
plasma 98, 100, 197, 199, 252–53, 255, 329
platelet aggregation, strokes, and heart attacks 196, 329
platelets 196, 199, 314, 329
play viii, xvi, 108, 121, 131, 139, 332
poisoning: by heavy metals (lead, mercury, etc.) 98; by water and oxygen 171, 210
poisons: in urban air 25; vitamin C as antidote 239
polio 46
pollutants increase production of protective enzymes 93–94
pollution vii, 29, 56, 91, 92, 94, 239. *See also* air pollution
polyamine synthesis 253
polynuclear aromatic hydrocarbons, 24, 25, 70, 109, 172, 199, 205, 314, 319, 321, 329
polyribosomes 331
positive synergy 183, 333
postmenopausal women 145, 159, 160
potency of vitamins 180, 183, 184, 189, 190, 191, 192, 300, 302
potentiation, alcohol, of brain and spinal cord injury 31
PPM (parts per million) 94
practitioners 165
precipitator 56
precursors 311, 319, 330, 331
predictor 18, 143

pregnancy 239; in mice and BHT 207
pregnant and lactating women, professional nutritional advice available 301
prescription drugs 4, 6, 7, 8, 11, 20, 21, 23, 32, 33, 38, 39, 41, 50, 55, 62, 63, 66, 99, 111, 121, 126, 131, 140, 144, 145, 166, 224, 239
preservatives viii, 60, 151–152, 201, 202, 203, 205, 206, 207, 230, 303, 304
preservatives may be preserving you 201, 207
pressures, career 3
preventive medicine xi, xiv
primates 95, 238
professional assistance xviii, 3, 101, 104, 234, 241, 301, 309, 310
profilers 237
project, clinical research, sickle cell anemia, free radicals and treatment via high dose Hydergine® 134
promoters 87, 143, 169, 170, 188
prophylaxis 134, 135–36, 330
protectants 60
protective mechanisms 26, 334
protoporphyria 89
psoriasis 153
psychobiochemistry 102, 330
psychomotor 43, 115
psychoneuroendocrine 29, 61
psychopharmacology 124, 125, 330
psychosis 42, 122, 141, 210
psychotherapy 11
psychotropic 117, 152
puberty 7
pulse 22, 332
pumps, vitamin C 18, 237
purity 65, 126, 190

quality xiv, 93, 126, 148, 180, 185, 191, 301, 308
questionaire 154, 228

rabbit alveolar macrophages 198, 203
rabbits 15, 50, 128, 198, 199, 203
race 40
radiation 16, 49, 79, 81, 83, 91, 92, 93–94, 95, 127, 172, 173, 196, 321
radiation sickness 16, 49, 81, 127, 196, 321
radioactivity 172, 173, 253
radiodurans 196
rags, oily, free radicals and spontaneous combustion 314, 316
rancidity 49, 50, 71, 78, 85, 92, 119, 120, 128, 142, 175, 188–89, 195, 196, 198, 199, 202, 203, 205, 314, 315, 326
rapid eye movement (REM) sleep 41, 121
rats 13, 16, 17, 29, 30, 43, 51, 55, 56–57, 66, 80, 81, 82, 91, 114, 125, 147, 148, 183, 196, 254
RDAs (FDA's Recommended Daily Allowances) 219
reaction time 39, 145, 232
reactive hypoglycemia 75
reactors 197
receptors 21, 26, 37, 38, 43, 86, 91, 103, 110, 115, 139, 149, 253, 312, 315, 316, 326, 330

redwood trees 207
refereed journals 234, 331
referrals, professional 228, 229, 310
register, experimental life extension subjects
and clinical research physicians (SAVES
DATA) viii, 218, 221, 222, 226, 227
regulating 48, 69, 110, 119, 236
regulation 10, 59, 66, 86, 115, 125, 145, 236,
256, 317
regulations 107, 126, 171, 182, 236
regulatory 107
rehabilitation 305
rejuvenation 83, 148
REM (rapid eye movement) 41, 121;
deprivation 123; sleep (dreaming) 121,125
remission 60, 153, 204
replete 48
replication 53
reproduction 101, 175, 219
reptile brain 102, 103
reptiles 5, 139; brain, 102–03
research subject physician authorization form
(SAVES DATA) 225
resetting 10, 108, 114
resorption 238
respiration 156, 253
respirators 171
rest 18, 19, 86, 127, 160
restlessness 110
restore 53, 159
retinas 317
rheumatism 239
rheumatoid arthritis 98, 99, 314
ribosomes 253
RNA synthesis 253
rock music 201
rotifers 98, 100
royalties i, 207
ruptures 18

safety x, 66, 122, 165, 166, 168, 170, 171, 172,
173, 210, 237, 299
sarcomas 53, 55
satiation 66
satiation signal 66
SAVES, Study of Aging Volunteer
Experimental Subjects ix, 218, 219, 220,
221, 222, 223, 225
SAVES DATA 218, 219, 225
SAVES subject register 219, 221, 222, 225
scalp 78, 320
Schizophrenia 34, 48, 99, 111, 139, 239, 316
sclerosis 151, 314
Scottish deerhounds 55
scurvy 18, 20
sedation 25, 27, 36, 104, 105, 110, 118, 143
seeds 175, 178
self-administering 99, 219, 221, 226
self-experimentation 213, 218, 219, 220, 232
senility 41, 133, 195, 210
sensations 105, 143
sensitivity, Hydergine® 42, 210
serial learning 38, 43
serum xiii, 60, 61, 86, 142, 155, 159, 186, 194,
196, 251, 323
serum C levels as predictor of 5-year survival
18
severe overwork 6

sex viii, 33, 137, 139, 144, 146, 148, 149, 158,
159, 160, 223, 312, 321, 327
sex flush, Masters and Johnson 139
sexes 254
sexism 32
sexual 39, 139, 146, 148, 160
sexual activity 141, 317, 320
sexual rejuvenation 6, 139
shampoos 78
shock 17, 19, 20, 123
sickle cell anemia, free radicals, and high
dose Hydergine® therapy vii, 67, 133,
134, 135, 136
side effects xi, 9, 27, 33, 39, 58, 146, 232, 239
skin 8, 22, 23, 24, 58, 78, 80, 84, 85, 86, 87,
88, 89, 91, 191, 205, 304, 312, 318, 319,
320, 321, 326, 329, 331
skinfold measurements, for body fat
determination 305
sleep viii, 36, 55, 108, 109, 110, 113, 114, 117,
119, 120, 121, 122, 123, 124, 125, 250,
251–52, 315, 323, 331
sleepwalking 120
Slim Guide®, skin fold thickness caliper 305
slow growing hair 76
smoking 11, 13, 14, 18, 24, 29, 56, 57, 58, 75,
80–81, 82, 83, 87, 89, 158, 159, 160, 316
smoking, lung cancer, and beta carotene 14,
58
sobriety 64, 69
solar ultraviolet light, cancer danger 329
solvents 65, 127, 319
sparganum 254
spasms 20, 40
spawning 315
specific metabolic rate 95
spectrometer 126, 131
spin 131
spinal cord 16, 18, 33, 85, 97, 131, 196, 205,
236, 317
spirometer, for self-measurement of
respiratory function 305
spirometra 254
spleen 45, 121, 324, 325
spontaneous combustion, and free radicals
314, 316
sports 126, 127, 129
Sprague-Dawley rats 205
stamina 17, 146
standard deviation 216–17, 218
starvation 66
statistical significance 217
Statistical variation 214, 216
stethoscopes 11, 21
stimulate 8, 21, 50, 75, 81, 96, 112, 159–60,
248, 254 315, 316, 327, 329, 330, 336
stimuli 11, 12, 39, 55, 110, 119, 332
stimulus barrier 11, 332
stomach 9, 33, 55, 99, 104, 109, 140, 143,
152, 154, 189, 323
stomach cancer, possible reduction by BHT
206
storage 54, 92, 191, 314
strains 55, 63, 151, 206, 207, 238, 315
strength 17, 144, 300, 305, 318
stress 4, 14, 3, 4–6, 7, 10, 11, 12, 17, 19, 20,
24, 25, 26, 29, 101, 148, 150, 152, 219,
239, 323

stressors 11, 13, 22, 29
strokes 16, 30, 41, 86, 133, 209, 239, 314
Study of Aging Volunteer Experimental
  Subjects (SAVES) ix, 218, 219, 223, 225
success vii, 3, 32, 33, 42, 97, 101
sudden death 3, 20, 103
suicides 36, 41, 143, 210
sulfur containing 53, 75
sunglasses 11
sunlight, cancer danger 22–23, 58, 63, 80, 89.
  See also tanning
suntan, cancer danger 22–23, 89
supercoiled DNA 317
supernutrition 237–38
supplementation 51, 239
supplements xiv, 4, 7, 8, 9, 10, 17, 26, 27, 28,
  36, 50, 53, 62, 70, 78, 80, 82, 86, 88, 99,
  110, 113, 118, 122, 143, 171, 199, 219,
  221, 223, 225, 226, 228, 235, 239, 300,
  301, 304
suppliers 9, 13, 19, 85, 191, 299, 304
suppository 159–60
suppressants 92
surgery 18, 18, 19, 30, 59, 124
surveillance, immune system 50, 112
surveys 70, 101, 239
survival xvi, 29, 59, 80, 82, 83, 202, 312
survivors 7
susceptibility 70, 87
sweating 104
sweet 124
sweetening 170
swelling 127, 130, 329
swimming 17, 147
symptoms of vitamin A overdosage 51
synapses 35, 317, 332
synergy 143, 172, 176, 183, 332–33
synovial fluids 98
synthetics viii, xii, xiii, xiv, 39, 55, 63, 66, 99,
  111, 120, 143, 145, 174, 176, 177–78,
  179, 180, 181, 182, 183, 184, 185, 186,
  187, 188, 189, 190, 191, 192, 199, 203,
  205, 300, 305, 313, 315
systolic blood pressure 333

T-cells 7, 45, 52, 122, 314, 333, 334
tablets xiii, 23, 99, 160, 176, 191, 209, 210,
  301, 302, 303
tanning 22–23, 24, 56, 63, 84
tarry 371
technology xii, xiv, 29, 186
teenagers 16, 101, 301
tension 22, 39
testicular degeneration, from natural
  estrogens 176
throat 13, 56
thrombogenic substances 50, 120, 142, 195,
  334
thymocyte 334
thymoma 59, 83
thymotropic 30, 59, 124, 334
thymus 26, 27, 45, 49, 50–51, 53, 54, 60, 80,
  121–22, 124, 171, 324, 325, 334
tissue culture 94, 152, 334
tolerance 124, 300
toxicity 14, 13, 24, 29, 42, 60, 71, 72, 82, 83,
  94, 135, 151, 152, 157, 195, 319, 323, 334
tranquilization 105

trauma 29, 31, 131, 323
travel 10, 21, 110, 112–13, 242
Trends In Pharmacological Science® 43, 69,
  115
tricarboxylic acid cycle 17, 317, 334
tumorigenesis 199, 334
tumors 47–48, 53, 55, 61, 73, 80, 199, 205,
  208, 254, 314, 329, 334
twins 318

ulcers 25, 239, 299
ultraviolet light 22–23, 58, 84, 89, 126, 150,
  152, 205, 208, 316, 319, 331
unapproved drugs and uses viii, 64, 69, 134,
  155, 165–66, 232
uncontrolled free radicals can do serious
  harm 202
unicorn 241
unneutralized acidic vitamins (niacin and C)
  and ulcers 299
unpaired electrons 16, 49, 71, 78, 92, 97, 127,
  195, 321
unsaturated fats viii, 85, 86, 89, 175, 181, 183,
  184, 196, 322, 328, 329–30
upper (stimulant) 40
urethra 144
urinary bladder, cystine stones 9, 13, 24, 27,
  53–54, 78, 99–100
urinary tract infection, cystine stones 9, 14,
  24, 27, 53–54, 78, 99–100
urination 121, 232
uterus 55, 159
utilization 166
utilize 240
UV ultraviolet light and skin cancer danger
  58, 89

vagina 144, 159, 160
vagus nerve 20
vascular disease 209
vegetables 15, 50, 96, 181, 184, 188, 189, 190,
  191, 198, 206–07
venereal disease 150
ventricle 333
ventricular fibrillation 20
verbal abilities 39, 40
violence, reduction with tryptophan 36, 143
viruses 6, 45, 51, 53, 55, 60, 71, 80, 112, 122,
  150, 151, 152, 154, 157, 238, 313, 314,
  324, 325, 333
vision 23
visualization 121
visual abilities 40, 121
vitalistic nonsense 191, 192
vitamin C pumps 18, 237
volunteers 30, 53, 59, 169, 218, 219, 220, 225,
  254
vomit 210
vulcanization 76, 202, 319

waking 108, 315
warmed-over flavor 208
water soluble 9, 13, 24, 27, 54, 78, 100, 334
weaning 207
weight 50, 65, 66, 248, 251, 253, 303
white blood cells 7, 19, 45, 49, 50, 51, 80,
  122, 151, 197, 198, 203–04, 314, 324,
  325, 333, 334

windshield wiper, free radical deterioration
318
wired 33
withdrawal, narcotics and stimulus barrier
drugs 305, 332
wound healing 251
wounds 20, 143, 239
wrinkling 24, 80, 86, 89, 312, 318

x-rays 16
xeroderma pigmentosa 89

yeast 176, 300

zero tolerance concept violates Second Law
of Thermodynamics 171

INDEX TO SUBSTANCES:
FOODS, NUTRIENTS, DRUGS, AND CHEMICALS

IMPORTANT NOTICE:

Do not use any information from our *Life Extension Companion* or our *Life Extension. A Practical Scientific Approach* without first checking the Safety Indexes for both books for the supplement, drug, or action that you plan to take. Also check the Safety Indexes for any illness that you might have and for any drugs that you are now using, since this may influence the safety of your intended actions. It is important that you heed these warnings.

Live Long and Prosper,

Durk Pearson & Sandy Shaw

Leading Numbers:
2-deoxy-5-iodouridine (idoxuridine) 151
5-HIAA (5-hydroxyindoleacetic acid) 25, 36, 143, 323
5-HT (serotonin, 5-hydroxytryptamine) 249
5-hydroxyindoleacetic acid (5-HIAA) 143, 323
6-OH-dopamine (6-hydroxy-dopamine) 316

acetaldehyde 13, 16, 24, 29, 56, 57, 60, 80–81, 82, 83, 311, 312
acetate 56, 181, 186, 191
acetyl coenzyme A 17, 146, 317
acetylcholine (ACH) 11, 39, 110, 119, 139, 141, 144, 146, 148, 311, 317, 327
ACH. *See* acetylcholine
acids 28, 80, 82, 99, 119–20, 142, 150, 151, 152, 186, 189, 305, 312, 317, 318, 321, 322, 323, 328, 334
ACTH 328
Acyclovir® 151
additives 55, 178, 202, 206, 301, 333
adenosine diphosphate (ADP) 326
adenosine triphosphate (ATP) 17, 19, 146, 314, 317–18, 326
ADP. *See* adenosine diphosphate
adrenaline (epipnephrine) 6, 21, 33, 102, 103, 110, 311, 315, 327
agonists 312
alcohol 11, 12, 15–16, 24, 30, 37–38, 41, 56, 80–81, 156, 184, 224, 311, 312, 321, 331, 332
aldehydes 24, 25, 81, 311, 312, 319, 325

alkaloids 43, 44, 115, 209, 210
allergens 176
aloe vera 300
alpha agonists 21
alpha tocopherol (vitamin E) 60, 182, 183, 184, 187, 188. *See also* vitamin E
alpha tocopherol acetate (vitamin E) 183
aluminum 187, 204
amine 312, 323
amino acids 6, 7, 8, 13, 16, 25, 26, 33, 36, 48, 49, 53, 55, 57, 60, 62, 66, 72, 75, 76, 86, 93, 97, 99, 109, 110, 111, 115, 122, 125, 127, 128, 140, 143, 149, 174, 196, 197, 202, 300, 302, 303, 305, 312, 313, 322, 329, 331, 332
aminoacetic acid. *See* glycine
amphetamines 34–35, 48, 110–11, 122–23
amyl acetate 321
analgesics 128
androgens (male sex hormones) 312
anti-cancer compounds 50, 54
anti-clotting hormone 19, 80, 159
anti-free radical 50, 209
anti-mutagen 54
antibacterials 304
antibodies 45, 80, 121–22, 151, 313, 314, 318, 324
anticholinergics 117
antidepressants 6, 34, 48, 60, 111, 115, 140, 149
antigens 313, 323
antiinflammatories 100

antimicrobials 304
antioxidant nutrients 24, 236, 302
antioxidant vitamins 13, 142
antioxidants (free radical scavengers) xiv, 8, 9,
    13, 15, 24, 27, 50, 54, 55, 56, 57, 60, 62,
    63, 71, 78, 79–80, 86, 87, 88, 89, 92–93,
    97, 100, 120, 127, 128, 129, 134, 151,
    159, 174, 175, 183, 185, 186, 187, 188,
    189, 190, 195, 196, 197, 199, 202, 203,
    204, 205, 206, 207, 208, 209, 219, 220,
    232, 300, 301, 302, 304, 305, 313, 315,
    316, 319, 328, 330, 331, 333
Anturane® 20, 21
aphrodisiacs 324
apomorphine 249
apples 129
arachidonic acid 119, 142
arginine 8, 9, 30, 53, 59, 124, 252, 254, 313
aromatics 109
artificial sweeteners 170
ascorbate (vitamin C) 30, 59, 61. *See also*
    vitamin C
ascorbic acid (vitamin C) 20, 29, 30, 59, 60,
    61, 83, 178, 200, 319. *See also* vitamin C
ascorbyl palmitate (fat soluble ester of
    vitamin C) 188, 190, 204, 205, 235, 300,
    303, 304
Aspartame® 305
aspartic acid 99
aspirin 62, 98
atherogens 92
atoms 16, 71, 77, 92, 127, 194, 318, 321, 329,
    332
ATP. *See* adenosine triphosphate
autoantibodies 314

B-1. *See* vitamin B-1
B-2. *See* vitamin B-2
B-3. (niacin-nicotinic acid, nicotinamide) 26
B-5. (pantothenic acid, calcium pantothenate)
    16, 25, 26, 49, 86, 88, 89, 93, 97, 110,
    119, 127, 141, 142, 146, 174, 196, 197,
    202, 313
B-6. (pyridoxine) 7, 9, 13, 16, 25, 26, 35, 36,
    49, 78, 86, 93, 97, 110, 118, 127, 143,
    159, 160, 174, 196, 197, 202, 313
B-12. *See* vitamin B-12
bananas 21, 117, 129, 321, 331
barbiturates 156
bases xvi, 218, 219, 301
beets 63
benactyzine 106
benzene 126
benzoalphapyrene 55, 205, 313
benzodiazepine 26, 37, 38, 43, 115, 313
beta blockers 21, 43, 103, 104, 107
beta carotene 9, 14, 15, 23, 25, 27, 30, 56, 58,
    63, 86, 89, 97, 300, 302, 303, 304, 313,
    316, 331
BHA (butylated hydroxyanisole) 55, 157, 187,
    196, 303, 304, 313, 315
BHT (butylated hydroxytoluene) 55, 56, 60,
    63, 152, 153, 154, 155, 156, 157, 187,
    196, 199, 202, 203, 204, 205, 206, 207,
    235, 300, 303, 304, 313, 315, 328
binders 301
biochemical pathways 79
bioflavonoids 174, 176, 235

biogenic amines 124, 149, 250
Biosnax 65
biotin (vitamin H) 89, 300
birth control pills 158, 159, 160, 175
blockers 21, 103
blood 7, 11, 18, 19, 20, 21, 22, 28, 33, 34, 45,
    48, 49, 50, 51, 66, 72, 80, 81, 97, 98, 102,
    103, 107, 111, 120, 122, 129, 133, 140,
    142, 151, 155, 159, 195, 197, 198, 203,
    204, 209, 236, 238, 255, 314, 319, 323,
    324, 325, 329, 330, 333, 334
body fat 49, 305
bones 7, 18, 25, 45, 121, 122, 314, 324, 329
bread, whole wheat 176
bromelain 330
bromocriptine (Parlodel®) 140, 141, 144, 145,
    149
brussels sprouts 96, 97, 206
butter viii, 194
butylated hydroxyanisole. *See* BHA
butylated hydroxytoluene. *See* BHT

caffeine 41, 42, 210, 332, 334
calcium 98
calcium ascorbate (vitamin C)
calcium pantothenate (vitamin B-5) 16, 17,
    38, 39, 88, 89, 110, 146, 148, 235
calming neurotransmitter 36
cannabis 62
canthaxanthin 23–24, 58, 63, 87, 89, 300, 303
carbohydrates 26, 114, 116, 118–19, 317, 323
carbon 193, 194, 312, 321, 326, 329
carbon dioxide 16, 146, 193, 314, 318, 326
carbon monoxide 24
carboxylic acid 85, 326
carcinogens 55, 56, 70, 71, 78, 85, 87, 92, 151,
    168, 169, 170, 171, 172, 188, 200, 201,
    205, 206, 207, 311, 312, 315, 325, 388
carotene. *See* beta carotene
carotenoids. *See* beta carotene
carrots 14, 15, 23, 58, 89, 97, 316, 332
catalases 49, 79, 86, 93, 97, 128, 316, 328
catalysts 19, 129, 314, 316, 320
cataract 332
catecholamines 121, 125, 316, 320
CCK. *See* cholecystokinin
cereals 60, 190
chapparal herb extract. *See* NDGA
charcoal 329
chelate 96, 99
chelated copper 99
chelators 99
chloromethylating agents 184
chlorophyll 96
chocolate 114, 180
cholecystokinin (CCK0) 65, 66, 317
cholesterol xiii, 194, 197, 200, 238, 314, 324,
    329
cholesterol epoxides 321
cholesterol, itself is an antioxidant 197
choline 12, 39, 43, 110, 119, 141, 142, 147,
    300, 301, 311, 317
choline chloride with B-5 300
cholinergic 115, 119, 142, 317
chromium 300, 304
cigars 11
cigarettes 10, 13, 56, 61, 83, 172, 311, 312,
    316, 332

citrate 98
citric acid 99
citric acid cycle 17, 317, 334
Clonidine® 21
clot 19, 92, 159, 188, 189, 197, 198, 314, 324, 330, 331, 334
cloves 202
coal 172
cocaine 35, 39, 110–11
    cofactors 115–16
cold pressed wheat germ oil 175–76, 181, 182
collagen 17–18, 24, 80, 83, 84, 85, 91, 236
combustion tars 25, 56, 329
complement 45, 80, 121, 318, 324
complexes 100
conjugated estrogens (female sex hormones) 159
contraceptives 158, 159, 160
cookies 206
cooking oil 203
copper 19, 96, 97, 98, 99, 100, 129, 131, 314, 316, 332
copper salicylates 98, 99, 100
corn oil 196
corticosteroids 6
cortisol 254–55
cortisone 324
cosmetics 85, 165, 180, 301, 304
cosolvents 85
cream 180, 302
creosote bush (chapparal bush extract). See NDGA
cross-linkers 24, 85, 311, 312, 319, 321, 325
cruciform vegetables 206
cumin 115
cysteine 5, 8, 9, 13, 16, 24, 25, 27, 49, 53–54, 57, 59, 61, 62, 63, 72, 75, 76, 78, 80, 81, 82, 83, 86, 93, 97, 99, 100, 127, 128, 174, 196, 197, 202, 235, 299, 302, 313, 332
cysteine hydrochloride monohydrate 75
cystine 9, 13, 24, 27, 54, 78, 82, 100

d-alpha tocopherol. (vitamin E) 182, 183, 184, 186, 187, 188, 191
d-alpha tocopheryl acetate. (vitamin E) 191,193
d-alpha tocopheryl acid succinate (vitamin E) 190, 191
d-beta tocopherol (vitamin E) 184
d-gamma tocopherol (vitamin E) 184
d-penicillamine 97, 98, 99, 100
DA. See dopamine
dairy products
dandruff 78, 92, 127, 196
Deaner® 235
decarboxylase 253
dehydroascorbic acid 61, 319
delta tocopherol 184
deoxyribonucleic acid. See DNA
depressants 188
DES (diethylstilbesterol) 176
Diapid® 39, 40–41, 55, 66–67, 111, 121, 145, 232
diethylstilbesterol. See DES
dihydroergocornine. See Hydergine®
dihydroergocristine. See Hydergine®
dihydroergotoxine. See Hydergine®
dihydrolysergic acid compounds. See Hydergine®

dilators 323
dilauryl thiodipropionate 300
dimethyl sulfoxide. See DMSO
dimethylbenzanthracene 55, 56, 319
dimethylsulfide 126
dimethylsulfone 126
disulfide 128, 318, 319
disulfide bonds 75–76, 81, 318, 319
disulphide 83
diuretics 21
dl-alpha tocopherol (vitamin E) 182, 183, 184, 186
dl-alpha tocopherol acetate (vitamin E) 181, 183, 184, 191
dl-alpha tocopheryl acetate (vitamin E) 181
DMAE. See dimethylaminoethanol
DMSO (dimethyl sulfoxide) viii, 63, 64, 65, 126, 127, 128, 129, 131, 196, 319
DNA (deoxyribonucleic acid) 18, 22, 47, 50, 54, 58, 71, 72, 80, 85, 92, 97, 120, 127, 142, 150, 151, 175, 195, 253, 313, 315, 317, 318, 319, 322, 326, 330, 331
DOPA. See L-DOPA
dopamine (DA) 121, 139, 140, 149, 249, 252–53, 316, 320, 326, 327
dopaminergic stimulants 140, 144, 253
dopaminergic system 125, 249, 320
downers (sedatives) 156

EDTA 96, 98, 99, 100
EGF. See epidermal growth factor
eggs 9, 13, 16, 24, 27, 54, 62, 73, 75, 76, 78, 99
EGTA 98, 99
electrons 127, 131, 187, 328, 331
enhancers 39
enzymes 17, 18–19, 54, 71, 79, 80, 92, 93, 94, 97, 99, 128, 151, 152, 153, 157, 175, 186, 197, 202, 206, 238, 312, 316, 317, 320, 322, 326, 328, 330, 332, 334
epidermal growth factor (EGF) 86, 91, 320
epinephrine. See adrenaline
epoxides 56, 321
epoxy 321
ergot 43, 44, 115, 140, 209, 210
ergotamine 209
esters 58, 180, 182, 187, 188, 189, 191, 300, 321, 331
estradiol (female sex hormone) 160
estrogens (female sex hormones) 159, 160, 161, 175, 176, 182, 321
ethanol 31
ethoxyquin 186
excitatory neurotransmitters 25
extract of rosemary 202
extractables 176

fats (lipids) ix, 8, 18, 49, 50, 54, 56, 71, 77, 78, 85, 86, 88, 92, 97, 128, 151, 159, 175, 189, 190, 194, 195, 196, 198, 199, 200, 201, 202, 203, 204, 205, 207, 208, 253, 313, 314, 315, 316, 317, 325, 326, 329–30, 331, 334
fatty acids 151, 175, 196, 253, 321
feces 52
female sex hormones. See estrogens
FFA. See free fatty acids
fibroblasts 51, 321, 325

357

fillers 188, 189, 190, 191, 301
fluorine 128, 175
fly ash 172
folic acid 239, 299
food additives 63, 96
food preservatives viii, 60, 151, 201, 205, 230
foods 17, 114, 143, 146, 168, 174, 178, 190,
    191, 201, 202, 203, 204, 205, 300, 314,
    315, 317
formaldehyde 24, 56, 184, 312
formulations 85, 190, 301, 302, 304
free fatty acids (FFA) 254, 255
free radical damage 18, 19, 78, 79, 86, 92, 97,
    129, 196, 205, 314
free radical disease 49, 92, 127, 196, 321–22
free radical pathology ix, 31, 132, 133, 231,
    236
free radical scavengers (antioxidants) 16,
    321–22
free radical theory of aging ix, xiii, 83, 92,
    127, 131, 152, 196, 199, 208, 226, 227,
    309
free radicals 16, 18, 19, 25, 30, 41, 49, 50, 54,
    56, 71, 72, 73, 77, 79, 80, 81, 83, 84, 86,
    89, 92, 94, 95, 96, 97, 98, 99, 127, 128,
    129, 131, 132, 133, 152, 171, 175, 187,
    195, 196, 197, 199, 201, 202, 204, 208,
    209, 233, 235, 238, 301, 311, 312, 313,
    314, 316, 319, 321–22, 324, 325, 326,
    328, 330, 332
FSH (a gonadotropin) 254, 255
fuels 10, 70, 315, 319, 329

GABA (gamma aminobutyric acid) 300, 305,
    322, 324, 327
gamma aminobutyric acid. See GABA
garlic 73
gasoline 172, 314
gelatin capsules 189, 190, 191, 306
GH. See growth hormone
gluconic acid 99
glucose 254, 255, 304
glucose tolerance factor (GTF) 300, 304
glutamate 25, 322, 331
glutamic acid 322
glutathione 49, 61, 83, 86, 196, 197, 202, 300
glutathione peroxidase 54, 71, 73, 79, 86, 93,
    94, 97, 127, 197, 202, 322
glycine (aminoacetic acid) 25, 26, 28, 36, 37,
    99, 300, 312, 322, 324
glycoproteins 323, 324
gonadotropin 249
growth hormone (GH) 45, 48, 49, 53, 54, 55,
    61, 112, 113, 115, 121, 122, 124, 125,
    219, 249, 250, 251, 252, 253, 254, 255,
    256, 313, 322, 323, 328
growth hormone release (GH release) 121,
    122, 249, 253, 254
growth hormone releasers (GH releasers) 54,
    55, 112
growth hormone secretion (GH secretion)
    viii, 59, 248, 250, 251, 255, 256
GTF. See glucose tolerance factor

hair 5, 8, 51, 62, 63, 75, 76, 77, 78, 87, 300
ham 202
HDL. See high density lipoproteins
Head and Shoulders® (shampoo) 78

health food 6, 26, 38, 62, 63, 64, 66, 75, 99,
    112, 117, 119, 126, 142, 168, 176, 179,
    182, 203
heavy metals 25, 96, 97, 98, 99
heavy metals poisoning 98
helium 171, 334
hemoglobin 133, 134, 135
HGH (human growth hormone). See growth
    hormone
high density lipoproteins (HDL) 200, 323, 325
histamine 19, 143, 144, 323
histidine 143
hormones viii, 39, 45, 60, 66, 67, 81, 86, 121,
    124, 144, 148, 158, 159, 160, 175, 181,
    253, 254, 256, 312, 315, 317, 320, 323,
    324, 327, 328, 329, 330, 334
HPRL (human prolactin) 254–55
Hydergine® viii, 41, 42, 43, 44, 55, 61, 67,
    115, 133, 134, 135, 136, 209, 210, 249,
    327
hydrocortisone 326
hydrogen 151, 312, 332
hydrogen peroxide 128, 316, 317, 323, 328
hydroperoxides 188, 189, 324
hydroxyl radicals 128, 324

idoxuridine (2-deoxy-5-iodouridine) 151
immune system stimulants 8–9, 53, 313
immune system stimulant nutrients 8, 9
immunosuppressive 195
inducers 60, 94, 124
inhibitors 7, 28, 83, 111, 203, 326
inhibitory neurotransmitters 25, 36, 117, 143,
    322, 324, 331
inositol 25, 26, 28, 36, 37, 38, 110, 128, 300,
    326
insulin 62, 81, 82, 118, 251, 252, 254, 255,
    323
insulin hypoglycemia 251
interferon 45, 51, 80, 121, 324, 325
intravenous ascorbate 305
ions 96
iron 19, 96, 97, 129, 131, 314, 316
irritants 78, 94, 311
Isocarboxazid® 326
isolysergic acid compounds 249
isomers 182, 183, 184
isotopes 172

JB-329 117
Jell-O® 85
jojoba 207

1-alpha tocopherols. (vitamin E) 183
L-DOPA 8, 9, 26, 27, 55, 115, 122, 125, 140,
    149, 249, 250, 251, 252, 254, 255, 300,
    303, 319
1-gamma tocopherols 183
1-penicillamine 98
laetrile 68
lard 196
laxatives 148
LDL. See low density lipoprotein
lead 24, 25, 98, 99
leather 84
lecithin 119, 120, 141, 142, 147, 300
leftovers 205
LH (a gonadotropin) 254, 255, 328

LHRH 24
Librium® 26, 37, 38, 110, 315
ligands 43, 115
linoleic acid hydroperoxide 60, 207
lipid antioxidant 200
lipid peroxides 159, 329
lipid soluble 300, 325
lipid coated viruses 151–52
lipid containing viruses 60
lipids (fats or oils) viii, 18, 50, 60, 61, 73, 78,
    88, 98, 100, 136, 151, 153, 155, 157, 175,
    178, 198, 200, 210, 301, 313, 316, 318,
    321, 325, 328, 329, 330
lipoproteins 60, 325. *See also* high density
    lipoproteins; low density lipoproteins;
    very-low-density lipoproteins
Loniten® 21
low density lipoproteins (LDL) 325
lubricants 128, 301
lymph 45, 325
lysergic acid compounds 249

malonaldehyde 189, 312, 325
manganese 332
MAO (monamine oxidase) 7, 28, 111, 326
MAO inhibitor (monamine oxidase inhibitor)
    34, 48, 140
meats 143, 202, 205, 208, 329
medications viii, xi, xii, xiii, xiv, 3, 11, 21, 103,
    161, 189, 213, 222, 226, 227, 236, 240,
    243, 309
membrane stabilizers 326
menhaden oil 196
meprobamate 104
mercaptoethanol 53
mercury 99
metabolites 6
metals 96, 99, 317
methionine 72, 99, 128, 235
Methotrexate® 299
methylphenidate (Ritalin®) 249
milk 117, 253, 304, 330, 331
minerals 8, 25, 49, 54, 70, 78, 86, 93, 97, 127,
    174, 196, 197, 202, 300, 313, 362
moisturizers 85, 326
Moloney sarcoma virus (MSV) 53
monamine oxidase (MAO) 7, 28, 111, 326
monamine oxidase inhibitors (MAO
    inhibitors) 326
monoclonal antibodies 66, 318
monounsaturated fats 194, 199, 326
morphine 213, 329
MSV. *See* Moloney sarcoma virus
mutagens 52, 53, 56, 78, 85, 92, 151, 201,
    311, 312, 325, 326

Na-PCA 84, 85, 300, 302, 303, 304, 326
narcotics 68
natural antioxidants 128, 143, 188, 190, 300
natural form vitamin E 180, 188
natural tocopherols 188, 189. *See also* vitamin E
natural vitamin C 176, 177
natural vitamins 174, 176, 177, 178, 179, 180,
    181, 184, 186, 187, 188, 189, 192
natural-source vitamin E 181, 184, 186, 187,
    188
NDGA 300
NE. *See* norepinepherine

nerve growth factor (NGF) 41, 327
neurochemicals 11, 48, 327
neuromodulators 25, 327
neurotransmitters 11, 25, 33, 39, 48, 54, 109,
    110, 112, 115, 116, 119, 121, 123, 139,
    140, 148, 239, 249, 311, 316, 317, 320,
    322, 323, 326, 327, 330, 332
neutrons 79, 127
NGF. *See* nerve growth factor
niacin (nicatinic acid, vitamin B-3) 144, 300,
    327
niacin flush (like Masters and Johnson sex
    flush) 144
niacinamide. *See* vitamin B-3
niacinamide ascorbate 26, 28, 300, 303
nicotine 11, 12, 332
nicotinic acid (niacin, vitamin B-3), 182, 200,
    327
nicotinyl alcohol 182
nitrogen 119, 142, 187, 253
nitrogen oxides (NOX) 24, 25, 49, 126
non-d-alpha tocopherols 184
noradrenaline. *See* norepinephrine
norepinephrine (noradrenaline, NE) 6, 7, 20,
    25, 33, 35, 48, 110, 111, 113, 115, 121,
    123, 139, 244, 249, 311, 315, 317, 326,
    327, 332
nucleases 151, 328

oils (lipids) xiii, 18, 50, 54, 78, 84, 88, 92, 97,
    157, 172, 175, 179, 181, 183, 184, 187,
    188, 189, 190, 191, 198, 199, 201, 202,
    203, 204, 205, 207, 208, 301, 316, 325
olive oil 196
opiates 305
oranges 21
oregano 202
organic peroxides 19, 50, 54, 71, 78, 80, 85,
    94, 97, 120, 142, 195, 198, 300, 311, 324
ornithine 8, 9, 53, 253
oxidants 49, 60, 71, 128, 175, 194, 207, 313,
    323, 325, 328
oxidation 8, 16, 17, 54, 56, 77, 78, 81, 85, 86,
    88, 96, 127, 159, 174, 175, 178, 191, 196,
    201, 202, 203, 236, 253, 314, 317, 318,
    326, 328
oxidizer 328
oxidizers 49, 128, 175, 194
oxprenolol 103, 104
oxygen 3, 19, 41, 49, 78, 128, 133, 171, 173,
    189, 191, 194, 209, 210, 252, 312, 313,
    314, 316, 321, 324, 326, 328, 330, 331,
    334
Oxygen Free Radicals and Tissue Damage
    100
ozone 24, 25, 49, 94, 319, 321, 328
PABA (p-aminobenzoic acid, para-
    aminobenzoic acid) 16, 25, 27, 58, 93,
    174, 196, 197, 300, 326
PAH. *See* polycyclic aromatic hydrocarbons;
    polynuclear aromatic hydrocarbons
paint 314
pantothenate. *See* vitamin B-5
pantothenic acid. *See* vitamin B-5
Parlodel® (bromocriptine) 55, 144, 145
pathways 17, 20, 115
penicillamine. *See* d-penicillamine; l-
    penicillamine

peptides 253, 254, 329
peracetic acid 311
peristaltic stimulants 148
peroxidases 49, 132, 328
peroxides 189, 190, 301, 322, 328
peroxidized fats (lipid) 50, 85, 86, 120,
    127–28, 142, 195, 198, 312, 321–22, 330
peroxyacetylnitrate 94
peroxyacetylnitrile 94
pesticides 126
petroleum 184
PGI$_2$. See prostacyclin
Phenelzine® 326
phenols 157
phenylalanine 6, 7, 28, 33, 34, 35, 36, 48, 110,
    111, 1i4, 115, 139, 140, 302
phosphate 146, 314, 318
phosphatidyl choline 119, 300
Phylan 100® (phenylalanine) 302
pigment 23
pineapple 330
pioracetam 142
Piribedil® 249
pituitary hormone 55, 111, 145, 146
placebo effect 11. See also Hawthorne effect
placebos 66, 213, 320, 328–29
plaques xvii, 6, 45, 51, 72, 98, 112, 314, 324,
    329
plasma 98, 100, 197, 200, 252, 253, 255, 329
poisons 25, 171, 239
pollutants 49, 91, 92, 94, 172
polonium 173
polyamine 253
polycyclic aromatic hydrocarbons (PAH) 55,
    56, 200, 329
polymerase 253
polynuclear aromatic hydrocarbons (PAH) 24,
    25, 70, 172, 205, 315, 319, 321, 329
polypeptides 65–66, 312, 317, 323, 324, 329
polysorbate 80, 300, 304
polyunsaturated fats viii, xiii, 49, 50, 56, 119,
    142, 194, 196, 199, 202, 205, 326,
    329–30, 331
polyunsaturated fatty acids 119, 142, 200
polyunsaturated lipids (fats and oils) 18, 50,
    66, 97, 188, 196, 198, 199, 325
potassium 21
potato chips 202
potatoes 176
precursors 115–16, 311, 319, 330, 331
preservatives 201, 202, 203, 207, 303, 304
preservatives may be preserving you 201,
    207
pro-oxidant 319
pro-vitamin A. See beta carotene
progestin (female sex hormone) 160
prolactin (PRL, HPRL) 124, 144, 149, 250,
    254, 255, 330
promoters 87, 143, 169, 170, 188
propranolol 20, 21, 66, 103, 104, 105, 106,
    107
propyl gallate (PG) 196
prostacyclin (PGI$_2$) 19, 80, 159, 197–98, 328,
    330
prostacyclin synthetase 18–19
prostaglandins 99, 254, 330
proteases 330

protectants 60
protective antioxidant (free radical scavenger)
    49, 171, 197
protective enzymes 23, 49, 86, 93, 94, 97,
    127, 128, 169, 197
proteins 17, 18, 62, 72, 73, 80, 84, 85, 98,
    114, 119, 127, 151, 191, 196, 236, 253
    254, 313, 317, 318, 319, 320, 322, 325,
    329, 330, 331, 332

quenchers 331

radicals. See free radicals
radon 173
rags 314, 316
rancid fats and oils (peroxidized fats, lipids)
    49, 50, 71, 77–78, 85, 92, 120, 127–28,
    142, 175, 196, 197, 205
rancid oil (peroxidized fat, lipid) 50
reagent 126
reduced glutathione 93, 97, 304, 313, 322,
    332
retinoic acid. See vitamin A
retinoids. See vitamin A
ribonucleic acid. See RNA
Rimso-50® (50 percent DMSO in water) 63,
    126
Ritalin® (methylphenidate) 249
RNA (ribonucleic acid) 18, 71, 80, 97, 123,
    127, 196, 253, 299, 300, 313, 318, 331,
    334
rosemary 202
rubber 76, 80, 319

saccharin 169–70
safflower oil 189, 196
sage 202
salt 21, 85, 171, 210, 326
Santoquin® (ethoxyquin) 186–87
saturated fats 194, 196, 199, 205, 326, 331
scavenger 45, 128
secondary antioxidants 300
sedatives 26, 27–28, 36, 102, 104, 110, 118,
    143, 156
seeds 175
selenite. See selenium
selenium iv, 8, 9, 13, 16, 25, 27, 30, 49, 54,
    56, 59, 61, 70, 71, 72, 73, 74, 78, 86, 93,
    97, 127, 174, 196, 197, 202, 235, 300,
    302, 313
selenium sulfide 78
selenocystine 72
selenomethionine 72, 73
Selsun Blue® (selenium sulfide) 78
serotonin (5-HT, 5-hydroxytryptamine) 25,
    36, 54, 110, 112, 113, 114, 116, 117, 118,
    119, 124, 139, 143, 249, 323, 324, 326,
    327, 331
serum xiii, 18, 60, 61, 87, 142, 155, 159, 186,
    194, 197, 251, 323
serum levels of vitamin C were the single
    best predictor of five-year survival 18
shampoos 78
sidestream smoke 13, 56
singlet oxygen 331
sludge 19, 188, 193
smart pills 38, 41

Smartz® 42
smog 94, 311, 312
smoke 10, 11, 12, 13, 24, 29, 56, 61, 80, 81,
    83, 89, 158, 160, 311, 312, 329
SOD. *See* superoxide dismutase
sodium chloride 171
sodium hydrogen urate. *See* uric acid 334
sodium salicylate 99
sodium selenite 9, 54, 72, 73, 78, 300
solvent 65, 126, 319
Somacton® (GH, growth hormone) 249
somatomedins 253
somatotrophic hormone. *See* growth hormone
somatotropin. *See* growth hormone
soy 176, 188
soybean oil 181, 184, 188, 193
spices 202, 207
starches 201, 301
stereoisomers 183
steroids 181
STH (somatotrophic hormone, GH, growth
    hormone) 249
stimulants 19, 21, 53, 110–11, 122, 210, 249
stimulatory neurotransmitters 332
stimulus barriers 11, 12, 332
succinates 187
sugars 36, 38, 81, 170, 301
sulfa drugs 27
sulfa type A 27
sulfhydryl compounds 60, 75, 82, 332, 334
sulfone 128
sulfoxide 128
sulfur 29, 72, 75–76, 83, 99, 318, 319, 332
sunblock 58
sunscreen 300
suntan 22, 23, 89
superoxide dismutases (SOD) 49, 79, 86, 93,
    95, 97, 99, 100, 127, 128, 197, 202, 328,
    332
superoxide radicals 131, 332
suppository 159, 160
suppressants 92
surfactants 85
sweat 73
sweeteners 168, 170, 304, 305
synergist 205
synthetic vitamins 176–78
synthetics 196

tars 55, 56, 172
TBHQ 188, 190, 196, 203
tea 114
Test-Estrin® 160
testosterone (male sex hormone) 148, 160,
    323
thalidomide 237
theobromine 114
theophylline 114
thiamine. *See* vitamin B-1
thiodipropionic acid 300
thiol 53, 334
thorium 173
thrombogens 92
thromboxane 197, 329, 334
thymidine 151
Timolol® 20
tin 204

tobacco 11, 12, 29, 56, 70, 81, 224, 329
tocopheryl acetate. *See* vitamin E
tocopherols. *See* vitamin E
tomatoes 176
toxins 176
Trammamil® 67
tranquilizers 102, 104, 332
Tranylcypromine® 326
tricarboxylic acid cycle 17, 317, 334
triglycerides 200, 334
trimethylamine 39
triplet oxygen 316
tryptophan 25, 26, 27, 28, 30, 35, 36, 43,
    54–55, 109, 110, 114, 117, 118, 119, 143,
    300, 331
tyrosine 6, 7, 28, 33, 34, 35, 36, 43, 48, 110,
    111, 114, 139, 140

uncontrolled free radicals can do serious
    harm 202
unpaired electrons 16, 49, 71, 77, 92, 97, 195,
    321
unsaturated fats and oils (lipids) viii, 85, 86,
    89, 174, 175, 181, 183, 184, 321, 329–30
uranium 173
urea 185
uric acid 334
urine 25, 36, 51, 73, 98, 143, 145, 305
urine test 304

Valium® 26, 37, 38, 104, 110, 315
Valium® live 26
vanilla 180
vasoconstrictors viii, 209
vasopressin (Diapid®) 39, 40, 41, 43, 44, 55,
    66, 111, 121, 124, 145, 146, 149, 237,
    323, 328
vegetables 15, 50, 96, 181, 184, 188, 189, 190,
    191, 198
Velvet Bean Protein Plus™ 300, 303
velvet beans 300, 303. *See also* L-DOPA
vitamin A 8, 9, 15, 30, 50, 51, 54, 58, 59, 60,
    86, 87, 88, 331, 332
vitamin B-1 Thiamine 9, 13, 16, 24, 25, 26,
    49, 57, 78, 81, 86, 88, 89, 93, 97, 119,
    127, 141, 142, 174, 196, 197, 313, 332
vitamin B-2 (riboflavin) 26
vitamin B-3 (niacin, nicotinic acid,
    nicotinamide) 26, 28, 37, 38, 110, 182,
    200, 300, 327
vitamin B-5 (pantothenic acid, calcium
    pantothenate) 16, 17, 24, 25, 26, 29, 39,
    49, 86, 88, 89, 93, 97, 110, 119, 141, 142,
    146, 148, 149, 174, 196, 197, 202, 235,
    239, 300, 313, 317, 327
vitamin B-6 (pyridoxine) 7, 8, 13, 16, 25, 26,
    27, 35, 36, 49, 78, 86, 93, 97, 110, 118,
    127, 143, 159, 160, 174, 178, 196, 197,
    202, 313
vitamin B-12 123, 124, 178, 300
vitamin C 9, 13, 16, 17, 18, 19, 20, 24, 25, 27,
    51, 53, 54, 59, 78, 81, 98, 99, 100, 110,
    118, 159, 174, 176, 177, 197, 200, 205,
    235, 236, 237, 238, 239, 300, 304, 305,
    306, 309, 319, 323. *See also* ascorbate;
    ascorbic acid, ascorbyl palmitate
vitamin C pumps 18, 237

vitamin E viii, xiii, 8, 9, 30, 51, 52, 53, 60, 78,
    132, 175–76, 179, 180, 181, 182, 183,
    184, 185, 186, 187, 188, 189, 190, 191,
    192, 193, 198, 200, 235, 238, 305, 323,
    326, 328. *See also* alpha tocopherol
vitamin E acetate 191, 193
vitamin E esters 189, 190
vitamin E oil 187
vitamin H (biotin) 88
vitamins xiv, 7, 8, 9, 16, 25, 26, 35, 36, 38, 49,
    52, 53, 56, 57, 58, 62, 63, 78, 86, 87, 88,
    93, 97, 110, 113, 117–18, 119, 127, 128,
    141, 142, 143, 146, 159, 174, 175, 176,
    177, 178, 182, 183, 185, 190, 196, 197,
    198, 200, 202, 237, 238, 239, 300, 301,
    303, 304, 305, 313

warmed-over flavor 208
wheat 175, 176, 181
wines 143

xanthine oxidase 334
xenon 128

yeast 176, 300
yogurt 39

zinc 8, 9, 16, 25, 27, 49, 51, 54, 78, 86, 88, 93,
    97, 127, 174, 196, 197, 202, 313, 332
zinc pyrithione 78

INDEX TO NAMES:
PERSONS, ORGANIZATIONS, AND PLACES

IMPORTANT NOTICE:

Do not use any information from our *Life Extension Companion* or our *Life Extension. A Practical Scientific Approach* without first checking the Safety Indexes for both books for the supplement, drug, or action that you plan to take. Also check the Safety Indexes for any illness that you might have and for any drugs that you are now using, since this may influence the safety of your intended actions. It is important that you heed these warnings.

Live Long and Prosper,

Durk Pearson & Sandy Shaw

Advanced Research Health Products® 302
Africa 134, 135
Ahner, Neil A. 223, 225, 226
Ajinomoto 90
Ajlouni, K. 255
Alexander 83
Alfin-Slater 199
Alzheimer's Disease 67, 134
American Academy of Medical Preventics 100
American Aging Association (AGE) 208, 227, 228, 229, 309
American Heart Association xiii, 194, 228
Anastasi 199
Anderson 30, 59
Argonne National Laboratory 113

Bacall, Aaron 306–07
Bacq 83
Ballenger 44
Barbotin 135
Barbul 30, 59, 124
Beck, J. C. 255
Benditt 29
Benowicz, Robert J. 239
Berde 43, 210
Biggert 73
Birmingham, Alabama 91
Bjelke 59
Bjorksten 83, 100
Bonhomme 135

Borison 60, 115, 149
Botalla, L. 252
Boyd 125, 250
Braestrup 43, 115
Branen 157
Breslow 28
Bronson Pharmaceuticals 305
Brugh, M., Jr. 157
Burkitt's Lymphoma, 55, 150
Burnet 59

California 91, 126, 157, 244, 303, 304
Cameron 235–236
Campbell 59, 83
Canada 20, 23, 24, 54, 70, 89, 238, 305
Cartoonist's Guild 307
Chambless 160
Chan 208
Charman 200
China 91
Chinese 25, 27, 36, 110, 118, 143
Chiodini, P. G. 252–53
Chope 28
Ciba-Geigy® 100
Colussi, G. 252–53
Connelly, Bill 134
Coullet 135
Cowan 161
Cremascoli, G. 252–53
Criqui 161
Cuisinier 135

Cupp 157
Cutler 95

Dajean Gerontological Laboratories®
    299–300
Darracq 135
Data (Doctors' Registry For Treatment Of
    The Aging) ix, 218, 219, 220, 221, 222,
    223, 226, 227, 228, 229
Dean, Sandy 308
Debono 149
Dekker 131
Dela torre 130–131
Delaney Amendment 170, 171
Demopoulcs, H. B. 16, 31, 61, 95, 100, 119,
    131, 132, 136, 142, 189, 210
Dix 200
Doctors' Registry For The Treatment Of The
    Aging. See DATA
Drachman 115
Drake 28–29
Ducloux 135
Dumm 17, 29, 149
Dupre, J. 255
Durk i, xviii, 20–21, 35, 152–53, 181, 231,
    232, 235, 302, 310

Eddy, Dennis E. 199, 208
Edison, Thomas A. 3
Edmund Scientific® 305
Ehret, Charles F. 113–14, 116
Ehrlich Ascites tumor 61, 73
Elden 91
England 103, 184
Engle 160
Environmental Protection Agency (EPA) 170,
    171, 172
Ermini, Marco 310
Europe 11, 41, 42, 66, 103, 106, 141, 142,
    168, 210

FASEB. See Federation of American Societies
    For Experimental Biology
FDA. See Food and Drug Administration
Federation of American Societies For
    Experimental Biology (FASED) 30, 60,
    115, 149, 200
Feig, Seymour v
Fernstrom 114, 116, 118, 124
Finnish 16, 30
Fisher, Jeffrey A. 10–15 28
Flamm 31, 95
Food And Drug Administration (FDA) viii,
    20–21, 23–24, 42, 62, 63, 63–64, 65, 66,
    68, 69, 73, 85, 99, 103, 107, 126, 131,
    135, 151, 154–55, 165, 166, 167, 170,
    171, 182, 203, 232, 237, 239
Foundation For Experimental Ageing
    Research 310
Fowler 160
France 65, 142
Franklyn 60
Freeman 29, 59, 235–36
Friesen, H. G. 254
Fuller 125
Fund For Integrative Biomedical Research
    (FIBER) 161, 309

Gee 60, 207
Gelenberg 43
General Foods® 178
Georgieff 208
Germany 237
GM® 255
Goetzl 59
Goldzieher 161
Gonzales 29, 60, 83
Goodwin 44
Grace Slick (Jefferson Starship rock group)
    201
Greeder 61, 73
Greek 96, 174
Greenberg 160
Gregory 178
Griffin, Merv iii, 35
Gross 232
Growdon 115–16
Gutheil 125
Gutman 95

Hagen, T. C. 255
Harman, Denham ix, xiii, 83, 92, 127, 131,
    152, 178, 196, 199, 208, 226, 227, 228,
    309
Harris, Sidney 307
Hawn, Goldie 174
Hawthorne (effect) 213
Hayashi 82
Helmrich 160
Hendricks, Shelton 199, 208
Henkel Corporation® 7, 13, 179, 180, 181,
    182, 187, 188, 189, 192, 193
Hess 30
Hindmarch 43–44, 115
Hoekstra 73
Hoffmann-La Roche® 187
Hourani 100
Hulka 160
Hume 30, 200

Jacquet 173
Japan 13, 56, 76, 168, 172
Jerne 124
Jetten 91
Johns Hopkins 55
Julian 100

Kabara 157
Kalokerinos, A. 306
Karel 60
Karon 161
Kato, Y. 255
Kaufman 160
Kefauver 66, 237
Keith 157, 178
Keller 29
Kelner 237
Kettler 115
Khandwala 60, 207
Kielholz 43, 107
Kim 157
Kirk 178
Knott's Berry Farm® 105–06
Koppel 100
Korda 43
Koreh 61, 136, 210

Krebs 146
Krebs cycle 17, 146
Kuakuvi 135
Kugler 236
Kurokawa 61

Laboratory For The Advancement Of
    Biomedical Research iii
Laden 91
Lagarde 135
Landau, Richard L. 69, 236
Larner 82
Lasagna, Louis xii
Latshaw 73
Lattime 29
Laughlin 28
Lazarus, L. 251
Leake 131
Leavitt 115
Legros 43, 124, 149, 237
Lian, K. O. 255
Life Extension Foundation 225, 302, 306, 309
Life Extension Products® 301–02
Linus Pauling Institute Of Science And
    Medicine 309
Liuzzi, A. 252
Longevity Products, Inc. 303
Los Angeles, CA 91, 94, 108, 113, 235, 244,
    305
Lowrey 29
Luckey 95

Machlin, L. J. 253
Magellan 202
Malitz 149
Mann, John A. 233
Marnett 200
Martinson, D. R. 255
Marx, Jean L. 60, 124
Massachusetts Institue of Technology (MIT)
    38–39
Mattick 178
McBrien 73
McCord 31, 127, 128, 131
McKinley 115
Medawar, P. B. 47
Medical Hotline® 30, 69
Medical Preventics, American Academy of
    100
Medlars (National Library of Medicine
    computer literature search service) ix,
    xvi, xvii, 231, 237, 240, 241–43, 243, 248,
    251
Medline (National Library of Medicine
    computer literature search service) ix,
    240, 249
Meites 124, 149, 250
Merck 181
Miettinen 160
Milner 61, 73
MIT (Massachusetts Institute of Technology)
    38–39
Moehler 43, 115
Moloney sarcoma virus 53
Moncada 159
Monsanto® 186–87
Morehouse, Lawrence 232
Müller, E. E. 61, 252, 255

Multinational Nutrient Trading Company®
    303
Myers 149
Mytilna brevispina 98, 100

National Academy Of Science (NAS) 199, 206
National Cancer Institute (NCI) 199, 240
National Library Of Medicine (NLM) ix, 240
National Research Council (NRC) 172, 206
New Jersey 91, 92, 95, 115, 135, 149
New York University (NYU) 16, 119, 131,
    142, 189
Newark, New Jersey 91, 92
Newcastle disease 157
Newton 213
Niang 135
Nielsen 43, 115
Nightingale 200
Nockels 30, 60
non-profit research foundations 308
NRC (see National Research Council)

Occupational Health and Safety
    Administration (OSHA) 170–71, 173
Oeriu, Vochitu 82
Oliveros 124
Olwin 100
Ono 95
Oppizzi, G. 252
Oroville 172
OSHA. See Occupational Health And Safety
    Administration

Pan 94
Pao 29
Pardridge 115, 125
Parker 29, 60, 82, 83
Parkinson's disease 9, 26
Passwater, Richard 237
Pauling, Linus 59, 235–36, 236, 309
Pearson, Durk, i, xviii, 73, 82, 90, 100, 107,
    114, 124, 149, 152–53, 178, 181, 199,
    207, 225, 231, 235, 248, 302, 310
Pecile 61
Pegue 135
Pelletier 178
Peltzman, Sam 69, 236–37
Pennsylvania, PA 91, 131
Pieri 115
Pierredon 135
Pietronigro 95
Pinter, E. J. 254
Pittsburgh, PA 91
Pocidalo 173
Polc 115
Polish 157
Presse 135
Prinz 125, 250
Proxmire Act 63
Pryor 132, 200
Pularkat 157
Purdy 161
Pure Planet Products® 306

Radden 59, 83
Ralli 17, 29, 149
Reade 59, 83
Reichlin 59

Remington's Pharmaceutical Sciences 237
Repace 29
Research Foundation 300, 303, 304, 305, 306
Rifkind 161
Riley 29, 61
Rohrer 89
Rosenberg 160
Rosenfeld, Albert 236
Rosenshein 160
Russia 168
Rouser, George 151, 157
Rubinow 44
Rucinsky 157

Sachar 115
Sahara Desert 85
San Francisco, CA 29, 91, 228
San Francisco General Hospital Brain
    Trauma And Edema Center 131
San Mateo study 18, 28–29
Sandoz® 111, 121, 134, 144, 145, 232, 327
Sandy 35, 104–105, 106, 133, 134, 135, 153,
    232, 308, 310
Sandy Shaw i, xviii, 181, 231–32, 235, 302
Sankale 135
Sanosho 135
Sapienza 157
Saratoga 305
Sasaki 61
Sato 82, 208
Saul Kent 233, 234, 302
SAVES (Study Of Aging Volunteer
    Experimental Subjects) ix, 218–19, 219,
    220, 221, 223, 225, 226
Saves Data (*See* SAVES) 218, 219, 225
Saves Subject Register (*See* SAVES) 219, 220,
    221, 222, 225
Scanlon, Lynne Waller 114, 116
Schild 43, 210
Schottenfeld 160
Schrauzer 73
Scottish 55
Sebrell 17
Seibold ix, 199, 208
Seligman 61, 95, 136, 210
Shamberger 60, 73
Shapiro 160
Shaw, Sandy i, xviii, 28, 35, 42, 59, 69, 73, 82,
    90, 100, 104, 105, 106, 107, 114, 134–35,
    149, 153, 178, 181, 199, 207, 225,
    231–32, 235, 302, 310
Shekelle 30, 60
Sherrard 28
Sherwin 208
Shute, Wilfrid E. 200, 238
Shute Clinic 238
Sigma Chemical® 119, 142
Silvestrini, F. 252
Simic 60
Simonton, Carl xi
Sincock 98, 100

Sitaram 43
Slater 73, 200
Slick, Grace 201
Slone 160
Smallberg 44
Smith 29, 60, 74, 82, 83
Snipes 60, 152, 153, 157
Sourkes 116
Soviet 205
Spallholz 30, 59, 73
Spector 200, 237
Spitzer 91
Sprince, Herbert 29, 56, 60, 81, 82, 83
Stein 115
Steiner 200
Stolley 160
Stone, Irwin 238
Strausser 29
Study Of Aging Volunteer Experimental
    Subjects (SAVES) ix, 218, 219, 223, 225
Sulzman 125
Summers 44
Sundaram 60
Sunde 73
Sutton J. 251
Switzerland 310
Szent-gyorgyi 131

Tanzer 91
Tappel 132, 200
Tietze, Christopher 158, 160
Timex® 22
Tolis, G. 254
Tolmasoff 95
Tufik 125
Turner, M. R. 256
Tyroler 161

Ungar 29
United States 95, 172, 181, 190

Vane 159
Vecchi 183
Venn 210
Verzar 83, 91
Vitmain Research Products® 304
Vochitu 82

Walford, Roy, 125, 235, 302
Wallace 161
Wanda 157
Washington 125, 244, 309
Weber 183
Weingartner 44
Weiser 183
Wheeler, Jack v
Wholesale Nutrition Club® 305–06
Williams, Roger J. 239
Wilson, Gerald G. 179, 180–93
Wohler, Frederick 185
Wurtman 30, 43, 114, 116, 125

INDEX TO:
GENERAL TOPICS

ROMAN NUMERAL PAGE NUMBER SECTION

IMPORTANT NOTICE:

Do not use any information from our *Life Extension Companion* or our *Life Extension, A Practical Scientific Approach* without first checking the Safety Indexes for both books for the supplement, drug, or action that you plan to take. Also check the Safety Indexes for any illness that you might have and for any drugs that you are now using, since this may influence the safety of your intended actions. It is important that you heed these warnings.

Live Long and Prosper,

Durk Pearson & Sandy Shaw

accidents xi
acids, some vitamins are xvi, xviii
adaptation xxxii, xxxv
advertising xxxiii, xxxv
age ix, xviii, xxviii
aging clocks x
air xvii
alcoholism xvi
allergies xi
animal studies ix, xiii, xxii, xxvii
antidotes xvii
antisepsis xviii
antitumor agents xvii
appearance xxxi
appendices xii, xiii, xxiv, xxvii
artwork xxxii
arteries x
arthritis xi, xxviii
asthma xi
atherosclerosis xi, xvii
athletics xi

bacteria xviii
baldness x
bases xv
biochemical individuality xii

biochemistry xxi, xxix, xxxii, xxxiii
biomedical xii, xv, xxi, xxxiii, xxxiv, xxxvi
bioscience xxxii
bleeding xxiv
blindness x
boldface, for emphasis of warnings and
     cautions xxix
bone-growth device xxxiv
brain x, xxxiii

cancer xi, xv, xvi, xvii, xix, xxiv, xxviii, xxx
cardiovascular disease xi, xxvii
cartoons, credit for xxxi, xxxii, xxxiii, xxxiv,
     xxxv, xxxvi, xxxvii
case histories, use of xiii, xxii
cautions, general xvi, xxix
cautious, preventive medicine proposals xviii
caveat emptor xii
chemicals x, xvi, xvii, xxxv, xxxvi
childhood xxxv
children, this book not for xxiv, xxix
circulation xxii
clinical laboratory tests, vitally important xii,
     xvii, xxiv, xxvi
clocked cell cycle clocks xxxvii
clocks xxxi

communicable diseases xviii
computers xii, xxxiv, xxxv
consultation, with health professionals xxiv,
    xxvi, xxviii
controls xvi
coping xxix
coronary xix
coronary-care units xviii
corpses xxi
courtesy xxxi, xxxii, xxxiii, xxxiv, xxxv, xxxvi,
    xxxvii
creativity xxxix, xxxv
crosslinking x
cryonics xii
cults xxiii

daredevil, this book not for xxiv
depression, x
despair xxviii
diagnostics xxxvii
diet xi, xvi, xxii, xxxi
digestion xxx
diptheria xviii
disclaimers, very important information! xxiii,
    xxvi
diseases xi, xvii, xviii, xix, xxiv, xxvii
doctor, need for xii, xvii, xxiv
doses xii, xvi, xvii, xxiii, xxiv
doubling time for knowledge ix
dreams vii, xxi
duodenum, acid vitamins and ulcers xxiv

"Eat Starch Mom" (song) xxxii
elderly xxvii
environment xvii, xix
epidemiologists xvi
errors, by authors xxiii
esophagus, acid vitamins and ulcers xxiv
examinations, medical, frequency of xvi
exercise xi, xxvii

faddists xxx
family xxxiv
fantasy xi
fears ix
fever xviii
free radical theory of aging v, xxii
funds xxi
future xii, xviii, xxii

gerontologists vii
gerontology xxviii
glossary xiii, xv, xvi, xxvii, xxix
graphs xxxi, xxxii, xxxiii, xxxiv
greenness xvi
growth xvii

habits xvi
hands xvii
hearing xxix
heart xxxv
heart attacks xi, xxvii
heart disease xxiv
hepatitis xviii
hospitals xxvii
how-to-do-it-yourself xxii, xxx

illustrations, credit for xxxiii
immune system x, xi
immunization xviii, xxxv
immunology xxxiii
individuality, biochemical xii
individualization, of life extension program
    xxix
infallible, authors not xxiii
infection xvii, xviii
intelligence xxii, xxvi, xxviii

journals xiii

kidney disease, sodium in some supplements
    and xxiv

lethal disorders xv
life extension i, ix, x, xi, xii, xiii, xvii, xxii, xxiv,
    xxvi, xxvii, xxix, xxx
lifespan ix, xxiii, xxxiii
lifestyle xxvii, xxx
lipid antioxidant xi
longevity x, xi
lungs xvi, xxx

male pattern baldness x
measles xviii
mechanisms of aging x, xxvi, xxix, xxxi
media xv
Medlars xxxvi
megadoses xvi, xvii, xviii, xxiv
memorizing xxviii, xxix
middle-aged xxii, xxvii
moderation xvi, xxvii
mole, xxxii
molecules x, xv, xxxi
monitoring xxi

natural substances ix, x, xviii
nervousness xxxiii
neurochemistry xxxiii
nursing xviii
nutrients xii, xv, xvi, xvii, xviii, xxii, xxiv
nutrition xi, xxiii

occlusive vascular disease xvii
organs x
over-the-counter drugs (non-prescription
    drugs) xvii

parents xxxv
pathology xv, xix, xxiv
pathways ix
performance xi, xvii
periodic clinical laboratory tests, necessity for
    xvi
pharmaceuticals v, xxiii, xxxvi
pharmacology xxxiii, xxxiv
physician xxiv
physician, need for xv, xvi, xvii, xix, xxiii, xxiv
pioneers xvii, xxii, xxiii
pitfalls xxvii
plants xvi, xviii
polio xviii
pollution xi, xvii
precautions, seriousness of xxii, xxix
pregnant women, this book not for xviii, xxiv

prescription drugs xii, xxii, xxiii, xxiv, xxx
preservatives xi
protocols xvii
psychopharmacology xxxiii
puerperal fever xviii

quality ix, x, xxvi

radiation xvi, xvii
recommended daily allowances xi
records, medical, possession of xii
refrigeration x, xviii
regeneration x
regimen xvii, xxiii
responsibility for planning xxiii
risks xix, xxx

sanitation xviii
sedentary lifestyle xxii
self-administration xvii
self-experimentation xxii
senility xxviii
sequoia tree xxxi
sewage xviii
sex x
skin x

sleep x
smallpox xviii
smoking xi, xvi, xxx, xxxiv
stroke xi
supplements xii, xv, xvi, xvii, xviii, xxii
suppliers xiii, xxiii
surgery xviii
synthetics ix

technology xxii, xxviii, xxxii, xxxiii
teenagers xxix
tests, importance for monitoring your health
    xii, xvii, xxi, xxii, xxiv, xxvi
tetanus xviii
Trends in Pharmacological Science® xxxiii,
    xxxiv
tumors xvii

vaccinations xviii
vegetables xvi
viruses xviii

warnings, seriousness of xxix
weight xi
women xviii, xxiv
worldview xxii

INDEX TO:
GENERAL TOPICS

IMPORTANT NOTICE:

Do not use any information from our *Life Extension Companion* or our *Life Extension, A Practical Scientific Approach* without first checking the Safety Indexes for both books for the supplement, drug, or action that you plan to take. Also check the Safety Indexes for any illness that you might have and for any drugs that you are now using, since this may influence the safety of your intended actions. It is important that you heed these warnings.

Live Long and Prosper,

Durk Pearson & Sandy Shaw

abilities 29, 128, 134, 167, 178, 204, 236, 735
abnormalities 97, 102, 135, 204, 244, 271, 289, 293, 323, 339, 422, 446, 642, 643, 761, 764, 766, 785
abortion 202, 203
absenteeism 492
accelerated aging test 380
accelerometers 523
accidents 24, 30, 67, 100, 112, 128, 164, 173, 174, 183, 344, 350, 351, 561, 567, 577, 599, 614, 651, 746
aches 25, 300, 305, 730, 732, 760
acid indigestion 415, 487
acidic vitamins 246, 258, 281, 435, 468, 487, 488, 755
acidity 247, 249, 415, 426, 462, 487, 488, 491
acne 214, 215, 756
acromegaly 136, 662, 765
activated charcoal filter 315
active oxygen method (ACM) 378
adaptation 18, 39, 71, 72, 73, 104, 237, 415, 420, 430, 432, 632, 697
addiction 270, 271, 272, 277, 282, 293, 294, 621, 657, 669, 715, 718
addictive substances 162, 193, 278, 293, 564, 571
additives 97, 112, 163, 218, 249, 264, 274, 278, 283, 336, 338, 368, 375, 376, 383, 384, 389, 391, 416, 462, 465, 466, 471, 510, 569, 570, 573, 613, 620, 632, 685, 689, 802, 803

adipose tissue 372
adolescents 657, 659
adrenal glands 121, 140, 409, 413, 420, 634, 647, 649, 652, 656, 657, 662, 683, 686
adrenergic 673, 735
adrenocorticotropic 180
adult-onset diabetes 84
adulteration 274, 603
Adventurer's Guide 3, 629, 721, 733
advertisements 493, 495, 574, 590, 591, 592
advertising 52, 113, 143, 176, 493, 495, 496, 497, 498, 574, 590, 591, 592, 593, 636, 672, 689, 713
advisory agencies 305, 589, 590
aerobic 227, 784
aerosols 368
aflatoxin-caused cancer 383
African green monkey 105
aftereffects 127
aftertaste 374
age spots 102, 120, 121, 124, 127, 175, 211, 796
aggression 129, 176, 197, 251, 496, 736, 799
aging clocks 22, 58, 65, 67, 68, 69, 71, 74, 129, 136, 137, 138, 140, 142, 147, 153, 165, 170, 212, 213, 220, 221, 290, 461, 471, 506, 514, 517, 643, 653, 734, 784, 786, 795, 799
aging damage 23, 24, 38, 66, 67, 71, 74, 101, 120, 168, 208, 391, 734, 762

aging mechanisms 6, 7, 17, 23, 28, 29, 32, 33, 56, 59, 64, 66, 67, 69, 70, 76, 208, 210, 257, 319, 320, 391, 404, 429, 441, 464, 510, 536, 557, 558, 617, 619, 621, 770
aging mechanisms chart 155
agoraphobia 734
air 101, 104, 135, 146, 147, 163, 177, 209, 210, 252, 253, 254, 260, 261, 262, 263, 265, 266, 304, 313, 369, 377, 378, 382, 386, 417, 418, 476, 491, 503, 516, 615, 635, 665, 667, 705, 706, 732, 753, 774, 783, 803
air cleaners 253, 254, 263, 624, 666, 669
aircraft 344, 375, 753
airways 252, 673
albinos 700, 701
alcoholism 221, 224, 267, 268, 270, 271, 272, 273, 274, 277, 278, 279, 282, 525, 563, 606, 647, 663, 668, 669, 670, 676, 677, 694, 784
alertness 112, 126, 127, 168, 178, 273, 276, 277, 312, 421, 532, 663, 670, 717, 737, 740
alkalinity 241, 249, 256, 448, 451, 479, 488, 489, 777
allergenic substances 462, 619, 763
allergies 54, 89, 170, 254, 302, 303, 304, 305, 306, 350, 434, 462, 485, 620, 627, 673, 744, 745, 747, 758, 763
allergic conjunctivitis 304, 763
allergic reactions to tablet binders and fillers 305, 485
alopecia areata 660
alternative health care 24, 39, 49, 194, 561, 566, 582, 590, 657
altitude 228, 615
alveolar macrophages 634, 636, 664, 667, 668, 700
Alzheimer's disease 129
amelanotic 683
American Aging Association (AGE) 535, 552, 621, 638
amnesia 128, 164, 173, 320, 642, 649, 670, 677, 701
amnesiacs 128
amoeba 507
amputation 149, 150, 151, 506
amyloidosis 116, 636, 639
anaerobic, 227, 402, 784
analogs 168, 186, 421, 667, 681, 695, 699
anecdotal evidence 47, 302, 725, 785
anemia 165, 168, 207, 437, 453, 524
anesthesia 31, 150, 228, 345, 412, 414
angina pectoris 174, 204, 229
angiology 663, 695, 700
animal studies 17, 18, 19, 20, 25, 28, 29, 30, 31, 38, 54, 55, 56, 57, 58, 59, 63, 65, 66, 67, 69, 72, 73, 76, 82, 85, 86, 87, 88, 89, 96, 97, 98, 102, 104, 106, 107, 110, 122, 127, 136, 140, 141, 144, 147, 150, 165, 168, 170, 175, 180, 181, 182, 197, 202, 217, 227, 236, 241, 242, 251, 257, 261, 263, 273, 277, 287, 290, 291, 294, 303, 314, 332, 333, 338, 339, 341, 342, 345, 348, 351, 366, 368, 375, 376, 377, 378, 379, 398, 402, 403, 404, 405, 409, 410, 412, 415, 416, 417, 418, 419, 421, 433, 461, 464, 471, 473, 477, 478, 479, 480,

481, 483, 484, 491, 498, 502, 506, 507, 509, 511, 514, 517, 518, 519, 521, 524, 539, 560, 570, 608, 614, 616, 635, 669, 680, 685, 691, 721, 725, 741, 743, 744, 745, 751, 759, 766, 771, 776, 787, 788, 789, 792, 804
ankles 455
anoxia 318, 785
antacids, 244, 249, 345, 415, 426, 435, 462, 468, 488, 489, 613, 768
anterior lobe 794
anterior pituitary 484, 765, 766
Anti-aging News® 534, 535
anti-anxiety 282, 477
anti-capitalistic mentality 718
anti-proteolytic 403
anti-thrombic 403
antibiotic-resistant microbes 593
anticancer agents 636, 682
antidandruff agents 220
antifoam 436, 489
antifreeze 608
antiherpes agents 753
antiinflammatory agents 672
antimetastatic agents 683
antinociceptive agents 664
antiproteolytic agents 676, 679, 698
antipsychotic agents 334, 585
antistress agents 165
antithrombic agents 676, 679, 698
antithyroid agents 631
antitumor agents 680
antiviral agents 689, 702
anus 488, 489
anxiety 282, 373, 426, 667
AOM. *See* active oxygen method
aortas 89, 482, 674, 687
apes 398, 409
aplastic anemia 584
appetite 184, 251, 274, 284, 287, 288, 289, 290, 291, 295, 497, 498, 671, 795, 799
approval, drugs 7, 14, 98, 99, 124, 150, 219, 221, 305, 336, 350, 535, 566, 567, 572, 575, 576, 590, 591, 592, 748
approved uses, drugs 273, 457, 502, 592
aqueous solutions 475
aromas 179, 292, 377, 734, 792
arousal 494, 594, 648, 664, 667, 676, 699
arrhythmias 638, 680
art 41, 56, 268, 356, 527, 608, 653, 656, 747
arterial endothelial cell 109
arteries 70, 83, 91, 92, 96, 102, 103, 108, 124, 209, 242, 269, 275, 285, 299, 307, 308, 312, 313, 314, 315, 316, 317, 318, 319, 320, 322, 324, 325, 364, 368, 372, 404, 411, 424, 425, 478, 505, 523, 524, 638, 643, 674, 675, 677, 680, 687, 695, 777, 785, 786, 787, 790, 796, 800, 801
arteriosclerosis 177, 674, 676, 678
arthritis 74, 83, 84, 85, 102, 103, 104, 106, 161, 162, 190, 296, 297, 298, 299, 300, 303, 305, 347, 402, 438, 453, 455, 468, 474, 477, 485, 496, 557, 607, 638, 672, 673, 715, 747, 748, 749, 760, 762, 765, 786, 795, 803
artifacts 229, 777, 785
artists 299, 509, 747
ascites 242, 333, 633, 682

371

Aspergillis flavis 383
assays 100, 449, 518, 519, 520
asthma 254, 302, 303, 304, 482, 667, 673,
    744, 745, 756
asthma relief with PABA 756
astronauts 752
atherogenic 313, 314, 368, 674, 676, 678, 699
atherosclerosis 6, 66, 81, 82, 83, 91, 97, 100,
    108, 109, 144, 176, 241, 270, 275, 299,
    307, 312, 313, 314, 315, 316, 318, 320,
    323, 324, 330, 338, 363, 366, 368, 370,
    372, 406, 411, 467, 474, 505, 534, 674,
    675, 676, 677, 678, 687, 693, 785, 786
atherosclerotic plaques 81, 83, 107, 108, 129,
    190, 241, 312, 316, 317, 319, 320, 366,
    368, 373, 408, 474, 483, 677, 785, 796
athletes 223, 229, 237, 238, 509, 772, 775
athletics 165, 204, 223, 226, 227, 228, 231,
    237, 238, 290, 509, 515, 661, 736, 774,
    775
Atlantic bottle-nosed dolphin 616
Atlas Shrugged 717
atmosphere 104, 264
atoms 78, 102, 104, 107, 265, 297, 376, 385,
    403, 422, 471, 476, 789, 792, 793, 800,
    803, 804
atrophy 81, 84, 125, 202, 212, 213, 219, 796
attitudes 3, 5, 9, 184, 499, 714
auditory nerves 178, 522, 788
augmentor 509
aural sign of coronary-artery disease 679
auricle 326
autocatalytic process 787
autoimmune attack 123, 133, 759
autoimmune disease 72, 83, 85, 762, 784
autoimmunity 84, 85, 129, 161, 190, 297, 298,
    303, 304, 467, 525, 557, 762, 786
automobiles 9, 18, 19, 96, 164, 173, 253, 263,
    265, 316, 319, 351, 364, 413, 446, 562,
    690, 706, 718, 732, 746, 747, 783
autonomic nervous system 176, 446
autopsies 322, 575
autoxidation 111, 124, 133, 135, 165, 220,
    237, 244, 265, 270, 279, 280, 297, 311,
    338, 340, 341, 347, 368, 369, 371, 376,
    377, 391, 407, 413, 462, 475, 563, 636,
    637, 638, 642, 689, 690, 752, 758, 783,
    784, 786, 787, 788, 800, 802
average life span 27, 57, 68, 71, 108, 141,
    143, 404, 467, 521, 556
a very special thank you (about computers
    and word processing) 722
awake state 133, 189, 746
axial tomography 787
Axiomat® 527
axons 132, 642, 646

B-cells 85, 87, 303, 357, 405, 785, 786, 803
babies. See infants
baboons 105
bacillus 99, 340
backaches 761, 762, 767
bacon 31, 239, 292, 383, 384, 389, 437
bacteria 28, 57, 81, 82, 83, 85, 87, 88, 102,
    104, 106, 108, 161, 164, 190, 248, 250,
    253, 285, 296, 297, 336, 340, 356, 368,
    373, 376, 382, 384, 402, 405, 408, 410,
    411, 419, 477, 481, 482, 506, 511, 518,
    539, 566, 634, 636, 664, 667, 700, 740,
    761, 785, 796, 797, 798, 803
bactericidal 635
baldness 65, 68, 104, 137, 138, 139, 212, 213,
    214, 215, 217, 218, 219, 220, 476, 482,
    516, 659, 660, 742, 768, 784, 786, 801
ballet dancers 509, 653
ballistocardiography 330, 522
bans, FDA 497, 564, 571, 575, 595, 691, 720
benign breast disease 692
benzodiazepine receptors 193, 282, 477, 754,
    755
bibliography 51, 294, 543, 548, 549, 640, 652,
    712
bilirubin, total and direct 448
bioavailability 55, 106, 409, 632, 693
biochemical individuality 429, 430, 431, 432,
    459, 499, 696
biochemical pathways chart 79, 107, 115,
    118, 154, 155, 156, 417
biochemistry 5, 39, 40, 47, 53, 56, 58, 59, 66,
    69, 71, 75, 83, 89, 91, 121, 123, 167, 176,
    182, 188, 190, 194, 226, 230, 268, 273,
    280, 284, 297, 338, 349, 407, 425, 429,
    430, 431, 433, 434, 441, 442, 456, 462,
    466, 507, 514, 524, 557, 558, 559, 563,
    608, 624, 632, 641, 648, 652, 657, 697,
    698, 725, 729, 742, 748, 770
biofeedback 286, 329, 444, 446
biogenic 634, 641, 662, 671
biological clocks 141, 197, 517, 644, 660, 709,
    784, 786
biological gerontologists 174, 511, 551
biologists 11, 19, 65, 266, 331, 559
biology 11, 33, 113, 163, 504, 550, 551, 572,
    627, 630, 639, 646, 660, 666, 671, 685,
    693, 699, 703, 704, 720, 721, 735
biomedicine 223, 536, 541, 543, 544, 551,
    556, 559, 560, 563, 564, 591, 593, 619,
    628, 712, 713
birds 242, 333, 409
birth 9, 19, 37, 112, 121, 143, 183, 201, 202,
    269, 270, 277, 279, 318, 419, 429, 431,
    471, 474, 482, 506, 571, 585, 614, 727
birthmarks 175, 750
bitter taste 374
black lung disease 266
black market 180, 607, 715
bladder 217, 247, 298, 340, 348, 421, 482
bladder cancer 390
blastema 150
bleeding 92, 317, 344, 345, 351, 452
bleeding time 314, 447, 449, 452
blindness 315, 373, 420
blistering 422
blockers 328
blood count 437, 452
blood pressure 92, 110, 128, 129, 136, 172,
    173, 184, 185, 186, 191, 204, 221, 228,
    229, 243, 251, 273, 288, 289, 293, 294,
    316, 325, 328, 329, 345, 354, 406, 438,
    444, 446, 484, 488, 674, 676, 678, 697,
    734, 736, 750
blood pressure gauges 329, 444, 446, 624
blood tests 170, 336
blood urea nitrogen 447, 448, 451
blood-brain barrier (BUN) 111, 134, 204, 413,
    431, 475, 639, 740

bloodstream 24, 108, 111, 242, 243, 246, 270, 293, 315, 324, 364, 370, 466, 484, 496, 639, 740, 795, 804
body fat 233, 237, 671, 721, 772, 774, 775
bodybuilding 226, 230, 232, 509, 735, 736
boiled foods 369, 688
bonding 269, 784, 790, 792, 803
bonds, chemical 87, 92, 95, 163, 175, 209, 227, 242, 246, 264, 269, 298, 304, 373, 385, 467, 482, 656, 786, 789, 790, 800, 802
bone-growth device 151
bones 82, 85, 148, 150, 152, 236, 263, 264, 405, 408, 413, 434, 437, 451, 466, 477, 645, 646, 732, 735, 765, 786, 796, 802
botulism 31, 261, 383, 599
brain 20, 38, 40, 71, 86, 97, 98, 100, 102, 105, 106, 108, 111, 112, 119, 120, 121, 122, 123, 124, 125, 126, 127, 128, 129, 131, 132, 134, 135, 136, 137, 139, 140, 141, 143, 164, 165, 167, 168, 169, 170, 171, 172, 174, 175, 176, 177, 178, 179, 181, 182, 184, 186, 187, 188, 189, 190, 192, 193, 196, 197, 198, 202, 204, 209, 211, 221, 228, 229, 236, 240, 247, 249, 250, 251, 252, 256, 257, 263, 265, 267, 269, 270, 273, 274, 275, 276, 277, 278, 279, 282, 284, 286, 287, 288, 289, 290, 291, 292, 293, 295, 297, 309, 316, 317, 318, 319, 320, 323, 342, 348, 350, 351, 352, 354, 406, 409, 413, 414, 426, 431, 473, 474, 475, 477, 479, 481, 482, 483, 484, 497, 498, 508, 524, 525, 532, 534, 537, 557, 563, 626, 634, 638, 639, 640, 641, 642, 643, 648, 649, 650, 651, 652, 657, 663, 669, 670, 671, 676, 691, 719, 734, 735, 737, 740, 741, 742, 745, 754, 783, 788, 791, 792, 794, 795, 797, 798, 799, 803
brand names 112, 179, 255, 378, 488, 501
Brassica species 631
breakfast 53, 110, 177, 186, 251, 291, 399, 560, 747
breastbone 82, 85, 336, 804
breasts 199, 202, 213, 236, 339, 343, 405, 421, 478, 497, 524, 681, 702, 766
breathing 101, 119, 176, 261, 264, 265, 266, 290, 304, 352, 404, 472, 614, 732, 763
Brevispina 637
bristlecone pine 616
broiled foods 369
bromsulphalein retention (BSP) 451
bronchi 482, 667, 673, 681, 695, 756
bronchoconstriction 304
browning 382
bruises 237, 299, 300, 347, 740, 759
Bullworker® (exercise aid) 233
Burkitt's lymphoma 206, 308, 333
businessmen 610, 746
byproducts 260, 315

C-Strips® 621, 688
cadavers 269, 505
calories 106, 110, 140, 144, 222, 230, 265, 279, 284, 287, 291, 292, 313, 324, 364, 365, 374, 515, 570, 571, 595
cancer 6, 8, 28, 57, 59, 70, 72, 74, 81, 82, 83, 85, 87, 88, 89, 91, 92, 98, 100, 102, 103, 104, 106, 107, 108, 110, 127, 129, 136, 144, 146, 147, 152, 161, 162, 181, 183, 184, 190, 197, 199, 206, 219, 236, 241, 242, 243, 247, 249, 250, 252, 256, 258, 259, 260, 263, 264, 265, 266, 268, 269, 270, 278, 279, 284, 285, 296, 303, 307, 308, 315, 324, 327, 331, 332, 333, 334, 335, 336, 337, 338, 339, 340, 341, 342, 343, 357, 358, 363, 364, 366, 368, 373, 374, 376, 377, 383, 384, 386, 402, 404, 405, 408, 410, 411, 414, 419, 420, 421, 422, 424, 425, 437, 447, 451, 453, 467, 471, 476, 478, 479, 480, 481, 482, 515, 517, 518, 524, 531, 540, 557, 558, 559, 561, 563, 564, 565, 566, 569, 570, 571, 585, 595, 602, 626, 629, 633, 634, 635, 637, 645, 651, 660, 663, 664, 665, 666, 667, 668, 680, 681, 682, 683, 684, 685, 690, 692, 693, 694, 695, 698, 701, 702, 703, 705, 715, 720, 727, 728, 729, 730, 740, 764, 770, 785, 786, 787, 791, 793, 796, 797, 798, 800, 801, 803, 804
cancer incidence 339, 340, 516, 793
cancer-causing substances 24, 31, 87, 244, 246, 256, 265, 334, 338, 376, 419, 570. *See also* Carcinogens
cancer-prone rats 571
cans 368, 374, 391, 595
capillaries 103, 300, 309, 477, 483, 676, 678, 698, 740, 759, 790, 795
capsules 289, 305, 347, 407, 462, 485, 492, 619, 620, 737
capuchin monkey 616
carcinogenesis 162, 421, 471, 570, 638, 660, 664, 667, 668, 681, 682, 683, 695, 698, 699, 786
carcinogens 31, 144, 145, 211, 252, 253, 260, 261, 264, 279, 300, 308, 313, 333, 334, 336, 337, 338, 340, 341, 349, 364, 367, 368, 369, 376, 377, 378, 383, 384, 410, 475, 563, 573, 660, 704, 705, 706, 783, 784, 792, 797, 800, 802
carcinoma. *See* cancer
cardiac arrest 177, 318
cardiopulmonary resuscitation (CPR) 344, 351, 352, 685
cardiopulmonary resuscitation chart 353
cardiovascular system 104, 202, 222, 223, 224, 249, 315, 324, 328, 330, 338, 367, 372, 405, 444, 515, 666, 679, 684, 703
cardiovascular disease 8, 44, 59, 103, 110, 183, 241, 260, 268, 270, 278, 279, 284, 307, 313, 317, 322, 338, 339, 367, 373, 406, 425, 467, 474, 518, 557, 559, 677, 778, 779, 793
caries 371
carnivores 420, 476
carotid artery 177, 350
cartilage 501
cartoons 21, 48, 50, 58, 444, 456, 463, 472, 513, 599, 600, 601, 602, 603, 604, 605, 606, 607, 718
carvings 653
case histories 47, 48, 128, 162, 164, 205, 264, 304, 334, 721, 725, 726
castration 139, 141, 644, 659
CAT scans 524, 556, 719, 787
catalogs 492, 533, 553, 708

catalysis 103, 106, 299, 311, 759, 787, 792, 311, 793, 799
cataracts 270, 348, 363, 477, 483, 496, 635, 760, 803
catatonic 135
catecholamines 102, 107, 651
catnaps 194
cats 23, 113, 228, 275, 290, 300, 309, 318, 319, 348, 354, 420, 577, 638, 719, 744, 745, 759, 763, 764, 787
caveat emptor 179, 490, 493, 497, 503, 706
cavities (dental) 371, 498
CBC. *See* complete blood count
cells 5, 68, 72, 76, 87, 88, 97, 98, 106, 108, 111, 121, 122, 123, 133, 137, 138, 149, 152, 171, 174, 175, 176, 184, 196, 206, 210, 216, 218, 242, 244, 250, 254, 262, 264, 265, 269, 286, 303, 304, 307, 308, 311, 316, 320, 324, 332, 333, 336, 341, 351, 386, 404, 405, 411, 413, 417, 420, 447, 449, 470, 472, 473, 476, 518, 524, 534, 626, 629, 633, 634, 644, 645, 647, 648, 665, 675, 677, 681, 683, 693, 699, 700, 710, 720, 729, 740, 758, 759, 762, 770, 789, 790, 792, 796, 797, 798, 801, 802, 803, 804
cellular immunity 411
central nervous system 111, 282, 497, 498, 514, 638, 639, 642, 646, 648, 650, 690, 788, 793, 794
cerebral circulation 265, 638, 643
cerebral cortex 122, 290, 669, 735
cerebral palsy 112, 318
cereus, Bacillus 99
cervical carcinoma 184, 200, 206, 308, 333
Cessna 185® 527
chain reactions, free radical 83, 106, 107, 196, 261, 270, 279, 318, 332, 368, 793, 799
charts 27, 54, 73, 79, 105, 106, 107, 123, 130, 131, 145, 147, 153, 154, 156, 157, 203, 224, 353, 354, 355, 358, 359, 360, 379, 381, 390, 446, 460, 632, 657, 675, 689, 775, 777, 780, 781, 782
checkups 184, 750
chelation 96, 97, 99, 245, 247, 263, 264, 280, 299, 391, 419, 421, 465, 468, 612, 637, 674, 748, 749, 756, 788
chemistry 59, 166, 514, 551, 627, 666, 671, 682, 685, 689, 704, 718
chemists 627, 632, 659
chemoprevention of cancer 559, 664, 682
chemotactic 633, 694
chemotherapy 88, 89, 335, 336, 337, 729, 730
chest 204, 325, 352
Chicago BCG 343
chickens 82, 86, 192, 308, 382, 388, 389, 405, 477, 702
childbearing 39
childhood 258, 343, 356, 357, 505, 686, 744, 767, 770
children 4, 20, 81, 122, 135, 149, 150, 172, 176, 182, 183, 186, 190, 193, 261, 274, 277, 305, 313, 339, 340, 341, 350, 351, 354, 356, 357, 358, 360, 399, 420, 431, 451, 465, 468, 471, 485, 508, 571, 611, 614, 615, 621, 631, 651, 686, 718, 734, 747
chimpanzees 18, 20, 105, 146, 614, 616

chlorination 260, 315, 570, 705
choking 102, 344, 354, 355
cholinergic 131, 134, 135, 170, 171, 175, 190, 250, 641, 647, 649, 651, 788
chromatography 518, 527
chromosomes 84, 264, 338, 506, 507, 636, 663, 682, 693, 710, 769, 789, 793
chronogene 710
circadian rhythms 786
circulation 119, 197, 199, 201, 213, 273, 316, 317, 318, 324, 351, 372, 386, 406, 421, 514, 767
cirrhosis of the liver, 272, 274
citations 457, 543
claudication 406
claustrophobia 534
Clean Air Act 720
Clinical Guide to Undesirable Drug Interactions and Interferences 444
clinical laboratory tests 29, 90, 166, 430, 434, 435, 437, 439, 441, 442, 443, 447, 448, 455, 458, 459, 462, 463, 466, 467, 697, 730, 731, 737, 750, 757, 775, 776
clinical research 305, 457, 485, 538, 551, 658
Clinistix® 315
Clinistrips® 446
Clinitest® 688
clocked cell cycle clocks 644, 660, 709
clocklike 644, 660
clocks 9, 21, 65, 98, 137, 138, 139, 140, 141, 142, 147, 153, 213, 216, 220, 286, 515, 551, 629, 642, 644, 709, 710, 786, 790, 795
clones 86, 506, 507, 708, 722, 789
closed-chest cardiopulmonary resuscitation (CPR) 177
clot 70, 102, 108, 224, 311, 312, 317, 318, 327, 338, 366, 377, 786, 796, 800, 802, 804
clot-preventing 70
clots 103, 108, 279, 285, 307, 309, 311, 314, 316, 317, 318, 319, 322, 327, 329, 368, 386, 402, 403, 404, 415, 452, 642, 801
CNS. *See* central nervous system
coal burning power plants, radiation released by 264, 705
cochlea 175
cognitive abilities 112, 127, 175, 178, 469, 648, 664, 667, 676, 699
cold extremities 323, 766, 767
colds 408, 740
collagen injections 499
collapse, respiratory 206–207, 281
colon 339, 366, 683
coma 133, 442, 706
combustion 144, 279, 333, 336, 339, 364, 378, 406, 688, 705, 786, 787, 800
common cold 408, 531, 634, 693, 699
complete blood count (CBC) 447, 449 (PTO)
computer hacker 724
computer hackers 515
computer program 315, 519, 523
computer programmer 751, 752
computer systems 514, 625, 722
computers 78, 330, 373, 444, 508, 509, 510, 512, 513, 514, 515, 519, 523, 524, 527, 543, 551, 625, 675, 688, 722, 723, 724, 771, 787

Comtel® computerized image analysis
equipment 527
conception 103
concussion 350
conditioning 222, 223, 224, 254, 444, 515,
648
condom 202
confusion, mental 127, 187, 227, 273, 351,706
congestion 135, 179, 192
congestive heart failure 455
conjunctivitis 763, 764
connective tissue 88, 95, 103, 137, 336, 409,
635, 789, 792
consciousness 110, 193, 352
constipation 135, 180, 192
consultations, physician 14, 29, 166, 168, 194,
246, 258, 281, 288, 294, 296, 302, 316,
435, 443, 459, 467, 539, 635, 708, 726,
737, 767
Consumer Reports® 624, 716
consumers 274, 375, 561, 566, 579, 581, 582,
583, 586, 587, 588, 632, 689, 691, 714,
716, 720
Consumers Union® 563, 595, 715, 716
containers 379, 388, 417, 418
contaminants 369, 383, 667
contraception 203, 471, 656
contraceptives 313, 696
contraindications 170, 174, 257, 435, 455
controlled experiments 48, 49, 86, 104, 112,
128, 129, 131, 149, 190, 250, 273, 274,
284, 288, 292, 295, 302, 326, 332, 402,
411, 412, 470, 473, 481, 482, 507, 567,
569, 572, 574, 647, 666, 670, 679, 684,
687, 694, 701, 703, 785, 789, 795
contusion 639
convulsions 193, 194, 277, 706, 804
cooked foods 237, 294, 313, 314, 369, 377,
382, 474, 689
cookie shelf life test 388
cooking 260, 294, 313, 314, 337, 343, 368,
369, 379, 380, 382, 386, 387, 388, 417,
474, 688
cooking oil shelf life test 386
coordination 131, 226, 228, 484
copper bracelets for arthritis 298
corneas 348
coronary 108, 316, 322, 325, 638, 677, 679,
680, 686, 687
coronary thrombosis 70, 108, 307
corpses 95, 505
corpuscles 800
correlation 143, 146, 147, 260, 324, 325, 562,
645, 666, 684, 691, 700, 703, 709, 712
cortex 647, 657, 662, 686
cosmetic surgery 501
cosmetics 53, 163, 210, 211, 422, 493, 499,
577, 578, 587, 626, 627, 659, 672, 677,
696, 714, 741
cosmetics industry 741
cost-benefit analysis 569, 691, 719
cost-effectiveness 19, 27, 556, 559, 562, 610
coughs 162, 244, 257, 352, 357, 730
CPR (cardiopulmonary resuscitation) 177,
351, 352, 686
cracked lips 420
cramps 135, 174, 204, 229, 767, 768
craving 249, 258, 292, 425, 606

creativity 39, 180, 185, 363, 631
Creutzfeldt-Jakob disease 129, 334
crib death (SIDS) 304, 621
crises 38, 508, 524
cross-linkers 88, 96, 210, 265, 300, 368, 784,
790, 792
cross-linking 91, 92, 93, 94, 95, 96, 97, 98, 99,
100, 102, 107, 112, 115, 153, 163, 174,
177, 209, 211, 242, 243, 247, 269, 270,
279, 316, 319, 320, 325, 339, 373, 382,
385, 387, 405, 406, 481, 501, 615, 635,
658, 670, 675, 677, 710, 789, 790, 792,
796, 800
cruciforms 710
crushed 732
crushing injuries 31, 237, 300, 347, 348, 354,
414, 477, 525, 759
cryobiology 720
cryogenics 609
cryonics 608, 609, 610, 720
crystalline 498, 620, 622, 744
crystallization 473, 769
crystals 103, 170, 244, 247, 387, 388, 430,
462, 466, 488, 620, 749, 805
CT (computerized tomography, CAT scan)
533, 719
cults 49, 50, 631, 656
cutaneous 676, 678, 698
cuts 412
cybernetics 511, 514
cyborgs 508
cycles 78, 79, 176, 187, 201, 213, 227, 271,
304, 316, 425, 475, 479, 502, 534, 644,
650, 758, 789
cystic fibrosis 339
cystine stone formation 482
cysts 298, 348
cytoplasm 121, 123, 803

dancers 93, 509, 653
dandruff 220, 471, 472, 744, 757, 758, 768
data base 153, 393, 510, 527, 540, 543, 712
de-differentiation 150, 151, 421, 790, 804
deafness 178, 508, 733
death clock 98, 141, 515
death hormone 74, 98
deep vein thrombosis 327, 403
deer mouse 105
deficiency 78, 87, 119, 126, 132, 134, 165,
175, 186, 202, 217, 227, 248, 265, 279,
289, 312, 313, 319, 354, 360, 421, 436,
437, 453, 467, 470, 471, 474, 477, 482,
666, 671, 677, 685, 686, 704, 722, 763,
764, 768, 788, 795
deficiency of thyroid hormone effects 767
degenerative diseases 6, 11, 74, 334, 635
Delaney amendment 570, 571, 704, 705
delirium 761
delusion 511, 589, 704
dementia 125, 649
demodulation 524
dendrites 132
densimeter 446
dental caries 371
depigmentation 757
deplete 289
depletion 171, 172, 174, 181, 251, 287, 182,
431, 498, 745, 799

375

depletor 182
depolymerizing 297
depression 37, 126, 127, 129, 136, 170, 171,
    172, 174, 181, 182, 183, 184, 185, 186,
    187, 196, 202, 204, 278, 288, 292, 305,
    431, 459, 468, 485, 649, 651, 652, 669,
    672, 713, 727, 745, 755, 799
dermatology 627
detoxification 334, 337, 347, 795, 797
developmental clock control 515, 551
diabetes insipidus 173, 174, 762
diabetes mellitus 84, 96, 138, 165, 168, 173,
    207, 212, 246, 267, 286, 315, 325, 334,
    371, 373, 415, 416, 417, 420, 425, 438,
    442, 446, 450, 467, 476, 482, 675, 689,
    762
diabetic retinopathy 315
diagnosis 168, 189, 296, 438, 449, 450, 451,
    453, 510, 658, 697, 726, 727, 749, 762,
    766
diagnostics 316, 420, 591, 619, 787
diagonal ear-lobe crease, as a coronary risk
    factor 679
dialysis 192, 556
diaphragm 202
diarrhea 135, 164, 171, 187, 246, 276, 281,
    415, 435, 487, 488, 489, 621
diet 10, 31, 44, 55, 77, 78, 86, 89, 110, 111,
    112, 126, 170, 171, 227, 230, 244, 247,
    249, 251, 261, 265, 268, 277, 284, 286,
    288, 289, 291, 292, 294, 295, 308, 312,
    313, 314, 315, 322, 324, 338, 341, 342,
    363, 364, 366, 367, 368, 370, 371, 373,
    377, 383, 392, 393, 398, 404, 405, 409,
    412, 415, 416, 417, 420, 421, 426, 436,
    459, 462, 470, 474, 478, 479, 482, 488,
    515, 571, 619, 629, 632, 634, 638, 644,
    649, 652, 666, 672, 674, 675, 681, 684,
    687, 688, 696, 699, 702, 703, 750, 754,
    759, 768, 777
dietary restriction, 66, 98
dietetic 693
dieting 110, 284, 286, 293, 425
differentiation 138, 149, 150, 151, 152, 421,
    790, 802
diffusion 123, 325, 584, 790
diffusion-dependent biochemical reactions
    121
digestion 99, 294, 383, 411, 672
digestive tract 291, 488, 748
dilator 795
diploid 708
disability 170, 303, 317, 585, 588
disasters 38, 157, 342, 568, 572, 584, 585, 714
disclaimers 246, 281, 485
discontinue cautions 138, 178, 194, 258, 423,
    436, 455, 456, 469, 470, 474, 498, 640,
    661, 662, 748, 751, 753, 762, 766, 767,
    768, 803
dishwashing 254
disinfection 260
disinhibiting 269, 277
disorientation 241, 498
distillation 54, 260, 268, 274, 315, 407, 603,
    754
diving 505
dizziness 127, 177, 247, 732
DNA repair 20, 142, 146, 147, 515, 645

DNA Software Project 515
DNA synthesis 147
doctors 4, 29, 44, 48, 51, 82, 165, 168, 169,
    173, 177, 178, 179, 188, 189, 194, 207,
    215, 226, 246, 256, 257, 258, 263, 275,
    281, 302, 321, 325, 328, 329, 341, 350,
    352, 358, 363, 373, 393, 410, 422, 430,
    432, 435, 437, 438, 439, 440, 442, 454,
    455, 456, 457, 459, 460, 462, 469, 474,
    492, 502, 515, 535, 537, 539, 541, 551,
    572, 573, 575, 582, 587, 592, 595, 713,
    746, 765
dogs 113, 128, 254, 276, 290, 326, 351, 409,
    412, 608, 638, 680, 681, 694, 699, 701,
    744, 745
dolphins 508, 616
donations 535, 536, 619, 621, 640, 661
Doomsday Has Been Cancelled 708
dopaminergic stimulation 135, 140, 290
Dorland's Illustrated Medical Dictionary 457,
    697
dosimeter 516, 791, 792
double blind studies 47, 49, 302, 327, 482,
    514, 725, 762, 725, 791. *See also*
    controlled study
Double Helix 76, 550, 633, 707
doublethink 593
doubling time for knowledge 32, 630
Down's syndrome 20
dreams 37, 167, 189, 193, 194, 195, 484, 526,
    722
drinking 5, 13, 23, 24, 174, 176, 241, 242,
    260, 265, 267, 268, 270, 271, 272, 274,
    275, 277, 278, 279, 281, 282, 315, 338,
    340, 345, 374, 386, 390, 391, 399, 413,
    418, 491, 518, 525, 751, 754, 755
driving 33, 174, 277, 747
Drosophila Melanogaster 121, 506, 673, 692
drowning 112, 176, 182, 183, 257, 350, 525,
    608
drowsiness 193, 420, 426
drug approval 350
drug delivery system 214
drug interactions 283, 444, 455, 531, 669, 670
drug lag 593
drug regulation 566, 572, 573, 589, 593
drug rehabilitation kit 621
drugstores 4, 5, 83, 92, 97, 164, 192, 193, 208,
    217, 249, 315, 354, 393, 446, 447, 624,
    713, 714, 748
duodenum 258, 290, 488
Durk: allergies 763; bad back 761; case
    history 304, 745, 761; gout 769; and
    growth hormone releasers 771; hair-
    raising experiences 768; ignores nutrition
    and gets an awful stomachache 768;
    peculiar pituitary, polydipsia, and
    polyuria 762, 765; and sunburn, 770;
    total serum cholesterol, 367; varicose
    veins, 767
dwarfism 136
dynamic equilibrium 72
dysfunction 501, 658, 765
dyskinesia 134, 482
dystrophy 334, 451

E deficiency 78, 639, 692, 794
ear lobe crease 325, 326, 327, 679

earaches 485, 732
ears 64, 175, 177, 178, 179, 305, 325, 501, 726, 732
economics 283, 444, 455, 461, 492, 507, 508, 531, 533, 551, 557, 561, 567, 578, 579, 580, 581, 585, 609, 630, 657, 669, 697, 713, 715, 716, 717, 718, 719, 721, 723
Economics From a Biological Viewpoint 630, 721
economists 558, 565, 577, 579, 594
edema 237, 348, 455, 456, 765
EEG. *See* electroencephalogram
eels 141
efficacy 47, 98, 161, 441, 442, 555, 564, 572, 575, 578, 580, 582, 588, 589, 716, 730
Ehrlich ascites tumor 242, 333, 633, 682
EKG. *See* electrocardiogram
elasticity 93, 100, 103, 165, 208, 209, 269, 316, 330, 368, 385, 386, 406, 635
elderly 9, 16, 25, 110, 129, 152, 183, 557, 652, 661
electrical stimulation 150, 152, 290, 646
electrobiology 152
electrocardiogram 791
electrochemistry 150, 518
electrocution 257
electroencephalogram (EEG) 135, 176, 177, 194, 228, 240, 257, 269, 319, 320, 350, 522, 642, 643, 791
electron micrograph 88, 310
electron spin resonance (ESR) spectrometer 520, 527
electron transport 406
electronegativity 151
electronic precipitator 253, 254
electronic pulse rate counters 446
electrophoresis 448, 518
electrostatic precipitator 261, 263, 625, 666, 669
electrotherapy 152
elephants 63, 64, 145, 147, 153, 616
elevated serum cholesterol is an indicator of elevated free radical activity 367
elevators 292, 502
embalming 268, 269, 608
embryos 112, 149, 403
emergency medicine 257, 350, 351, 352, 354, 524, 525
emissions 527, 562
emotions 49, 56, 126, 129, 131, 176, 276, 791, 799
emphysema 102, 176, 177, 242, 254, 256, 265, 269, 406, 524
emulsification 478, 776
emulsion 352
encephalitis 133, 411
endocrinology 626, 627, 644
endothelial cell 108, 109
endothelium 96
endurance 8
energy 15, 23, 37, 38, 77, 78, 97, 100, 101, 111, 165, 172, 176, 177, 181, 187, 209, 226, 227, 228, 236, 263, 264, 280, 285, 315, 320, 341, 378, 402, 406, 414, 474, 475, 479, 481, 506, 508, 516, 560, 594, 632, 706, 708, 717, 735, 740, 741, 743, 746, 749, 750, 755, 786, 789, 792, 797, 801, 804

engines 391
enhancer 509
environment 18, 68, 71, 72, 76, 77, 92, 131, 144, 240, 259, 266, 269, 271, 272, 274, 325, 354, 405, 430, 475, 484, 519, 523, 537, 561, 562, 574, 583, 587, 616, 626, 666, 671, 681, 685, 703, 708, 741
enzymatic 72, 104, 270, 279, 297, 382, 403, 520, 674, 678
enzyme activity 72, 73, 776
enzyme adaptation 72, 73
epidemiology 242, 792
epidermal 138, 165, 210, 211, 644, 646, 647, 658, 660, 694
epigraph 556
epilepsy 258, 277, 642, 643; treated with antioxidants 642, 643
epileptiform 643
epilogue 504, 708
epiphyses 765
epistemology 44, 45, 792
epithelial 151, 247, 419, 420, 421, 801
EPR (electron paramagnetic resonance) 162, 521
equilibrium 630, 721
equipment 93, 144, 180, 200, 352, 520, 521, 522, 527, 556, 625
equivalents 502, 707
erosion 401
erotic self-image 654
eroticism 652, 653, 654, 656
erythema 146, 770
erythematosus 89, 296
erythrocyte sedimentation rate 449, 453
erythropoietic protoporphyria 743
Escherichia coli 506
Eskimos 44, 313, 314
esophagus 278, 340
ESR (electron spin resonance) 520, 521, 524, 527
ESR. *See* erythrocyte sedimentation rate
essential hypertension 244, 249, 345, 426, 436, 462, 488, 619
estrogenic 199, 201, 704
estrous 644
ethics 18, 306, 485, 502, 503
euphoria 224, 277, 293
evolutionary 18, 20, 55, 142, 286, 551
excitation 204, 205, 793
executives 39
exercise 5, 86, 110, 165, 174, 222, 223, 224, 225, 226, 229, 230, 231, 233, 284, 286, 289, 290, 315, 373, 444, 446, 459, 505, 515, 535, 538, 573, 580, 661, 672, 675, 688, 725, 735, 736, 741, 745, 766, 772, 774
exercises 224, 231, 735
exhaustion 182, 227, 479
exogenous 693
experimental formulations 210, 513, 619, 776
experimental subjects 302, 726, 729, 764, 770, 789, 791
experimental treatment 180, 299, 466, 631, 791
experts 13, 49, 50, 51, 52, 273, 409, 438, 455, 563, 572, 580, 582, 587, 727
extended cooked-chicken shelf-storage life test 388

377

extended life spans 20, 30, 38, 41, 42, 43, 140, 725
eyebrows 420
eyes 14, 37, 56, 76, 93, 128, 139, 174, 175, 193, 209, 219, 315, 348, 350, 422, 447, 494, 515, 522, 604, 715, 745, 760, 763, 790

face 14, 15, 134, 197, 204, 277, 325, 494, 499, 501, 556, 727, 729
facelifts 501
faddist 368
faddists 368, 438
falls 63, 72, 86, 129, 139, 153, 172, 175, 181, 189, 196, 212, 213, 286, 323, 337, 345, 421, 444, 487, 491, 498, 585, 587, 594, 640, 657, 759, 787
family 39, 66, 104, 138, 169, 188, 235, 252, 263, 271, 303, 332, 374, 387, 400, 437, 438, 518, 657, 769
famines 285, 286
fantasy 363, 504, 517, 658, 747
farms 332, 505, 515
FAS. See fetal alcohol syndrome
fasting 86, 229, 289, 373, 450
fatalities 420
fatfold measurements 774
fatigue 165, 172, 227, 228, 305, 485
fauns 653
fears 30, 37, 317, 328, 331, 378, 408, 454, 499, 573, 705
feelings. See emotions
feet 317, 731, 732, 734, 735, 749, 751, 760, 765, 767, 769, 770, 774
females 10, 19, 54, 65, 112, 136, 139, 141, 196, 197, 199, 213, 286, 325, 329, 407, 451, 471, 482, 484, 653, 654, 656, 721, 775, 792
fermentation 268
fertility 203, 657
fertility control 202, 657
fetal alcohol syndrome (FAS) 277
fetus 112, 122, 124, 137, 175, 211, 431
fever 86, 260, 307, 411, 453, 584, 730
fiber 122, 164, 265, 276, 291, 366, 368, 370, 371, 399, 412, 482, 536, 666, 684, 703, 788
fibrillation 344, 352
fibrinolytic 224
fibroblast 144
fibrocystic breast disease 405
fibrosis 242, 339, 405
fight or flight reaction 328, 735
fillers 273, 305, 306, 347, 407, 462, 485, 492, 619, 620, 621
film badge dosimeter 728, 792
filters 253, 254, 255, 260, 262, 269, 315, 712, 803
filtration 260
finger joint diameter, and excessive growth hormone 765
fingerprints 429
fingers 93, 149, 200, 219, 299, 385, 747, 748, 765
fires 169, 171, 524, 717, 801, 803
fishy smell 164
fitness 224, 532, 661, 662, 671
flamingos 97, 422

flatus 489
flavors 347, 377, 378, 382, 388, 476, 499, 689
flies 19, 28, 110, 121, 264, 404, 507, 753
flu 83, 408, 479, 531, 634, 699, 740, 742
fluorescence 121, 527, 750, 788
flushing 193, 204, 205, 244, 246, 247, 281, 282, 283, 426, 434, 435, 436, 463, 470
flying 135, 189, 328, 574, 667, 734, 735, 753
fog 164, 173, 277
folklore 653
follicles 139, 213, 219, 765
followup 540
food preparation methods, carcinogen production and 369
food safety regulations 691, 719
forgetfulness 127, 131, 168
foundations 33, 535, 538, 552, 619, 621
fractures 148, 150, 152, 408, 413, 645
Framingham Study 324, 679, 687
frauds 494, 499, 501, 502, 566, 591, 593, 713, 714
freckles 121, 124, 175, 750
free radical damage 100, 102, 103, 104, 110, 111, 112, 124, 142, 209, 221, 265, 297, 313, 314, 318, 320, 324, 338, 347, 406, 413, 417, 482, 518, 560, 642, 665, 696, 729, 740, 758, 759, 785
free radical disease 793
free radical pathology 100, 273, 277, 339, 457, 557, 559, 560, 636, 638, 643, 685, 752, 768, 770
free radical scavengers, epileptics and 642
free radical theory of aging 100, 103, 110, 146, 378, 496, 636, 637, 638, 639, 650, 690, 700, 702, 751
Free Radicals in Medicine and Biology 639
Free to Choose 533, 564, 714, 717
freedom of choice 555, 567, 573, 589, 590, 592, 595, 596, 691, 713, 714, 716, 718
Freedom of Choice legislation 590, 592, 593, 594, 595, 596
freezers 357
freshness 99, 110, 322, 347, 368, 371, 376, 382, 386, 388, 408, 492
frogs 56, 150, 151, 165, 227, 479, 507
fruit flies. See Drosophila Melanogaster
frying 368, 382
fuels 206, 227, 265, 324, 391, 479, 688, 800
funding 11, 24, 33, 42, 305, 502, 511, 514, 535, 536, 551, 552, 555, 556, 557, 559, 563, 604, 609, 610, 619, 621, 771
further information 42, 165, 193, 198, 211, 257, 263, 316, 320, 321, 405, 426, 484, 592, 593, 705, 745, 764
fusion 38
future 4, 6, 13, 17, 30, 32, 37, 38, 40, 86, 89, 148, 166, 180, 208, 221, 275, 336, 504, 505, 507, 511, 584, 596, 608, 609, 717

gadgets 723
Galapagos turtle 616
gamma rays 791
garlic breath, urine, and sweat (selenium overdose) 472
gasoline storage and BHT 391
gastric cancer 663, 683, 690
gastrointestinal cancer 666, 684, 703

gastrointestinal tract 97, 122, 135, 151, 164, 174, 204, 228, 229, 247, 290, 291, 340, 386, 403, 410, 419, 451, 464, 488, 489, 519, 672, 802
gender 657, 778
gene splicing 509
gene synthesizing machine 624
generic 179, 492, 501, 502, 503
genes 18, 19, 20, 21, 22, 141, 367, 507, 519, 534, 617, 630, 648, 718, 793
genetic defects 77, 104, 138, 252, 271, 339, 769
genetic diseases 289, 506, 693, 744
genetic engineering 21, 506, 507, 617
genetic programming 506
genetic read only memories (GROMS) 517, 658
genetically determined life span 71
genetics 11, 18, 20, 21, 22, 39, 40, 68, 71, 76, 81, 98, 101, 103, 106, 107, 137, 138, 139, 140, 145, 146, 149, 219, 221, 265, 271, 272, 293, 332, 429, 471, 472, 473, 506, 507, 524, 534, 551, 616, 617, 629, 632, 658, 669, 670, 710, 753, 762, 770, 786, 789, 790, 791, 793
genital herpes 205, 206, 752
geniuses 505, 550
genome 506, 514
geriatrics 327, 627
germs 54, 100, 403, 407
gerontologists 11, 65, 106, 174, 407, 461, 495, 511, 551, 557, 558, 560
gerontology 11, 49, 58, 66, 157, 511, 541, 557, 558, 560, 626, 627, 640, 641, 645, 652, 661, 664, 677, 685, 692, 701, 777
gestation 581, 583
GH. See growth hormone
giant anteater 616
giantism 765
giraffe 616
glands 57, 73, 82, 85, 86, 87, 89, 98, 131, 134, 137, 139, 140, 141, 164, 165, 172, 174, 190, 196, 223, 228, 229, 287, 290, 293, 305, 321, 323, 336, 342, 345, 373, 413, 419, 421, 432, 452, 475, 534, 565, 649, 726, 728, 735, 740, 741, 742, 763, 771, 786, 788, 794, 795, 796, 799, 804
glossary 783–805
glycolysis 227
goiter 631
Gompertz law 9, 70, 794
gonads 420, 644
gorillas 55, 105, 409, 616
gout 103, 169, 170, 267, 271, 305, 328, 429, 430, 435, 450, 465, 466, 473, 485, 487, 575, 592, 677, 762, 765, 769, 776, 805
government funds 604
government policies 526, 556
government regulations 560
grants 535, 538, 552, 558, 559, 619, 621, 656, 685, 717
graphs 72, 73, 105, 123, 145, 147, 780
graying hair 217, 473, 476
great Indian rhinoceros 616
GROMS. See (genetic read only memories)
growth hormone (GH) release 86, 134, 194, 223, 229, 236, 288. 289, 373, 432, 475, 509, 678

growth-hormone-releaser scandal 509
growth hormone (GH) secretion 633, 634, 641, 662
growth stimulants 213, 345
guinea pigs 26, 31, 56, 57, 59, 65, 123, 345, 398, 409, 410, 412, 414, 416, 441, 467, 481, 518, 640, 649, 658, 701
gut 164, 187, 291, 294, 336, 354, 384, 410, 421, 488, 671, 798, 801
guts 384
gynecologists 200, 201
gynecomastia 766

habits 5, 6, 24, 222, 256, 459
hacker 724
hackers 515
hair 8, 76, 81, 139, 175, 197, 212, 213, 214, 215, 216, 217, 218, 219, 220, 221, 382, 420, 473, 476, 479, 482, 516, 574, 659, 660, 742, 744, 745, 757, 758, 759, 768
hair follicles 139, 213, 214, 216, 742, 758
hair loss 212, 215, 217, 219, 220, 471, 472, 473, 476, 659, 757
hallucinations 426
hamburgers, hot dogs, and sausages, peroxidation and 369
hands 63, 93, 138, 182, 183, 226, 275, 299, 352, 385, 386, 526, 594, 745, 747, 767
hangovers 194, 270, 272, 603, 751, 752
hard work 44, 232
hardback 531
hardening of the arteries 209, 307, 316, 368
Harrison act 714
HDL/LDL ratios 312, 324, 365, 367, 450, 466, 780
head 7, 42, 104, 139, 173, 212, 214, 219, 220, 231, 240, 316, 350, 471, 502, 554, 555, 556, 557, 567, 651, 749, 757, 758
headaches 135, 177, 178, 179, 185, 188, 192, 229, 247, 251, 276, 288, 305, 373, 420, 485, 576, 751, 763
healing 99, 129, 148, 150, 152, 165, 237, 238, 345, 347, 348, 408, 412, 413, 416, 420, 470, 477, 481, 532, 602, 646, 673, 693, 694, 735, 790, 795
health food 5, 164, 192, 193, 208, 217, 239, 244, 389, 776
health food stores 55, 83, 87, 89, 92, 102, 127, 135, 164, 169, 171, 195, 238, 240, 243, 251, 259, 272, 298, 348, 462, 663, 670, 748
hearing lll, 178, 179, 239, 642, 726, 731, 732, 733
hearing loss 128, 178
heart 92, 105, 106, 121, 123, 216, 222, 224, 257, 279, 284, 285, 302, 326, 328, 329, 330, 331, 336, 344, 350, 352, 363, 366, 405, 406, 413, 450, 451, 452, 455, 476, 522, 532, 663, 674, 675, 676, 677, 678, 679, 687, 691, 692, 693, 694, 695, 697, 723, 735, 777
heart attacks 11, 25, 103, 124, 176, 224, 229, 257, 260, 285, 312, 314, 316, 318, 322, 323, 324, 325, 326, 327, 328, 350, 363, 366, 367, 402, 413, 426, 439, 451, 453, 467, 525, 575, 576, 592, 595, 602, 677, 679, 680, 717, 734, 786, 801

heart disease 6, 74, 225, 259, 285, 294, 308,
   315, 324, 325, 328, 363, 364, 365, 406,
   424, 450, 463, 585, 677, 679, 687, 777,
   794, 796
heartbeat 352
heartburn 487
heat 98, 209, 240, 285, 300, 377, 384, 387,
   417, 491, 508, 756
height 76, 236, 342, 477, 765
Heimlich maneuver (for choking) 355
helixes 789
helplessness 136, 170, 181, 182, 183, 184,
   278, 651
Hemastix® 447
hemoglobin level 447, 449, 453
hemolysis 106, 237, 403, 518, 759, 764, 777,
   786, 794
hemorrhages 92, 96, 102, 174, 317, 318, 319
HEPA filter 253, 254, 263, 624, 666, 669
hepatitis 333, 351, 352, 412
heredity 18, 22, 58, 146, 267, 268, 270, 271,
   285, 293, 341, 429, 438, 466, 762, 763,
   767, 769, 795
herpes 206, 308, 320, 333, 334, 411, 479, 573,
   752, 753
hexokinase method 246, 447, 448, 450, 467,
   777
hiccups 256
high blood pressure 92, 110, 136, 172, 185,
   186, 191, 204, 221, 224, 229, 251, 273,
   288, 293, 294, 325, 328, 329, 438, 444,
   450, 488, 659, 734, 736
high-energy radiation 127
high-nicotine and low-carcinogen cigarette
   563
high-pressure liquid chromatography 518,
   527
hirsutism 221
hives 305, 485, 763
Hodgkin's disease 730
homeopathic remedies 572
homeostasis 639
homocysteinemia 674, 676, 678
homocystinuria 674, 678
hormone replacement therapy 198
horse 54, 113, 117, 145, 289, 298, 505, 616,
   744, 745, 754, 767
hospitals 152, 277, 330, 334, 337, 343, 344,
   345, 348, 352, 554, 556, 573, 580, 657,
   685, 735
hot flashes 200, 201
humectants 163, 210
humoral 633, 681, 693, 699
hunger 176, 284, 286, 289, 291, 295, 425
hydrocephaly 524
hydroelectric power 705
hydrogenated oils 425
hydrolysis 407, 462
hydrophobic 215, 702
hygrometer 446
hyperactivity 140
hyperbaric 119, 516, 665, 696
hypercholesterolemia 367, 425, 438, 478, 663,
   695, 700, 795
hyperkinesis 135, 172, 186, 193, 274
hyperplasia 660, 758
hyperprolactinemia 766
hypersensitivity 743, 766

hypertension. See High blood pressure
hypervitaminosis A (overdose of vitamin A)
   419, 420
hypoascorbemia 693
hypochondria 456
hypoglycemia 176, 229, 289, 370, 373, 425,
   672, 678, 696
hypoglycemic 372, 373, 482
hyponatremia 706
hypophysectomy 236, 343, 478
hypothalamus 71, 131, 140, 236, 286, 290,
   292, 323, 343, 478, 497, 534, 641, 657,
   740, 765, 786, 788, 795
hypothermia 142, 720, 769
hypothyroidism 678, 721, 767
hypoventilation 265
hypoxia 112, 119, 124, 318, 320, 350, 351,
   354, 413, 482, 502, 524, 525, 674, 767,
   795
hysteria 571, 714

ice 285, 347, 351, 499, 767, 775
identical twins 53, 149, 429, 506, 789
ideology 537, 560
illness 182, 183, 185, 189, 436, 561, 631, 658,
   719, 760
immediate hypersensitivity reactions 673
immortal 6, 614
immortalist 11
immortalists 11
immortality 6, 26, 58
immune function 88, 308, 437, 449, 466
immune system 57, 59, 70, 73, 81, 82, 83, 84,
   85, 86, 87, 88, 89, 90, 100, 108, 110, 127,
   129, 161, 162, 165, 172, 183, 184, 190,
   206, 210, 223, 229, 263, 266, 270, 279,
   285, 296, 298, 303, 305, 307, 308, 313,
   316, 320, 323, 331, 332, 335, 336, 337,
   339, 340, 341, 342, 356, 357, 358, 370,
   405, 408, 409, 416, 419, 421, 452, 459,
   471, 483, 509, 559, 573, 602, 633, 634,
   635, 652, 672, 683, 686, 727, 729, 730,
   740, 741, 742, 762, 785, 786, 789, 794,
   796, 801, 804
immune system decline 86, 804
immune system function 83, 86, 88, 89, 127,
   139, 285, 303, 481, 771, 791, 804
immune system stimulant 87, 305, 323, 339,
   419, 421, 477, 481
immunity 28, 57, 66, 81, 85, 86, 87, 88, 89,
   112, 126, 129, 162, 181, 191, 262, 286,
   296, 304, 308, 319, 335, 337, 338, 340,
   341, 356, 357, 358, 368, 373, 377, 411,
   421, 448, 449, 477, 534, 633, 681, 693,
   699, 730, 800
immunization 340, 357, 358, 360, 686, 730
immunization schedules 358, 359, 360
immunocompetence 634, 652, 683
immunodeficiency 89, 634, 682
immunofluorescence 634
immunoglobulin electrophoresis 448
immunology 123, 351, 352, 449, 627, 633,
   634, 672, 681, 682, 699, 730
immunostimulation 730
immunosuppression 191, 727
immunotherapy 340, 357
impotence 202, 207
IND (investigational new drug) 553

Indian fruit bat 616
indicators 51, 312, 324, 325, 420, 437, 442,
    446, 453, 470, 635, 765
induction of protective enzymes 515, 516
indigestion 415, 487
industry 39, 253, 261, 308, 349, 375, 387, 476,
    492, 508, 509, 560, 561, 562, 593, 594,
    659, 672, 677, 696, 708, 714, 741
inertial confinement fusion 508
infants 20, 93, 149, 210, 289, 304, 341, 343,
    356, 358, 360, 387, 420, 508, 537, 608,
    621, 686, 706
infarction 318, 413, 451, 452, 674, 678, 693,
    796
infections 8, 28, 29, 72, 81, 129, 178, 181,
    200, 205, 206, 207, 285, 296, 305, 308,
    323, 334, 337, 339, 350, 351, 356, 360,
    402, 411, 421, 437, 447, 467, 479, 482,
    485, 573, 584, 634, 636, 682, 686, 700,
    732, 752, 756, 758, 765
inflammations 237, 298, 304
influenza 334, 412
information theory 45, 504, 514, 521, 551
injections 31, 87, 89, 170, 171, 173, 177, 199,
    214, 238, 297, 327, 340, 345, 350, 351,
    354, 358, 403, 405, 410, 412, 451, 477,
    496, 499, 743, 748, 759
injuries 31, 87, 98, 149, 162, 173, 210, 237,
    238, 173, 237, 299, 300, 318, 345, 347,
    348, 350, 354, 414, 419, 421, 477, 484,
    636, 638, 643, 664, 667, 686, 700, 719,
    732, 740, 746, 754, 759, 760, 769, 785
inoculations 633, 682, 730
insects 140, 404, 599, 644, 758
insomnia 172, 178, 185, 186, 188, 191, 192,
    193, 195, 251, 276, 288, 498
instrumentation and systems characterization
    techniques for measuring aging 511
intelligence 20, 29, 112, 128, 166, 167, 168,
    251, 276, 356, 482, 502, 535, 620, 656
intercourse 200
interferometer 527
intermittent claudication 406
International Unit (I.U.) 407, 491, 613
intervention in the aging process 646, 699
intestinal. See Gastrointestinal tract
intima 801
intoxication 136, 187, 281, 283
intramuscular 177, 411
intrathoracic 352
intravenous 173, 345, 348, 350, 410, 411, 484,
    496, 620, 638
intravenous ascorbate 410
intrinsic life span 10
in vitro studies 502, 638, 640, 673, 689, 701
in vivo studies 502, 518, 645, 659, 692
involution 161, 796
ionization 527
ionizing radiation 534
IQ 351, 524
irradiation 332, 694, 699
irritability 135, 136, 172, 185, 188, 189, 192,
    251, 288, 420, 431, 498, 706
irritants 103, 187, 218, 488, 515, 758
ischemia 639, 677, 686
ischemic myocardium 638, 680
itching 193, 206, 244, 246, 247, 281, 282, 305,
    426, 463, 485, 744, 745, 758, 763, 764

itchy eyes 744
itchy scalp 757, 758, 768
IUDs 202, 203

jaundice 422
jelly 479, 491
jitters 127, 176, 187
jogging 222, 223, 224, 229, 290
joint 83, 103, 104, 149, 161, 169, 170, 236,
    250, 296, 297, 298, 300, 305, 342, 430,
    466, 473, 477, 485, 747, 748, 749, 760,
    765, 769, 795, 805
joint diameters (and excessive growth
    hormone) 765
journals 46, 51, 527, 539, 540, 541, 560, 574,
    626, 628, 801

kayaks 775
Kefauver amendments 98, 578, 580, 581, 704,
    714
keratinocytes 124, 138, 644
kidneys 87, 169, 170, 191, 192, 217, 247, 294,
    316, 390, 410, 415, 420, 430, 435, 437,
    446, 447, 450, 453, 459, 466, 473, 482,
    487, 515, 611, 671, 691, 762, 769, 805
knees 63, 749, 765, 769
knuckles 386, 765
Korsakoff's psychosis 221, 273, 276, 669
Krebs cycle 79, 187, 227
kuru 129, 334

labeling 210, 387, 388, 389, 400, 401, 407,
    490, 497, 503, 566, 574, 590, 591, 592,
    593, 713, 714, 717
Laboratory Tests in Common Use 444, 697
lactation 202, 766
lambs 82, 86, 405, 768
large intestine 488
larvae 140
larynx 174, 236, 278, 340, 342, 477
law 9, 24, 70, 98, 400, 551, 562, 564, 569,
    570, 571, 574, 578, 584, 589, 590, 592,
    605, 630, 704, 714, 715, 716, 718, 721,
    794
lawyers 494, 509
learned helplessness 182
learning 20, 25, 29, 38, 42, 63, 126, 128, 129,
    148, 163, 164, 167, 168, 169, 170, 171,
    173, 176, 180, 186, 187, 204, 221, 228,
    251, 257, 273, 277, 320, 356, 454, 473,
    477, 482, 483, 582, 640, 642, 647, 649,
    652, 664, 670, 677, 701, 798
leftovers 369, 375, 382
legislation 401, 562, 563, 573, 576, 577, 579,
    590, 591, 594, 595, 596, 716
legs 31, 148, 149, 165, 300, 316, 345, 414,
    759, 766, 767, 768
lemur 105
lenses 348
lesions 290, 753
lethargica, encephalitis (sleeping sickness) 133
lethargy 706
leukemia 89, 340, 343, 358, 451, 683, 686
leukocytes 297, 304, 409, 413, 633, 674, 678,
    693, 694
Leydig cells 138, 221
libertarianism 534
libido 657, 766

381

library 393, 455, 508, 527, 539, 540, 541, 542, 543, 544, 545, 628, 718, 764
life extension formulas, cholesterol levels and 367
life extension and government conflict of interest 556
lifespan 13, 29, 66, 81, 83, 89, 105, 106, 108, 134, 141, 146, 147, 171, 370, 404, 416, 467, 473, 478, 479, 554, 635, 638, 645, 692, 716
lifestyle 24, 322, 433, 459
ligand 643
lighting 219, 232, 494, 495
lightning 350
limbic 131
limb regeneration 150, 646
limbs 17, 132, 148, 149, 150, 151, 285, 299, 300, 354, 406, 493, 506, 515, 645, 646, 801
limerence 727
linking 77, 87, 91, 92, 93, 98, 103, 163, 242, 269, 312, 325, 382, 481, 483, 517, 527, 635, 669, 710, 720, 789
lipid antioxidant 402, 637, 673, 679, 692
lipid coat 206, 479, 657
lipid-coated viruses 334
lipid-containing viruses 681
lipid soluble 414, 465, 475, 612, 796
lipolytic 481
lipophilic 199, 200
lipoprotein electrophoresis 448
lips 99, 237, 420, 753
literature 13, 46, 52, 174, 179, 204, 214, 219, 220, 319, 393, 398, 455, 457, 461, 462, 497, 499, 502, 510, 526, 529, 541, 543, 544, 560, 562, 582, 592, 593, 598, 630, 651, 712, 728, 729, 730, 734
litmus paper 249
liver 24, 54, 71, 72, 89, 92, 96, 105, 106, 112, 121, 122, 124, 144, 148, 149, 174, 178, 192, 209, 242, 260, 265, 269, 270, 271, 272, 273, 274, 275, 278, 279, 282, 294, 305, 307, 308, 313, 325, 333, 334, 340, 385, 409, 411, 419, 420, 421, 422, 435, 437, 450, 451, 452, 459, 466, 470, 475, 477, 478, 479, 481, 482, 485, 563, 570, 611, 646, 668, 680, 681, 691, 698, 747, 750, 751, 764, 776, 777, 783, 784, 796, 797, 800
lizards 149
lobbying 594
lobes 325, 327, 794
long bones 765
long-lived species 145, 614
longevity 20, 30, 65, 67, 143, 370, 438, 482, 554, 614, 629, 630, 636, 645, 688, 700, 701, 721
longitudinal studies 223, 229, 661
low cholesterol levels, high intake of other antioxidants and 339
lubrication 131, 200, 296, 297, 391, 748, 760, 765
lumps 462, 488, 727
lunch 177, 251, 291, 457
lungs 102, 104, 151, 177, 242, 243, 244, 247, 248, 250, 252, 256, 258, 259, 265, 266, 269, 278, 302, 337, 340, 350, 369, 404, 406, 419, 420, 421, 481, 633, 634, 636,

664, 665, 666, 667, 668, 680, 684, 691, 692, 695, 700, 703, 790, 801
lymph 410, 796
lymph nodes 57, 82, 85
lymphatic system 796
lymphocyte rosette 88
lymphocytes 85, 87, 88, 452, 527, 796
lymphoma 206, 308, 333
lysing 473, 794
lysis 794
lysosomal 473
lysosomal membranes 103, 106, 216, 473
lysosomes 106, 121, 216, 534, 673, 700, 797

macaque monkey 660
macromolecules 472, 744, 802
macrophages 81, 84, 88, 108, 212, 250, 285, 386, 481, 482, 634, 636, 664, 667, 668, 700, 740, 759, 797
macroscopic 213, 520
magazines 46, 47, 51, 52, 53, 493, 494, 495, 496, 497, 498, 499, 526, 534, 539, 540, 614, 664, 674, 676, 678, 687, 708, 713, 717, 722, 751
makeup 507
malaise 730
male pattern baldness 65, 68, 137, 212, 213, 214, 217, 220, 482, 659, 768
malformation 585
malignancy 336, 633, 680, 683, 726
malignant melanomas 342, 480, 481
malpractice 439, 454, 573, 574, 575, 591
mammary cancer 421. *See also* Breasts
marathon runners 224, 229
Marek's disease 308
marriage 39, 657
marrow 82, 85, 435, 437, 466, 786, 796, 802
masturbation 754
maturation 140, 634, 644, 683
maximum life span 11, 18, 19, 20, 57, 58, 65, 71, 106, 110, 137, 171, 404, 467
maximum species life span 58, 68, 146
meals 242, 244, 246, 249, 279, 280, 281, 283, 286, 291, 293, 372, 422, 426, 464, 468, 488
measles 334, 357, 411
measure the rate of aging and repair 511
mechanisms of aging 58, 59, 63, 64, 66, 74, 461, 632
medical devices 624
Medical Hotline® 535, 538, 706
medication 47, 293, 456, 459, 734, 748
medicine 100, 167, 219, 226, 303, 326, 329, 335, 354, 356, 373, 393, 412, 433, 437, 438, 515, 527, 531, 536, 538, 543, 551, 565, 566, 572, 573, 575, 592, 627, 628, 631, 639, 666, 671, 685, 703, 715, 720, 726, 787
Medlars (National Library of Medicine computerized biomedical literature search service) 540, 543, 544, 545, 546, 547, 712, 729
Medline (National Library of Medicine computerized biomedical literature search service) 543, 544
megadoses 30, 54, 108, 193, 249, 306, 371, 390, 407, 412, 415, 416, 435, 485, 755
melanocytes 758, 759

melanomas 136, 341, 411, 683
membrane damage 216, 518
memory 25, 38, 40, 95, 126, 128, 129, 163, 164, 167, 169, 170, 171, 173, 174, 176, 177, 186, 187, 204, 221, 228, 229, 251, 269, 273, 274, 276, 277, 320, 321, 473, 483, 484, 522, 535, 640, 641, 642, 647, 648, 649, 652, 670, 677, 698, 701, 723, 783, 788
menopause 20, 65, 68, 137, 138, 196, 198, 199, 200, 471, 784, 786
menstruation 136, 139, 140, 197, 237, 471
mental improvement 164
mental organization 163
Merck Index® 538
Merck Manual of Diagnosis and Therapy® 697
metabolic activation 518
metabolic defects 22, 268, 270, 271, 466
metabolism 55, 56, 58, 76, 77, 78, 92, 95, 101, 102, 103, 106, 110, 120, 121, 124, 130, 131, 133, 134, 143, 144, 165, 169, 171, 177, 178, 185, 187, 213, 227, 228, 269, 271, 273, 286, 289, 312, 315, 332, 334, 338, 341, 370, 385, 402, 409, 411, 414, 422, 424, 425, 426, 429, 431, 435, 436, 438, 442, 450, 470, 473, 474, 476, 480, 481, 484, 627, 632, 641, 645, 649, 651, 659, 665, 669, 670, 672, 675, 676, 678, 681, 682, 693, 701, 784, 792, 793, 796, 797, 800, 805
metastatic 236, 343, 478
Methuselah pill 500
mice 21, 24, 25, 31, 56, 58, 59, 85, 87, 88, 89, 105, 108, 110, 112, 117, 121, 134, 138, 140, 141, 147, 170, 171, 181, 192, 242, 264, 290, 293, 333, 336, 383, 404, 414, 415, 421, 473, 476, 478, 479, 481, 496, 507, 524, 565, 614, 617, 633, 634, 636, 638, 639, 640, 641, 644, 649, 660, 669, 672, 681, 682, 683, 699, 700, 701, 702, 708, 743
microbes 82, 99, 180, 378, 509, 593, 771
microcirculation 638
microcomputers 329, 722, 724
microelectronics 708
microorganisms 82, 96, 376, 383, 570, 744
micropathology 449
microscopes 82, 309, 349, 527, 640
microsomes 668, 691, 698
microwave cooking 369
microwaves 264
middle-aged 30, 252, 276, 780
migraine 135, 763
miners 266, 505
mining 505, 508, 561
miscible 215
misrepresentations 497, 501, 566
mitochondria 406, 506, 668, 698, 797, 803
mitosis 646
MLP (maximum lifespan potential) 105, 106
MLS (maximum life span) 20
moderation 5, 371
moisturizers 53, 163, 208, 210, 632, 647, 658, 659, 741
mold 261, 376, 382, 383, 384, 570
mole 660
molecular biology 113, 627, 693, 699

Moloney murine sarcoma virus (MSV) 421
monitoring 138, 139, 142, 176, 186, 337, 430, 441, 611, 619, 731
monkeys 59, 105, 123, 140, 206, 287, 290, 398, 409, 474, 478, 616, 653, 655, 687, 776
mononucleosis 412
monsters 708
moods 25, 32, 127, 180, 292, 459, 648, 653
morphology 122, 639, 648, 656
motorcycles 574, 605, 732
mountain chinchilla 616
mouth 82, 99, 162, 177, 205, 237, 241, 275, 278, 292, 340, 347, 599, 615, 752
mouthwash 371, 689
mucoepidermoid carcinoma 727
mucosa 199, 200, 201
mucous 420
mucous membranes 131, 198, 205, 275, 419
mules 505
multiple sclerosis 84, 85, 129, 334, 522, 525, 786
multivitamins 431, 442, 468
mumps 334, 357, 451
muscle tone 129, 228
muscle 15, 95, 121, 134, 135, 149, 165, 187, 216, 222, 223, 226, 227, 228, 229, 230, 231, 233, 238, 279, 284, 286, 288, 289, 290, 298, 347, 373, 432, 435, 451, 452, 475, 476, 477, 479, 515, 661, 670, 673, 675, 677, 735, 736, 738, 741, 767, 768, 774, 783, 788
muscular output 165, 226, 783
mutagenesis, 319, 320
mutagenicity 88, 144, 300, 313, 339, 367, 376, 377, 410, 479, 645, 682, 689, 700, 792, 800
mutations 19, 20, 72, 99, 100, 102, 103, 106, 107, 139, 142, 144, 145, 147, 197, 221, 241, 264, 265, 279, 339, 377, 404, 405, 410, 479, 630, 637, 645, 668, 692, 701
myasthenia gravis 85
myelination 642, 646
myocardial infarction 451, 452, 674, 678, 693
myocardium 638, 680

nasal 164, 168, 173, 174, 179, 190, 192, 204, 229, 288, 320, 465, 613, 763
nasopharyngeal cancer 206, 308, 333
national health insurance, aged population and 719
natural antioxidants 162, 367, 371, 424, 484, 639, 666, 684, 690, 703
natural form 407
natural source 482, 759
natural vitamins 52, 53, 55, 490
NDA (new drug application) 589
nebulizer 756
NEC-5520 Spinwriter® 723
neck 204, 350, 494, 737
negative synergy 803
nematodes 19, 110
neoplasia 634, 652, 683, 727. See also Cancer
Nepalese erotic bronzes 653
nerves 84, 111, 112, 121, 122, 123, 124, 125, 127, 128, 129, 132, 133, 138, 149, 151, 169, 171, 172, 174, 175, 176, 178, 184, 188, 197, 211, 221, 228, 250, 251, 274, 276, 282, 299, 320, 326, 413, 474, 479,

482, 488, 502, 524, 639, 641, 646, 648, 649, 700, 712, 727, 740, 783, 784, 788, 791, 796, 798, 803

nervous system 111, 122, 123, 129, 131, 139, 176, 190, 192, 282, 348, 481, 483, 497, 498, 514, 525, 638, 639, 642, 646, 648, 649, 650, 690, 727, 728, 784, 788, 791, 793, 794, 798

neural-tube defects 695, 697

neurites 127, 128, 176, 178, 276, 320, 482, 524, 798

neurobiology 670

neurochemistry 169, 180, 639, 642, 648, 798

neuroelectronics 768

neuroendocrine function, and sexuality 652

neuroendocrine system 471, 516, 517, 644, 653, 654, 658, 795

neurology 314, 354, 557, 651, 669, 686, 770

neuromuscular 228, 783

neuronophages 125

neurons 85, 112, 121, 122, 124, 126, 135, 152, 157, 169, 170, 171, 176, 477, 522, 639, 640, 646, 648, 649, 701, 711, 796, 798, 802

neuropharmacology 733

neurosurgery 639

neurotransmitters 126, 127, 129, 132, 134, 157, 169, 170, 171, 179, 186, 190, 192, 193, 202, 228, 236, 274, 278, 287, 291, 295, 431, 474, 481, 498, 652, 669, 741, 783, 788, 791, 793, 794, 796, 798, 799, 802

neutralization 244, 247, 249, 345, 411, 415, 426, 435, 462, 487, 488, 755

neutrophils 411

new drug application (NDA) 218, 573, 575

newborns 252, 277, 289

newsletter 535, 536, 708

niacin, reduction of paraquat toxicity in rats 665, 696

nightmares 193

nipples 387

nitrogenous 76

No Time to Confuse 717

noise 240, 254, 269, 512, 521, 522, 712, 726, 731, 732

nomograms 671, 721, 774, 775

non-FDA-approved uses 454, 455, 591, 592, 593, 594

nonsmokers 202, 203, 247, 252, 259, 266, 278, 664

noradrenergic 176

Normanskii interferometer 527

Northstar® computer 723

nose 378, 381, 386, 501, 734, 743. See also Nasal

nostrils 173, 241

nuclear power plants 264, 705

nuclear transplant 507

nucleated cells 519

nucleosomes 710

nursing 183

nutrient manufacturers 622, 623

nutrient mix 210, 464, 467, 619, 742, 743, 750, 756, 759, 760

Nutrient Requirements of Nonhuman Primates (National Research Council) 398, 691, 693

nutrient suppliers 618, 619, 620

nutrients 5, 41, 80, 87, 92, 126, 127, 162, 164, 165, 172, 175, 182, 186, 193, 196, 240, 243, 246, 251, 261, 272, 274, 277, 280, 287, 288, 290, 298, 347, 349, 368, 371, 393, 398, 402, 409, 430, 435, 436, 441, 467, 470, 477, 479, 490, 597, 620, 642, 643, 688, 691, 757, 758, 764, 783

nutrition 10, 44, 46, 47, 48, 49, 51, 52, 53, 54, 83, 125, 164, 184, 202, 207, 220, 224, 230, 275, 284, 341, 361, 369, 390, 392, 393, 399, 400, 401, 403, 409, 430, 441, 466, 490, 497, 499, 534, 535, 537, 539, 540, 559, 566, 600, 618, 621, 626, 627, 628, 633, 637, 641, 648, 649, 652, 663, 666, 670, 671, 681, 685, 689, 691, 693, 698, 699, 700, 704, 737, 764, 765, 768

nutritional requirements 429, 768

nutritionists 86, 322, 370

Obedience to Authority 719

obesity 23, 224, 229, 249, 250, 251, 265, 279, 285, 289, 290, 293, 325, 338, 370, 414, 524, 570, 595, 671, 672, 794

Occam's razor 45

occlusive vascular disease 316

occult blood 447, 449

occupation 17, 266, 301, 551, 561

odors 175, 220, 239, 253, 254, 262, 347, 368, 376, 378, 379, 384, 389

offprints 533, 632, 633, 634, 641, 644, 661, 669, 681, 687

offspring 18, 19, 26, 39, 112, 138, 147, 197, 286, 505, 506, 638

old wives' tales 170, 190, 298

oligodendrocytes 642, 646

olivary nucleus 123

Olympic GH (growth hormone) releaser scandal 509

Olympic GH (growth hormone) use scandal 509

Olympics 508, 509, 775

oncologists 341, 729

ophthalmologists 522

ophthalmology 635

Opt-Out form 573, 574, 591, 713

optimization of the experimental protective formulations 520

Opting Out 569, 574

orangutan 105, 616

organoleptic 387

orgasm 196, 204, 205, 282, 484, 754, 795

orthomolecular 656, 695, 698

Orthomolecular Psychiatry 656, 695, 698

Orwell's doublethink 593

Osborne-1® 724

osteogenesis 646

OTC drugs. See Over-the-counter drugs

ova 197

ovaries 71, 197, 199

ovens 264, 380, 688, 731

over-the-counter (non-prescription drug) 171, 256, 289, 348, 488, 489, 753, 799

overdoses 97, 172, 192, 229, 354, 420, 421, 423, 442, 476, 571, 756

overeating 23, 293

overexertion 762

overgrowth 258

overstimulation 178, 199, 240
overweight 108, 284, 285, 289, 294, 324, 371, 374, 751. *See also* Obesity
overwork 99, 172, 744
oxidation 24, 55, 66, 68, 88, 95, 101, 104, 106, 107, 110, 111, 118, 135, 162, 170, 175, 216, 217, 227, 244, 246, 247, 248, 250, 257, 269, 270, 273, 285, 297, 299, 304, 308, 312, 313, 314, 319, 338, 339, 348, 366, 367, 376, 378, 381, 382, 386, 391, 402, 403, 404, 414, 417, 418, 421, 425, 453, 481, 482, 491, 492, 520, 636, 688, 689, 692, 764, 769, 783, 786, 789, 790, 792, 793, 797, 799
Oxygen Free Radicals and Tissue Damage 673

packaging 19, 255, 377, 378, 389, 534, 590, 591, 592, 713, 789
packagers 407
pain 21, 25, 34, 47, 49, 83, 103, 136, 170, 174, 186, 200, 202, 229, 240, 288, 296, 298, 299, 300, 305, 325, 349, 430, 455, 466, 473, 474, 485, 488, 715, 725, 729, 730, 732, 746, 747, 748, 749, 760, 762, 766, 767, 768, 769, 770, 791, 800, 805
painkilling 414
paint 165, 261, 299, 747, 786
pallor 229
palpation 766, 767
palpitations 735
palsy 112, 318
pancreas 290, 337, 370, 372, 451
Pap-smear 184, 200, 201
paralysis 238, 318, 351, 354, 356, 357, 567, 596, 727
paramedics 344, 348, 350, 351, 342, 354, 525, 562
paraplegia 348, 557, 759
parasites 303, 314, 340, 796
parenchymal cancer 266
Parkinson's disease 127, 132, 133, 134, 229, 236, 237, 414, 431, 432, 435, 474, 475, 522, 766, 788
parotid cancer 728
parotid tumor 726
patents 305, 319, 336, 377, 502, 551, 564, 575
pathobiology 629, 645
pathologists 514, 563, 727, 728
pathology 91, 96, 100, 101, 162, 273, 277, 339, 457, 501, 524, 557, 559, 560, 627, 636, 638, 643, 667, 685, 693, 752, 765, 768, 770
pathways 20, 23, 56, 79, 107, 115, 118, 130, 131, 154, 155, 156, 176, 223, 271, 417, 466, 480, 632, 635
PDR (*Physicians Desk Reference*®) 455, 456
Pearson, Durk. *See* Durk
penis 197
peptide synthesizers 624
percent body fat 772, 774, 775
perception 111, 175, 363, 387, 499, 555, 652, 729
peristaltic 187
permeability 96, 477, 676, 678, 698
peroxidation 103, 108, 140, 175, 209, 366, 369, 388, 403, 404, 405, 470, 478, 636, 638, 667, 668, 678, 691, 692, 698, 776, 799

peroxidized 66, 88, 102, 106, 107, 108, 111, 112, 119, 121, 133, 140, 174, 285, 308, 312, 318, 325, 332, 347, 363, 367, 368, 369, 370, 376, 377, 379, 385, 386, 403, 481, 492, 619, 639, 682, 689, 704, 740, 784, 793, 796, 797, 799, 800, 801, 802
perspiration 209
pesticides 349
pH 249, 489, 491
pH paper 489
phagocytes 81, 212, 308, 410, 668
pharmaceutical innovations 533, 555, 568, 578, 580, 581, 593, 594, 691, 704, 706, 716
pharmaceuticals 41, 124, 180, 201, 298, 305, 306, 308, 348, 455, 485, 492, 501, 502, 537, 541, 544, 551, 558, 566, 570, 573, 574, 577, 578, 590, 591, 592, 593, 595, 618, 620, 627, 628, 650, 651, 707, 713
pharmacists 200, 215, 305, 390, 537, 542, 544, 572, 573, 589, 590, 591, 592, 593, 594, 595
pharmacology 566, 573, 628, 641, 650, 664, 676, 677, 685, 701
pharmacopeia 173
Phaseolus vulgaris 671
phenylketonuria (PKU) 136, 252, 289, 341
phlebitis 786
phobias 328, 734, 735
photo micrographs 122, 309, 310, 311, 312, 449
photos, of Durk 94, 230, 231, 232, 654, 772, 773; of Sandy 233, 234, 235, 655, 738, 739
photochemical 261, 518, 744, 770, 771
photomutants 712
photons 264
photoreceptors 175, 648
photosensitivity 97, 420, 422, 476, 764
photosynthesis 402, 423, 787
Phycomyces 712
Physician's Desk Reference® (PDR) 454, 531, 697
physicists 550, 751
physiology 224, 430, 626, 661, 787
piezoelectric 150
pigment 81, 97, 102, 112, 120, 121, 122, 123, 124, 127, 128, 136, 174, 175, 176, 187, 208, 211, 212, 341, 342, 451, 480, 484, 639, 648, 692, 750, 757, 758, 759, 770, 784, 788, 796
pigmented malignant melanoma 127, 341
pigs 26, 31, 56, 57, 59, 65, 123, 145, 345, 398, 409, 410, 412, 414, 416, 441, 467, 481, 518, 609, 640, 649, 658, 701
pinch test, skin elasticity 94, 385
pipes, lead 261
pituitary gland 71, 73, 86, 98, 129, 134, 137, 139, 140, 141, 142, 164, 165, 174, 180, 190, 194, 196, 221, 223, 229, 288, 290, 293, 321, 323, 345, 373, 432, 475, 484, 680, 702, 735, 740, 741, 742, 762, 763, 765, 766, 771, 786, 788, 794, 799
PKU (phenylketonuria) 136, 341, 342
placebo, 47, 49, 249, 302, 405, 411, 514, 642, 647, 649, 725, 762, 791, 800
placebo effect 47, 762
planned obsolescence 18, 67, 142

plants 53, 54, 55, 76, 89, 102, 123, 137, 208, 263, 264, 375, 376, 378, 402, 403, 420, 423, 429, 464, 616, 631, 643, 705, 787, 793, 797
plasma 96, 97, 327, 403, 410, 634, 652, 662, 667, 680, 681, 683, 685, 687, 695, 800
plastic milk bottle test 387
plastic surgery 499
platelet aggregation 285, 683
platelets 108, 109, 309, 310, 311, 312, 316, 317, 324, 638, 639, 676, 678, 691, 699, 786, 800
plaque 82, 308, 312, 318, 319, 326
plaques 81, 83, 107, 108, 129, 190, 241, 307, 312, 314, 315, 316, 317, 319, 320, 366, 368, 373, 408, 474, 483, 674, 677, 785, 786, 796, 800
play 99, 142, 175, 282, 342, 345, 364, 366, 378, 422, 515, 519, 630, 638, 673, 721, 745, 746, 803
Playboy® 751
pneumonia 412, 761
poisons 52, 54, 102, 120, 244, 250, 271, 285, 335, 354, 375, 376, 383, 384, 413, 479, 570, 631, 665, 696, 797, 804
poisonings 350, 352, 354, 383, 412, 420, 524, 631, 665, 696
polio 356, 357, 411, 730
pollen 54, 253
pollutants 144, 263, 265, 340
pollution 31, 104, 146, 177, 253, 259, 260, 261, 263, 265, 266, 561, 569, 665, 667, 706, 720
polydipsia 762
polymerization 103, 165, 758
polymorphonuclear 297
polyribosomes 472, 802
polyuria 762
porpoises 616
positive synergy 381, 803
postamphetamine depression 204
posterior pituitary 129, 228, 763
postmenopausal 136, 197
postoperative period 345, 403
postsynaptic membrane 132
potency 72, 92, 96, 102, 133, 186, 194, 201, 273, 285, 298, 304, 339, 347, 358, 368, 369, 371, 377, 393, 400, 403, 407, 411, 442, 468, 475, 491, 492, 519, 520, 594, 619, 653, 683, 760, 766, 784
potentiation 178, 669, 683
poultry 55, 308, 367, 376, 560, 702
ppm (parts per million) 470
practitioners 538, 580
precancerous 151, 191, 221
precipitation 169, 204, 215, 430, 805
precipitator 253, 254, 261, 262, 263, 625, 666, 669
precursors 111, 145, 185, 186, 520, 641, 650, 766, 783, 796, 799, 800, 802
prediction of body density and total body fat from skinfold measurements 671,721, 775
predictors 336, 339, 414
pregnancy 112, 237, 277, 431, 451, 465, 468, 474, 475, 579, 611
preoptic gland 141
prescriptions 350, 492, 576, 595, 677, 713, 714, 716

preservatives 163, 195, 206, 332, 333, 371, 375, 376, 377, 378, 382, 384, 389, 414, 478, 499, 551, 663, 683, 689, 690, 752
preservatives may be preserving you 52, 375
presynaptic membrane 132
preventing cancer 332, 421, 476, 602, 651, 682, 685
preventive medicine 537, 681
privacy maintained by mathematical laws 509
professional athletes 509
profiling 10, 712
progeria 104, 146, 518, 801
programmed aging 65, 71, 402
prophylaxis 217, 242, 312, 343, 559, 651, 744, 762, 801
prostate 190, 191, 202, 453, 762
protectants 264, 265, 404, 421, 502, 664, 670, 679, 694, 700
protective mechanisms 69, 140, 280, 316, 403, 519, 753, 804
protein-digesting (proteolytic) 99, 163, 216, 237, 384
proteinaceous 112
proteolytic (protein-digesting) 99, 163, 216, 237, 384
protoporphyria 743
protozoans 507
Proxmire bill 400
pseudoarthrosis 150
psychiatrists 182, 565
psychiatry 11, 557, 648, 651, 656, 669, 695, 698
psychoactive 240, 669
psychobiochemical aspects of aging 658
psychobiochemical events involved in love, limerence, pair-bonding, and lust 516
psychobiochemistry 243, 426, 516, 517, 658; aspects of aging 658; events involved in love, limerence, pair-bonding, and lust 516
psychology 3, 38, 179, 223, 239, 240, 555, 557, 629, 712, 800
psychologists 182, 249
psychomotor 648, 664, 667, 676, 699
psychoneuroendocrine 634, 652, 683
psychopharmacology 179, 463, 516, 641, 648, 651, 652, 657, 664, 671
psychosis 175, 182, 187, 257
psychotherapy 565
psychotomimetic use of tobacco 664
puberty 9, 70, 82, 104, 763
pulmonary macrophage sputum test 449
pulse 92, 148,150, 329, 351,444, 446, 523, 803
pulse rate counters 329, 446, 624
pulsed field emission x-ray machine 527
Puma® (Unimate® lab robot) 527
pumps (vitamin c, in blood-brain barrier membrane) 111, 413, 639, 740
pupil 522
purification 294, 671
purifier 253

quadraplegia 557
quantum chemistry calculations 514
quantum electronic instrumentation 520

rabbits 89, 145, 308, 312, 315, 320, 348, 474, 483, 674, 687, 760

rabies 334, 412, 694
race 268, 271, 297, 562
racehorses 748
racemization of aspartic acid 615
radiation 92, 96, 100, 101, 102, 103, 110, 127,
    146, 178, 237, 253, 264, 265, 336, 337,
    341, 342, 387, 477, 480, 481, 482, 515,
    516, 534, 556, 560, 628, 705, 726, 728,
    729, 730, 731, 787, 791, 792, 793
radiation sickness 474, 793
radiators 96, 319
radicals. See free radicals
radioactivity 244, 253, 264, 265
radiodurans 106, 518
radioimmunoassays 765
radiologists 341, 342, 726, 728, 729
radiometer 524
radioprotective 728
radiotherapy 342
rads 637, 645, 668, 692, 701, 726, 729, 731
rags 786, 787
rancid fats 92, 101, 102, 285, 308, 332, 370,
    386
rancid oil 386
rancidity 106, 220, 363, 368, 369, 375, 376,
    377, 378, 379, 381, 382, 386, 387, 388,
    389, 403, 407, 462, 476, 492, 758, 786
random damage 58, 67, 70, 71, 378, 770
random damage aging 67
rashes 385, 485, 747
rational formulation of free radical
    modulating regimens 513
rats 25, 31, 56, 57, 59, 66, 71, 72, 73, 78, 83,
    86, 87, 92, 98, 104, 110, 111, 117, 122,
    127, 129, 131, 134, 138, 140, 142, 144,
    147, 148, 150, 162, 165, 169, 170, 171,
    175, 182, 183, 187, 227, 236, 240, 243,
    261, 265, 272, 275, 277, 327, 333, 341,
    351, 366, 374, 384, 403, 404, 405, 414,
    415, 430, 470, 473, 475, 477, 479, 481,
    482, 484, 506, 519, 571, 595, 599, 636,
    642, 644, 646, 648, 649, 650, 654, 659,
    662, 663, 664, 665, 668, 669, 672, 674,
    676, 678, 680, 681, 692, 696, 698, 699,
    701, 702, 741, 764
rattlesnake 412
RDA (FDA's Recommended Daily Allowance
    of nutrients) 242, 392, 393, 394, 395, 396,
    397, 398, 399, 416, 569, 600, 690, 691,
    694
reaction time 164, 174, 484
reactive hypoglycemia 373
reactivity 83, 280, 788
reactors 100, 106, 518, 705
reagents 214, 349, 624
reanimation 177, 350
recalcified 327, 403
receptors 88, 132, 133, 134, 135, 165, 168,
    169, 184, 193, 210, 213, 282, 293, 320,
    323, 328, 354, 431, 477, 642, 643, 647,
    650, 656, 658, 662, 663, 667, 673, 680,
    687, 694, 701, 735, 754, 755, 767, 788,
    797, 801
Recommended Daily Allowances. See RDAs
recreational drugs 256, 274, 275, 564
red blood cell count 447
red blood cell hemolysis model 518
red eyes 763

redifferentiation 559
refereed journals 45, 801
reflexes 522
reformulation 580, 707
refrigeration 351, 369, 376, 379, 389
refrigerator 350, 368, 389
regeneration 148, 149, 150, 151, 152, 176,
    188, 192, 221, 317, 348, 477, 506, 645,
    646, 790, 801, 804
regenerator 148
regrowth 148, 149, 150, 213, 214, 217, 218,
    219, 515, 801
regulation of carcinogenic hazards 706
regulatory agency 565, 590, 594, 713
regulatory bureaucracy 589
rehabilitation 621
reincarnation 36
rejuvenation 44, 495, 635, 674, 693
releasers 192, 218, 233, 236, 286, 290, 342,
    477, 478, 483, 509, 515, 640, 661, 662,
    741, 765, 771, 774
REM sleep 192, 193, 194, 342
remineralized 371
remissions 411, 642, 692
replication 46, 335
reproduction 19, 20, 42, 55, 138, 140, 142,
    147, 161, 196, 331, 507, 517, 630, 734
reptile brain 131, 735
resetting biological clocks 644
resistance 25, 29, 31, 145, 146, 152, 200, 208,
    270, 300, 350, 402, 416, 422, 480, 519,
    570, 593, 729, 759, 761, 770, 771
resistance to sunburn 743, 756, 761, 770
respirable particles 264
respiration 193, 206, 281, 339, 351, 352, 514,
    747, 756
restlessness 135, 190
resuscitation 177, 344, 350, 351, 352, 353,

retinas 420, 522, 788
retinopathy 315
revitalizing 40, 89, 167, 187, 257, 348, 648
Rhesus monkeys 105, 206, 287, 290, 478, 655,
    776
rheumatic fever 453
rheumatism 299, 300
rheumatoid arthritis 106, 190, 296, 297, 299,
    303, 438, 557, 748, 762, 786
rheumatology 634
rhinoceros 616
rhythms 190, 326, 328, 644
risk-free 26, 569
risks 6, 25, 26, 71, 91, 202, 203, 229, 239, 240,
    241, 243, 249, 250, 254, 255, 256, 266,
    270, 277, 278, 279, 284, 312, 313, 325,
    326, 329, 352, 357, 363, 365, 369, 390,
    405, 415, 424, 425, 430, 436, 450, 463,
    467, 563, 568, 569, 570, 571, 573, 575,
    579, 584, 585, 586, 592, 595, 605, 630,
    651, 657, 665, 666, 669, 682, 684, 703,
    705, 706, 734, 777, 778, 779, 794, 796
RNA synthesis 160, 170, 477
rock music 653, 718, 731
rodents 123, 139, 140, 290, 333, 339, 571. See
    also mice; rats
roentgens 694, 699
role of cholesterol in heart disease 363
rot 95, 96

rotifers 97, 637
roundworms 19
rubella 357
runners 224, 229
running 222, 223, 224, 229, 708, 723, 724, 735
rupture 106, 403, 470

safety regulations 561, 569, 585, 691, 705, 718, 719
salamanders 149, 151, 507
salivary gland 726
salivation 256
salmon 137, 140, 141, 644, 657, 786
salmonella 599
salty 372
Sandy's clinical laboratory test findings 775; broken foot and an experimental bodybuilding technique 735; phobias 734; hearing 726; total serum cholesterol 367
sanitation 303, 354, 356
sarcoma 421
satiation 290, 292, 672
scalp 212, 213, 214, 215, 216, 217, 218, 219, 220, 479, 659, 757, 758, 768, 791
scanners, CAT 556, 719, 787
scanning electron microscope 309, 527
scarring 121, 347, 358, 384, 412
scavenging 263, 271, 279, 300, 339, 406, 484, 685, 751, 759, 760, 773, 793, 800
Schaal Oven Test 380
schizophrenic 184, 185, 204, 278, 499, 640, 661, 662, 788
schizophrenics 134, 135, 426, 466, 640, 643, 661
sclerosis 84, 85, 129, 334, 522, 525, 786
scorpion 412
screening of candidate free radical modulating agents 511
scurvy 408, 410, 416, 417, 436, 470, 602, 682, 694
seal 382, 420
seamen 408
sedentary lifestyle 223, 224, 230, 233, 285, 289, 750, 751, 774
sedimentation 449, 453
seismographs 527
seizures 258, 277
self-defense 82, 336
self-experimentation 302, 514, 725, 726
self-image software 517
selfish gene 19, 630, 718
senescence 30, 67, 152, 170
senile dementia 125, 649
senility 125, 126, 127, 129, 161, 168, 170, 180, 276, 320, 438, 468, 557, 635, 640, 649, 650, 651, 700
senses 15, 508
sensory 111, 128, 175, 178, 190, 276, 277, 413, 484, 508, 803
sensory input 131, 783
septicemia 411
serial learning 170, 640, 642, 647, 649, 664
serum ratio of reduced cholesterol to oxidized cholesterol 339
servomechanism 522

sewage 356
sex 54, 126, 127, 131, 139, 181, 196, 197, 198, 199, 200, 201, 202, 204, 205, 214, 220, 407, 469, 494, 495, 653, 655, 656, 657, 658, 749, 750, 784, 792, 799
sex flush 204, 205
sexual activity 198, 205, 517, 752, 788
sexual behavior 129, 274, 517, 653, 656, 721, 765, 791
sexual rejuvenation 494, 658
sexual self-image 516, 653
sexuality 198, 468, 507, 652, 657
sexually precocious 765
shampooing 219
shampoos 218, 219, 220, 472, 758
sheep 87, 88, 336, 409, 449
shingles 391
shock 176, 182, 345, 354, 414, 442, 651, 685, 716, 774
short screen for toxic effects 447
short-lived species 19, 28, 59, 69, 145
shoulders 150, 204, 268, 495, 736, 747
sickle cell anemia 524
sickness 133, 159, 408, 657, 658, 721. See also illness.
side effects 28, 53, 128, 134, 135, 175, 177, 164, 171, 178, 185, 192, 197, 204, 206, 214, 215, 218, 219, 221, 229, 237, 244, 246, 256, 275, 276, 281, 282, 287, 288, 289, 303, 305, 329, 334, 338, 340, 358, 373, 406, 415, 426, 431, 432, 434, 435, 436, 438, 454, 455, 456, 470, 471, 474, 485, 498, 569, 726, 735, 747, 751, 754, 755, 799
SIDS (sudden infant death syndrome) 358, 360, 386, 621
sinuses 135, 179
skeleton 121, 451
skiing 740, 741, 746, 759, 761, 775
skin 8, 17, 53, 76, 82, 91, 92, 93, 95, 97, 98, 99, 102, 104, 112, 120, 121, 124, 127, 138, 146, 149, 151, 162, 163, 165, 174, 175, 208, 209, 210, 211, 215, 218, 236, 238, 242, 246, 247, 263, 264, 265, 268, 269, 270, 281, 316, 327, 337, 340, 342, 345, 347, 349, 350, 358, 366, 384, 385, 386, 406, 412, 419, 420, 421, 422, 426, 434, 452, 474, 477, 479, 499, 501, 515, 613, 615, 632, 635, 647, 659, 660, 740, 741, 742, 743, 744, 745, 750, 753, 757, 758, 759, 761, 770, 771, 784, 790, 791, 796, 800, 801, 802
skin irritation 745
skin pinch snap-back test for cross-linking 94, 385
skinfold measurements for body fat percentage 671, 721, 774, 775
sleep 86, 126, 131, 133, 134, 135, 179, 180, 186, 189, 190, 192, 193, 194, 195, 229, 274, 289, 299, 300, 373, 426, 455, 459, 498, 571, 640, 652, 661, 760, 786, 794, 802
sleeplessness 133, 189
sleepwalking 190, 363
slender 285, 286
slender-tailed cloud rat 616
slow virus 334

small intestine 488
smallpox 356, 357, 730
Smarts® 723
smell 111, 125, 128, 164, 178, 179, 368, 378, 386, 387, 388, 417, 471, 733, 734
smog 31, 473
smoke 91, 92, 96, 162, 202, 209, 239, 240, 241, 242, 244, 247, 248, 249, 250, 252, 253, 254, 257, 258, 261, 263, 265, 266, 279, 314, 337, 339, 340, 350, 364, 369, 378, 385, 392, 404, 406, 413, 475, 481, 482, 664, 665, 666, 667, 684, 703, 706, 783, 784, 800
smoking 5, 13, 14, 23, 162, 177, 202, 229, 239, 240, 241, 243, 244, 245, 246, 247, 249, 250, 252, 253, 254, 255, 256, 257, 258, 259, 265, 266, 275, 277, 278, 279, 313, 325, 337, 338, 340, 378, 386, 390, 391, 406, 413, 424, 425, 459, 474, 475, 487, 518, 532, 562, 647, 663, 665, 666, 668, 670, 676, 677, 684, 694, 703, 780
SMR (specific metabolic rate) 105, 144
snacks 291, 371, 398, 691, 752
snakes 63, 149
snapback test, skin 93
sneezing 744
sniffers 387
social gerontologists 11, 551
social security 40, 42, 556
socialism 718
sociobehavioral 223
sociobiology 516, 517, 630, 658, 718
sociochemistry 517
SOD (superoxide dismutase) versus lifespan graphs 105
software 515, 517, 524, 625, 722, 723, 724
solar heating 706
solar ultraviolet 515, 729, 753, 761
solvents 214, 215, 220, 348, 349, 624, 714, 791
soreness 96, 99, 200, 206, 237, 244, 752
sores 411, 752, 753
sour 382, 388
space colonies 37, 507
spaceships 508
spasms 174, 677
spawning 137, 140, 141, 644, 786
specialists 729
specific metabolic rate (SMR) 106, 143, 144, 645
spectrometer 162, 520, 521, 527
spectrophotofluorometric 640, 644
spectrophotometer 349, 520
speech 328, 727, 731
sperm 139, 142, 147, 197
spermatagonia 138
spiders 28, 123
spina bifida 419, 431
spinal cord 111, 134, 209, 238, 300, 340, 351, 354, 409, 413, 431, 475, 525, 557, 638, 740, 742, 759, 769, 788
spine 350, 522, 639, 686, 761, 762
Spinwriter® 723
spleen 57, 82, 85, 88, 149, 192, 307, 420, 796
split labels 574, 591, 713
spoilage 376, 383
spontaneous combustion 786, 787

sports medicine 226
Sports Medicine Research Institute 515
spotted hyena 616
Sprague-Dawley rats 71, 111
squirrel monkey 105
stainless steel 80
staleness 253, 254, 375, 377
stallions 754
stamina 29, 165, 204, 226, 227, 479, 732, 741
staphylococcus 635
starvation 86, 285, 290, 294, 705
statistical significance 575
stem cells 89, 802
sterculia trees 241
stereospecific 663
stiffness 64, 91, 102, 163, 209, 269, 298, 299, 319, 375, 737
stimulus barrier 240, 243, 249, 250, 256, 269, 274, 803
stomach 127, 172, 179, 185, 186, 192, 244, 245, 246, 247, 249, 251, 252, 258, 277, 281, 283, 288, 289, 333, 426, 434, 462, 464, 468, 477, 487, 488, 496, 735, 748, 768, 795
stomach cancer 110, 337, 376, 377, 681
stomachache 187, 768
stool guaiac test 447, 449, 453
strains 99, 108, 339, 478, 539, 595
stress 9, 25, 31, 70, 72, 78, 96, 165, 172, 181, 187, 223, 227, 228, 251, 319, 347, 409, 413, 416, 436, 459, 518, 519, 537, 644, 645, 652, 675, 683, 688, 795
strokes 74, 108, 112, 124, 176, 257, 273, 285, 299, 307, 317, 318, 319, 320, 329, 350, 402, 426, 467, 482, 525, 676, 786, 801
subcellular 157, 403
subclinical 436, 470
subconscious 5
subcutaneous 635
sudden death 182, 328, 677
sudden infant death syndrome (SIDS) 304, 358, 360, 621, 686
suicide 24, 281
sulfation 366
sulfur-containing substances 93, 162, 373, 413, 471, 475, 576, 481
Sumatran orangutan 616
sunburn 146, 422, 743, 744, 753, 756, 757, 761, 770, 771
sunlight 91, 92, 97, 98, 99, 124, 208, 209, 211, 263, 385, 387, 391, 402, 422, 423, 476, 743, 744, 753, 756, 757, 761, 764, 770, 773
suntan 97, 98, 211, 743, 744
supernutrition 532, 663, 674, 678, 687
supplements 5, 48, 53, 54, 77, 78, 83, 89, 90, 102, 110, 125, 134, 136, 162, 164, 165, 168, 196, 197, 202, 204, 205, 217, 220, 240, 247, 263, 265, 284, 285, 308, 314, 332, 340, 341, 371, 377, 390, 393, 398, 400, 401, 406, 409, 410, 411, 412, 420, 421, 422, 431, 441, 446, 462, 464, 466, 473, 474, 481, 482, 487, 490, 559, 600, 619, 725, 726, 754, 755, 756, 764
suppliers 207, 210, 345, 618, 619, 620, 741
suppository 201

suppressants 88, 263, 308, 323, 338, 339, 377, 497, 498
suppressors 303, 306, 573, 762
surgeons 305, 341, 342, 495, 576, 727, 728, 732
surgery 8, 194, 236, 290, 337, 341, 343, 345, 478, 499, 501, 633, 645, 662, 671, 677, 685, 700, 727, 728, 730, 761, 787
susceptibility 76, 96, 135, 139, 266, 323, 478, 524, 562, 638, 680, 691, 776
swallowing 53, 177, 194, 275, 354, 748
sweating 735
sweet 241, 371, 374
sweetening 374, 498, 571
sweets 371, 425
swelling 96, 351, 455, 474, 730, 747, 800
swimming 25, 127, 134, 165, 182, 187, 209, 227, 236, 264, 479, 481, 741, 772, 775
swine 117, 768
symptomology 640, 661, 662
synapses 128, 132, 169, 171, 184, 788, 803
synaptic vesicles 132
synergistic 263, 381, 414, 416, 471, 477, 480, 803
synovial fluid 297
synovial membranes 297
synthetic 52, 53, 54, 55, 80, 102, 107, 112, 264, 276, 312, 333, 337, 351, 352, 407, 408, 409, 412, 478, 484, 490, 491, 631, 632, 667, 681, 693, 695, 699, 754, 763
Syrian wild horse 616
systemic lupus erythematosus 89, 296

T-cells 82, 83, 85, 87, 89, 112, 161, 191, 303, 336, 405, 786, 803, 804
tables (of data) 177, 281, 295, 315, 330, 358, 359, 360, 372, 373, 379, 380, 381, 476, 522, 582, 583, 631
tablets 135, 162, 177, 178, 190, 194, 201, 237, 244, 246, 258, 273, 305, 350, 393, 418, 431, 442, 462, 464, 485, 487, 488, 489, 492, 496, 498, 569, 619, 621, 623, 707, 748, 749, 754, 758, 760
tabletting 407, 462
tamarin 105
tanning 91, 95, 96, 97, 98, 99, 124, 163, 208, 211, 263, 422, 613, 757, 770, 771
tardive dyskinesia 134, 482
taste 111, 125, 175, 241, 256, 260, 292, 301, 315, 347, 369, 373, 374, 375, 376, 377, 382, 388, 389, 399, 434, 467, 471, 476, 499, 601, 688, 729, 732
tasteless 369, 379, 388
TB. See tuberculosis
teenagers 236, 289, 290, 342, 478, 658, 732, 736, 765, 766, 771, 801
teeth 8, 149, 371, 615
temperature 19, 77, 142, 144, 300, 323, 351, 387, 418, 476, 520, 539, 608, 609, 615, 688, 720, 767, 795, 796
tensile strength of wounds 412
tension 478, 489, 501
teratogenic 669
terminal cancer patients 89, 334, 335, 408, 411, 517, 569
testable hypothesis 709
testes 54, 71, 197, 202, 221, 691, 765, 766

testicular cancer 337
testosterone-producing cells 139
tetanus 357, 730
thalidomide ban 571
thermodynamics 571, 704
thermometer 323
thighs 235, 760
thinning hair 220, 516
thirst 33
thorax 352, 482
thoroughbred 754
thresholds 570, 731
throat 162, 244, 247, 256, 354
thrombogenic 367, 368, 674, 676, 678, 699
thrombosis 70, 108, 307, 309, 312, 327, 403, 804
thumb 45, 93
thymocytes 87, 804
thymoma 633, 683
thymotropic 633, 662, 671, 685, 700
thymus 57, 82, 85, 86, 87, 89, 161, 172, 190, 286, 297, 303, 305, 336, 342, 405, 419, 421, 534, 565, 634, 683, 728, 741, 796, 804
thyroid 73, 141, 142, 236, 288, 323, 343, 452, 478, 613, 767
Tibetan and Mepalese erotic bronzes 653
Tice strain BCG 343
tick 220
tinnitus 177, 178, 648, 726, 731, 732
tissue cultures 165, 242, 332, 333, 477, 479, 642, 646, 804
Tissuemat® 527
toes 93, 747
tolerance 171, 192, 195, 198, 283, 415, 416, 425, 426, 442, 737, 770
tomography 787
tongue 134, 138, 162, 190, 202, 244
tonsils 149
torso 728, 791
total cholesterol 325, 448, 450
total fatty acids 448
total lipids 448, 450, 478
total serum cholesterol 367, 368, 424
toxicity 24, 29, 31, 97, 103, 119, 120, 178, 185, 197, 206, 215, 218, 227, 241, 242, 243, 252, 263, 270, 282, 304, 404, 406, 411, 413, 420, 423, 424, 435, 436, 441, 442, 447, 448, 454, 455, 462, 472, 473, 478, 481, 491, 511, 519, 559, 564, 565, 673, 647, 663, 664, 665, 667, 668, 670, 676, 679, 694, 696, 698, 700, 714, 736, 744, 775, 790, 795, 797, 804
toxicology 461, 514, 566, 626, 628, 667
tranquilization 136, 282, 754, 755
transfusions 352, 524
transmutation 205
transplantation 139, 212, 213, 216, 507 633, 642, 646, 683
traumas 174, 229, 318, 345, 348, 351, 414, 484, 557, 639, 685, 693, 695, 795
tree shrew 105
trees 64, 241, 260, 374, 518
tremors 127, 132, 133, 236
Trends in Pharmacological Sciences® (TIPS) 312, 538, 628, 680, 702, 717
tricarboxylic acid cycle 789

trogoderma 140
tropics 99, 285, 383
tuberculosis (TB) 322, 323, 340, 343, 357, 358, 411, 584, 585, 762
tumorigenesis 660
tumors 83, 87, 107, 108, 129, 151, 152, 178, 242, 266, 307, 308, 312, 315, 316, 319, 331, 332, 333, 337, 341, 357, 366, 405, 477, 478, 498, 559, 633, 637, 660, 668, 680, 702, 727, 729, 785, 790, 800
turkeys 82, 86, 240, 405
turtle 616
twins 53, 149, 429, 506, 789
typhoid 260, 584, 730

ulcers 99, 237, 249, 258, 426, 487, 768
ultrasonic doppler blood velocimeter 316
ultraviolet light 68, 92, 96, 97, 121, 146, 208, 209, 210, 211, 260, 263, 264, 332, 385, 387, 422, 474, 518, 615, 637, 668, 683, 743, 744, 750, 753, 761, 770, 771, 790, 802
Unapproved Uses 257, 535, 538, 572, 575
unconsciousness 3, 194
underfeeding 142
underground economy 717
underwater 774, 775
unesterified 491
Unimate Puma® (laboratory robot) 527
unpaired electrons 83, 102, 106, 107, 118, 265, 297, 376, 403, 793, 804
unsaturated 96, 103, 116, 121, 175, 279, 366, 391, 740, 742, 793, 799, 800
unwrinkling 163, 750
upset stomach 246, 276, 281, 305, 485
urinary bladder 247, 340, 390, 482
urinary urgency 190, 191
urination 173, 190, 278, 391, 409, 447, 762, 763, 769
urine densimeter 446
urologist 190
uterus 199, 228
UV (ultraviolet light) 97, 146, 147, 208, 263, 264, 770, 771, 787

vaccinations 343, 356, 357, 358, 683, 686, 730
vagina 196, 197, 199, 200, 201
vagus nerve 326
Varian® Q-band esr spectrometer 521
varicose veins 766, 767
vascular disease 312, 316
vascular elasticity 316
vasomotor instability 200, 201
vegetables 110, 334, 366, 368, 371, 376, 377, 378, 379, 381, 666, 684, 703
vegetarians 505
veins 307, 316, 327, 403, 415
venereal disease 205
vertigo 732
vesicles 169, 171
virility 653
virilization 199
virtues 15, 52
virulent 585
viruses 28, 57, 76, 81, 82, 83, 85, 87, 88, 101, 102, 104, 161, 129, 190, 205, 206, 250, 253, 285, 296, 308, 314, 320, 333, 334,

351, 356, 368, 373, 402, 405, 408, 410, 411, 412, 419, 421, 477, 479, 482, 573, 633, 657, 676, 681, 701, 740, 753, 785, 796, 797, 803
viscoelastic physical properties of the vascular system 522, 523
vision 111, 259, 420
vitality 9, 29, 172
vitamin c content of your urine test 390
vitamin c pumps 111, 413, 639, 740
voice 197, 236, 342, 477
volunteers 112, 127, 178, 227, 256, 289, 339, 410, 633, 670, 681, 693, 699
vomiting 241, 420, 488
vulcanization 95, 790

walking 72, 222, 732, 767
warmed-over flavor 377, 689
warts 501
water bed 231, 300, 301
water chlorination 570, 705
water-soluble vitamin loss test 390
WBC (white blood cell count) differential 452
weak 15, 271, 604, 651, 755, 761
weakness 9, 167, 351, 373, 420, 515
weaning 112
weight 20, 31, 87, 89, 106, 108, 143, 144, 237, 249, 250, 251, 277, 284, 285, 286, 287, 288, 290, 291, 292, 293, 294, 300, 301, 345, 348, 364, 373, 376, 386, 388, 409, 412, 414, 421, 425, 473, 481, 482, 484, 497, 498, 671, 672, 736, 750, 752, 766, 774
weights 87, 345, 412, 414, 774
whales 616
white blood cell (WBC) 87, 88, 405, 759, 796, 797, 804
white blood cell count with differential 447
white blood cells (WBC) 57, 82, 85, 88, 129, 250, 285, 297, 308, 336, 337, 351, 386, 405, 413, 421, 452, 481, 511, 519, 634, 740, 742, 786, 796, 803
white faced capuchin monkey 616
white footed mouse 617
wholesomeness 382, 400, 401, 573
whooping cough 357, 730
WI-38 fibroblasts 137, 138
Wiener analysis 511, 512, 516, 521, 522, 524, 527, 709
windshield wipers 91, 243, 269, 387, 790
withdrawal symptoms 240, 257, 258, 277, 293, 621, 671
wolfhounds 405
word processing 625, 722, 723
workload 768
workouts 222, 232, 743
worms 110, 314, 340
wound healing 345, 408, 412, 477, 735
wounds 151, 327, 344, 345, 412, 685, 694, 710
wrestling 739, 755, 774
wrinkle removal 499
wrinkled 8, 17, 91, 92, 95, 104, 162, 208, 209, 242, 247, 268, 269, 270, 384, 385, 494, 784, 790, 801
writer's block 172, 736

X-ray 146, 178, 265, 332, 516, 527, 728, 729, 770, 787, 793
xeroderma pigmentosa 146, 744

YAF (Young Americans for Freedom) 716
yeast 242, 305, 333, 472, 473, 485, 619, 666, 671, 685, 701, 703, 704, 737

zebra fish 708
Zeiss Axiomat® microscope with phase contrast 527
zero tolerance environmental pollution concept violates the Second Law of Thermodynamics 704

INDEX TO SUBSTANCES:
FOODS, NUTRIENTS, DRUGS, AND CHEMICALS

ROMAN NUMERAL PAGE NUMBER SECTION

IMPORTANT NOTICE:

Do not use any information from our *Life Extension Companion* or our *Life Extension, A Practical Scientific Approach* without first checking the Safety Indexes for both books for the supplement, drug, or action that you plan to take. Also check the Safety Indexes for any illness that you might have and for any drugs that you are now using, since this may influence the safety of your intended actions. It is important that you heed these warnings.

Live Long and Prosper,

Durk Pearson & Sandy Shaw

acidic vitamins xii, xxiv
acids xviii
Adriamycin® xvii
air xvii
alcohol xi, xxxiv
alpha tocopherol xvii
amino acids xvi, xviii
antibiotics xvii, xviii
antidotes xvii
antioxidant xvi, xvii, xxxv
ascorbic acid (vitamin C) xvi, xvii, xxxv
ascorbyl palmitate (fat soluble vitamin C ester) xvi, xxxv
aspirin xvii

bases xv
blood xxiv
brown spots x
butter xxii

carotenoids xvi
chicken xxxi
cholesterol xi, xxii
cigarette xvi
cysteine xvii

DNA xxxii, xxxiii

fats xi, xvi, xxii, xxvii, xxviii
food preservatives xi
free radicals v, x, xix, xxii
fruit xvi

Hydergine® v

interferons xvii
iron xxxiv

L-DOPA xvii, xxiv
lead xxiii
lipid antioxidant xi
lipids xxviii
lipoprotein pigments xxxiii

meats xxii
milk xxii
minerals xvi, xviii

niacin (vitamin B-3) xi
nutrients xi, xii, xv, xvi, xvii, xviii, xxii, xxiii, xxiv

oil xxxv
oxidants xvii
oxygen xxviii

PABA xvii
para-aminobenzoic acid (PABA) xvii
pyridoxine (vitamin B-6) xvii

radium vii
retinoids xvi

sewage xviii
smoke xxx
soup xxxi
spices xi
starch xxxii
sugar xi
sulfa xvii

tocopherols (see vitamin E)

vegetables xvi
vitamin A xi, xvi
vitamin B-3 xi
vitamin B-6 xvii, xxiv
vitamin C xi
vitamin E xi
vitamins xvi, xviii, xxiv

wastes x
water xviii
wine xxi

INDEX TO SUBSTANCES:
FOODS, NUTRIENTS, DRUGS, AND CHEMICALS

IMPORTANT NOTICE:

Do not use any information from our *Life Extension Companion* or our *Life Extension, A Practical Scientific Approach* without first checking the Safety Indexes for both books for the supplement, drug, or action that you plan to take. Also check the Safety Indexes for any illness that you might have and for any drugs that you are now using, since this may influence the safety of your intended actions. It is important that you heed these warnings.

Live Long and Prosper,

Durk Pearson & Sandy Shaw

Leading Numbers:
2-6-ditertiary butyl p-cresol (BHT) 391
2-pyrrolidone-5-carboxylic acid (PCA) 53, 163, 210
2-tertiary butylhydroquinone (TBHQ) 381
5-HIAA (5-hydroxyindoleacetic acid) 131
5-HT (5-hydroxytryptamine, serotonin) 131
5-HTP (5-hydroxytryptophan) 131
5-hydroxytryptamine (serotonin) 131
5-hydroxytryptophan 131
6-ethoxy-1-2-dihydro-2-2-4-trimethylquinoline (ethoxyquin) 114
6-GPD (6-glucose-phosphate dehydrogenase) 79, 448
6-hydroxy-dopamine 133
6-OH-dopamine (6-hydroxy-dopamine) 788
7-12-dimethylbenz-a-anthracene (DMBA) 700

acerola 55
acetaldehyde 24, 92, 147, 162, 178, 209, 242, 243, 250, 256, 265, 269, 270, 271, 272, 273, 275, 278, 279, 282, 325, 340, 341, 413, 475, 481, 483, 525, 563, 647, 663, 664, 668, 670, 676, 677, 679, 694, 700, 752, 783, 784
acetaldehyde dehydrogenase 271
acetate 130, 261, 270, 271, 491, 492
acetic acid 53, 270
acetone 179, 214, 734
acetyl co-enzyme A 79, 130, 479, 789

acetylcholine 126, 128, 129, 130, 131, 170, 186, 187, 193, 197, 198, 228, 250, 274, 431, 475, 484, 641, 649, 650, 733, 737, 783, 788, 798
acetylcholinesterase 130, 443
acid phosphatase 448, 453
acid vitamins 468, 488
acidic vitamins 246, 258, 281, 435, 487, 488, 755
acids 79, 92, 98, 101, 106, 123, 130, 131, 169, 175, 204, 206, 227, 242, 249, 345, 348, 415, 422, 426, 436, 446, 462, 479, 487, 488, 489, 492, 615, 647, 663, 676, 694, 721, 748, 769, 785, 789, 790, 792, 793, 795, 805
ACTH 168, 180, 644, 799
activated charcoal 254, 260, 315, 354
acyl radicals 279
additives 163, 249, 274, 278, 283, 338, 368, 375, 376, 383, 384, 389, 391, 416, 462, 466, 471, 510, 569, 570, 620, 632, 685, 689, 803
adenine 76
adenosine diphosphate (ADP) 797
adenosine triphosphate (ATP) 78, 130, 227, 710, 786, 797
ADH (antidiuretic hormone, vasopressin, Diapid®) 204, 484
ADP (adenosine diphosphate) 797
adrenaline 202, 328, 734, 735, 799
aflatoxin 31, 383, 384, 570, 680, 704, 764

age pigment (lipofuscin, ceroid, amyloid) 102, 112, 120, 121, 122, 124, 127, 128, 176, 187, 211, 484, 750
age spots (age pigment) 102, 120, 121, 124, 127, 175, 211, 796
air 101, 104, 135, 146, 147, 163, 177, 209, 210, 252, 253, 254, 260, 261, 262, 263, 265, 266, 304, 313, 369, 377, 378, 382, 386, 417, 418, 476, 491, 503, 516, 615, 624, 635, 665, 666, 667, 669, 705, 706, 720, 732, 753, 774, 783, 803
alanine 622
albumin 146, 297, 446, 447, 448, 449, 450
albumin, serum 450
alcohol 5, 13, 14, 24, 91, 92, 96, 136, 174, 178, 179, 187, 193, 206, 209, 214, 242, 255, 265, 267, 268, 269, 270, 271, 272, 273, 274, 275, 276, 277, 278, 279, 280, 281, 282, 283, 325, 340, 385, 406, 407, 413, 414, 474, 475, 481, 532, 563, 564, 571, 603, 606, 669, 670, 734, 751, 752, 754, 755, 783, 784, 792, 801, 803
alcohol dehydrogenase 269, 270, 271, 282, 752
aldehyde dehydrogenase 270
aldehydes 68, 96, 121, 209, 210, 243, 257, 265, 270, 325, 326, 385, 413, 475, 481, 482, 483, 783, 784, 790, 797
aldols 477
alfalfa 334, 643
alkaline phosphatase 448, 479, 777
alkalinity 241, 249, 256, 488, 489
alkaloids 240, 501, 640, 648, 664, 667, 676, 699, 707, 733
alkanolamine 495
alkyl radicals 279
alkylaminoalcohols 484
allergens 303, 745
allopurinol (Zyloprim®) 769
alpha tocopherol (vitamin E) 261, 339, 406, 491, 692
alpha-methyl-para-tyrosine 182
aluminum 96
amines 31, 244, 261, 336, 384, 410, 784, 785, 795, 798
amino acid 20, 24, 53, 82, 87, 92, 93, 98, 102, 107, 112, 127, 134, 135, 136, 162, 165, 172, 179, 184, 186, 190, 192, 195, 197, 202, 205, 217, 229, 243, 246, 250, 251, 252, 265, 272, 273, 278, 282, 287, 288, 289, 290, 291, 295, 313, 314, 326, 332, 341, 367, 371, 373, 413, 431, 453, 465, 467, 471, 474, 475, 479, 481, 510, 525, 550, 612, 613, 615, 649, 651, 665, 670, 672, 696, 701, 735, 740, 745, 749, 755, 759, 784, 785, 793, 794, 796, 802, 803
amino acids 76, 77, 78, 86, 87, 89, 95, 102, 107, 127, 162, 168, 179, 182, 184, 192, 202, 218, 229, 242, 251, 289, 298, 308, 332, 333, 341, 342, 345, 374, 384, 465, 474, 477, 615, 620, 622, 623, 640, 661, 662, 726, 764, 784, 785, 800
aminoacetic acid, 794
ammonia 179, 734
amphetamines 168, 171, 172, 174, 180, 278, 287, 289, 295, 497, 498, 799
amyl acetate 792
amylase 294, 448, 451, 672

amyloid 115, 123, 784, 796
Ananase® (bromelain) 237. See also proteolytic enzymes
androgens (male sex hormone) 199, 200, 214, 656, 657, 784
antacids 244, 249, 345, 415, 426, 435, 462, 468, 488, 489, 613, 768
anti-clotting hormone (PGI₂, prostacyclin) 102, 311, 320, 404
anti-mutagens 88
antibiotics 180, 323, 337, 349, 350, 584, 634, 682
antibodies 57, 82, 85, 87, 112, 351, 357, 634, 785, 786, 796
anticarcinogens 88, 369, 502, 565
anticoagulants 283
antidepressants 172, 184, 185, 649, 651, 670, 672, 701
antidiuretic hormone (ADH, vasopressin, Diapid®) 204, 228, 229, 484
antifoam 436, 489
antifreeze 608
antigens 449, 785, 794
antihistamines 282, 304, 347, 745
antimicrobial 689
antioxidant mineral 471
antioxidant nutrient 196, 759, 764
antioxidant vitamins 162, 246, 314, 563, 762
antioxidants 50, 55, 71, 99, 102, 104, 106, 107, 110, 111, 112, 113, 115, 116, 117, 118, 119, 127, 133, 134, 135, 142, 144, 146, 161, 162, 163, 165, 169, 175, 195, 202, 206, 209, 216, 217, 220, 237, 244, 247, 248, 250, 257, 263, 264, 265, 273, 277, 278, 279, 285, 298, 299, 300, 302, 303, 304, 308, 313, 314, 315, 316, 318, 319, 320, 324, 326, 327, 332, 333, 337, 338, 339, 341, 347, 348, 349, 351, 354, 360, 363, 365, 366, 367, 368, 370, 371, 376, 377, 378, 379, 380, 381, 382, 386, 387, 388, 389, 403, 404, 405, 406, 407, 414, 415, 416, 417, 421, 422, 442, 443, 446, 462, 471, 472, 473, 474, 475, 476, 477, 478, 479, 480, 481, 482, 483, 484, 491, 495, 499, 502, 518, 519, 525, 551, 559, 563, 619, 622, 636, 637, 638, 639, 643, 651, 663, 665, 668, 671, 678, 681, 682, 683, 685, 686, 689, 690, 691, 692, 693, 696, 700, 702, 726, 728, 729, 740, 742, 743, 744, 745, 751, 756, 758, 759, 760, 761, 769, 773, 785, 787, 790, 799, 800, 801, 802, 803
antiproteolytic 676, 679, 698
antipsychotic 334, 585
antithrombic 676, 679, 698
antithyroid 631
antitumor 680
antiviral 689, 702
Anturane® 326, 328, 439, 575, 576, 592, 595, 677, 769
AP (ascorbyl palmitate) 381
aphrodisiacs 131, 197, 205, 795
apples 284
arachidonic acid 642
arecholine 642, 647, 649
arginine 87, 89, 162, 192, 229, 288, 298, 308, 315, 320, 332, 345, 477, 483, 509, 620, 622, 633, 640, 661, 662, 671, 678, 685,

700, 735, 736, 741, 742, 752, 763, 771, 774
aromatics 130, 131, 144, 341, 342
arsenic 244, 599
artificial sweeteners 364, 374, 498
asbestos 266, 668
ascorbate (vitamin C) 31, 261, 410, 415, 488, 620, 633, 681, 682, 693, 694, 699
ascorbic acid (vitamin C) 249, 336, 339, 340, 341, 345, 366, 369, 388, 389, 408, 409, 411, 415, 417, 465, 475, 487, 488, 491, 611, 620, 632, 633, 637, 664, 668, 670, 673, 674, 675, 676, 677, 678, 679, 690, 692, 693, 694, 700, 755, 790
ascorbyl palmitate (a fat soluble ester of vitamin C) 369, 377, 378, 379, 381, 382, 388, 389, 414, 465, 475, 483, 612, 622, 637, 673, 690, 692, 700
ash 241
Aspartame® 374
aspartic acid 374, 615
asphalt 391
aspirin 110, 298, 321, 329, 680, 748, 749
atoms 78, 102, 104, 107, 265, 297, 376, 385, 403, 422, 471, 476, 789, 792, 800, 803, 804
ATP (adenosine triphosphate) 78, 130, 187, 227, 424, 425, 710, 786, 789, 797
autoantibodies 85, 786
auxin 123
avidin 217

B-1 (thiamine) 24, 55, 93, 99, 110, 133, 135, 162, 163, 175, 209, 243, 246, 250, 252, 265, 272, 273, 278, 280, 281, 298, 300, 314, 318, 320, 324, 326, 332, 347, 348, 367, 371, 373, 390, 413, 467, 475, 481, 491, 525, 563, 665, 696, 755, 785, 800
B-2 (riboflavin) 162, 246, 247, 390, 464, 763, 764
B-3 (niacin) 162, 246, 249, 390, 463
B-5 (calcium pantothenate, pantothenic acid) 55, 93, 99, 102, 110, 133, 135, 165, 175, 187, 246, 250, 273, 274, 278, 280, 291, 298, 300, 314, 318, 347, 348, 367, 371, 390, 422, 476, 479, 483, 785, 800
B-6 (pyridoxine) 55, 93, 99, 102, 110, 134, 135, 162, 165, 172, 186, 192, 202, 204, 205, 246, 250, 273, 278, 280, 288, 298, 314, 318, 320, 324, 347, 348, 367, 371, 390, 426, 431, 466, 474, 483, 785, 800
B-12 (cyanocobalamin) 78, 170, 195, 477
bacon 31, 239, 292, 383, 384, 389, 437
baking soda 244, 249, 345, 415, 426, 435, 436, 462, 488, 489, 613
bananas 102, 135, 179, 192, 375, 734, 759, 792, 802
barbiturates 193, 194, 206, 281, 354, 571, 643
bases 76, 153, 199, 200, 205, 214, 345, 393, 435, 510, 527, 540, 543, 693, 753
BCG (Bacillus Calmette-Guerin vaccine) 340, 343, 357, 358
beans 294, 671
beef 54, 367, 369, 375, 382, 509, 763
beets 373
benzene 349, 562
benzodiazepines (such as Librium® and Valium®) 193, 282, 426, 477, 754, 755

benzoic acid 382
berries 55
beta blockers (such as propranolol) 110, 328
beta carotene (pro-vitamin A) 53, 97, 208, 211, 245, 258, 261, 264, 420, 422, 423, 465, 468, 476, 483, 612, 620, 622, 665, 666, 684, 695, 702, 703, 743, 744, 756, 758, 771, 787, 801, 802, 804
beta lipotropin 236, 288, 290, 343, 478, 481, 484
BHA (butylated hydroxyanisole) 102, 107, 110, 144, 163, 264, 265, 332, 333, 337, 347, 368, 369, 371, 376, 377, 379, 380, 381, 389, 404, 479, 653, 685, 687, 785
BHT (butylated hydroxytoluene, 2-6-ditertiary butyl p-cresol) 102, 107, 108, 110, 112, 144, 163, 195, 206, 207, 264, 265, 298, 320, 332, 333, 334, 337, 338, 347, 367, 368, 369, 371, 376, 377, 378, 379, 380, 381, 382, 386, 387, 388, 389, 391, 404, 462, 465, 476, 478, 479, 483, 573, 574, 613, 620, 653, 681, 685, 687, 689, 690, 701, 751, 752, 753, 757, 776, 785, 799
bicarbonate of soda (baking soda, sodium bicarbonate) 249
bile 366, 451
bile acids 290, 291, 411, 679, 687, 694, 701
bilirubin 447, 448, 451
binders 273, 305, 306, 462, 485, 619, 620, 621
bioflavonoids 53, 54, 102, 300, 409, 411, 465, 477, 612, 674, 676, 678, 694, 699, 743, 758
biogenic amines 634, 641, 662, 671
biotin (vitamin H) 217, 218, 390, 743, 758
birth control pills 201, 202, 474
bleach 750
bleomycin 565
blood 57, 70, 76, 82, 85, 87, 88, 92, 95, 96, 99, 102, 103, 106, 107, 108, 110, 111, 119, 124, 128, 129, 135, 136, 170, 172, 173, 177, 184, 185, 186, 191, 204, 221, 224, 228, 229, 237, 242, 243, 244, 247, 249, 250, 251, 272, 275, 277, 279, 282, 284, 285, 288, 289, 293, 294, 297, 299, 300, 307, 308, 309, 310, 311, 312, 313, 314, 315, 316, 317, 318, 319, 323, 234, 325, 327, 328, 329, 330, 332, 333, 336, 337, 338, 345, 347, 350, 351, 352, 354, 363, 364, 366, 367, 368, 369, 372, 382, 386, 390, 402, 403, 405, 406, 410, 411, 413, 414, 415, 421, 424, 425, 426, 434, 437, 438, 444, 446, 447, 449, 450, 451, 452, 453, 463, 470, 473, 481, 484, 488, 506, 511, 518, 519, 520, 524, 525, 584, 624, 634, 644, 670, 674, 675, 676, 678, 679, 687, 694, 695, 696, 697, 706, 734, 735, 736, 740, 742, 750, 759, 764, 767, 769, 777, 778, 780, 785, 786, 794, 795, 796, 797, 800, 801, 803, 804
blood sugar 176, 187, 315, 324, 372, 415, 416, 425, 442, 443, 520, 762, 785
blood urea nitrogen (BUN) 447, 448, 451
body fat 233, 237, 671, 721, 772, 774, 775
bones 82, 85, 148, 150, 152, 236, 263, 264, 405, 408, 413, 434, 437, 451, 466, 477, 645, 646, 732, 735, 765, 786, 796, 802
booze. *See* alcohol

botulism toxin 383
brandy 268
bread 91, 294, 375, 382, 717
broccoli 334
bromelain (Ananase®) 87, 89, 99, 163, 237, 384, 801. *See also* proteolytic enzymes
bromocriptine (Parlodel®) 133, 136, 139, 140, 190, 191, 197, 202, 229, 237, 288, 339, 465, 471, 483, 613, 640, 643, 656, 661, 662, 766, 771
bronchoconstrictors 304
bronchodilators 756
brown spots 120, 121
brownies 371, 476
brussels sprouts 334, 797
BSP 449, 451
BUN (blood urea nitrogen) 447, 448, 451
burnt fat 369
Butazolidi® (phenylbutazone) 455, 456
butter 24, 312, 367, 371, 388, 476, 484
butylated hydroxyanisole (BHA) 381, 685
butylated hydroxytoluene (BHT) 206, 381, 478, 657, 701
butyric acid 53, 202

C-AMP (cyclic AMP, cyclic adenosine monophosphate) 502
C-GMP (cyclic GMP, cyclic guanosine monophosphate) 316
cabbage 334, 338
cadmium 96, 413, 599
caffeine 127, 168, 176, 178, 188, 276, 292, 498, 571, 769, 803, 805
calcium 24, 97, 99, 371, 420, 488, 494, 689
calcium ascorbate 415
calcium carbonate 244, 249, 345, 435, 436, 488, 489
calcium pantothenate (vitamin B-5) 24, 31, 162, 165, 170, 187, 204, 227, 246, 247, 264, 414, 465, 469, 479, 483, 492, 612, 755
calcium propionate 382, 383
cannabis 242, 264
canthaxanthin (Orobronze®) 97, 98, 261, 264, 422, 613, 623, 635, 743, 756, 771
carbohydrates 77, 78, 103, 165, 291, 370, 382, 409, 475, 476, 477, 689, 789, 794
carbon 243, 674, 784, 792, 800
carbon dioxide 79, 165, 227, 436, 489, 786, 789, 797
carbon monoxide 177, 244, 257, 275, 314, 350, 352, 406, 413, 524, 562
carbon-14 264
carcinogens 24, 87, 88, 144, 145, 243, 250, 252, 265, 279, 285, 308, 315, 324, 326, 333, 334, 336, 337, 338, 340, 366, 367, 369, 383, 386, 404, 410, 421, 475, 479, 570, 573, 660, 664, 680, 681, 683, 688, 695, 698, 704, 705, 783, 784, 787, 797, 800
carotene. *See* beta carotene
carotenoid. *See* beta carotene
carrots 97, 261, 420, 422, 476, 743, 787, 802
cartilage 501
casein 116
catalases 103, 106, 297, 518, 787, 799
catalysts 107, 312, 369, 382, 786, 787, 792
Catapres® (clonidine) 221, 273, 293

catecholamines 128, 129, 130, 131, 136, 297, 414, 479, 641, 649, 788, 791
catechols 102, 127, 237, 480
catsup 503
cauliflower 334, 338
cayenne pepper 218
CCK (cholecystokinin) 287, 290, 292
celery 334, 377
centrophenoxine (Lucidril®, meclofenoxate, dimethylaminomethanol p-chlorophenoxyacetate) 123, 124, 175, 640, 649
cereals 55, 110, 292, 371, 377, 399, 478, 560, 600, 663, 683, 690
cerebral-spinal fluid (CFS) 111
ceroid 103, 121, 122, 788, 796. *See also* age pigment
charcoal 254, 262, 369
cheeses 127, 184, 195, 202, 205, 251, 288, 291
chelated minerals 468, 748, 749
Chicago BCG (BCG vaccine) 343
chicken 192, 308, 382, 388, 389, 477, 702
chloramphenicol 583, 584, 585
chlorinated organics 259, 260, 705
chlorinated water 260, 705
chlorine 259, 260, 315
chlorohydrins 279
chlorophyll 423
chlorphenteramine 295
chocolate 292
cholecystokinin (CCK) 287, 290, 672
cholesterol 53, 83, 89, 213, 219, 243, 291, 307, 308, 312, 315, 318, 322, 324, 327, 338, 339, 363, 364, 365, 366, 367, 368, 408, 411, 425, 434, 435, 438, 442, 450, 463, 466, 478, 482, 483, 484, 659, 674, 676, 678, 679, 680, 687, 692, 694, 695, 696, 701, 750, 776, 777, 778, 779, 785, 795, 800
cholesterol epoxides 338, 366, 792
cholesterol, esterified 448, 450
cholesterol, free 448
cholesterol hydroperoxides 338
cholesterol is low because free radicals are being effectively scavenged 339
cholesterol is subject to peroxidation 366
cholesterol is the only major antioxidant we know of that humans can make without dietary trace elements 338
cholesterol oxidation products 366
cholesterol peroxides 366
cholesterol, total 448
choline 126, 130, 134, 135, 164, 168, 170, 171, 186, 187, 193, 198, 228, 245, 247, 250, 251, 256, 274, 280, 300, 475, 483, 640, 641, 642, 647, 649, 664, 737, 783, 788
choline acetylase 130
choline bitartrate 135, 164, 171
choline chloride 135, 164, 171, 465, 468, 613
choline hydrochloride 135, 164, 171
cholinergics 131, 134, 135, 170, 171, 175, 190, 250, 641, 647, 649, 651, 788
cigarettes 5, 91, 92, 96, 162, 239, 240, 241, 242, 244, 247, 248, 249, 252, 253, 254, 255, 256, 257, 258, 265, 269, 277, 325, 340, 364, 385, 404, 413, 475, 481, 563, 665, 666, 684, 703, 783, 784, 803

citrate 97
citric acid 79, 227, 368, 369, 380, 475
citric acid cycle 78, 79, 227, 425, 479, 789
citrus fruits 97
Clinistix® 315
Clinistrips® 446
Clinitest® 675
clonidine (Catapres®) 221, 273, 293, 671
clot 70, 102, 108, 224, 311, 312, 317, 318,
    327, 338, 366, 377, 786, 796, 800, 802,
    804
cloves 377
co-dergocrine mesylate (Hydergine®) 667,
    673
CoA (coenzyme A) 130, 227
coal 264, 266, 337, 364, 705, 706
cobalt 494
cocaine 171, 174, 745, 746
cod liver oil 305, 485, 747
coenzyme A (CoA) 130
coenzyme Q (ubiquinones) 406
cofactors 53, 54, 474
coffee 121, 176, 178, 187, 188, 276
colas 178, 188, 276
colchicine 769
cold pressed wheat germ oil 54, 407
collagen 93, 95, 96, 99, 103, 104, 146, 297,
    382, 409, 412, 416, 499, 534, 635, 658,
    659, 670, 675, 789
combustion tars 144, 800
Compazine® 283
complement 57, 82, 789, 796
complexes 298, 672, 710, 748, 784
conalbumin 53
contraceptives 313, 696
cookies 292, 388
cooking oil 368, 380, 386, 387
copper 78, 96, 107, 110, 237, 297, 298, 299,
    300, 311, 312, 319, 338, 347, 369, 382,
    417, 643, 672, 749, 759, 786, 787, 803
copper bracelet 298
copper gluconate 749
copper salicylates 298, 673, 745, 749
corn 305, 383, 485, 619, 621
corn oil 380
corticoids 634, 652, 683
corticosteroids 351, 756
cortisone 747, 795
cosmetics 53, 163, 210, 211, 422, 493, 499,
    501, 577, 578, 587, 626, 627, 659, 672,
    677, 696, 714, 741
CPK (creatine phosphokinase) 448, 451
creatine phosphokinase (CPK) 451
creatinine 447, 448, 453
cross-linkers 88, 92, 96, 210, 242, 265, 300,
    368, 475, 784, 790, 792, 797
cruciforms 710
CSF (cerebral-spinal fluid) 111
cyanocobalamin (vitamin B-12) 465, 477,
    612
cyclamates 374, 499, 570, 595
cyclic AMP (C-AMP, cyclic adenosine
    monophosphate) 176, 304, 502, 534, 650,
    758
cyclic GMP (C-GMP, cyclic guanosine
    monophosphate) 316, 758
Cylert® (magnesium pemoline) 168
cystathione 313, 474

cysteine 24, 53, 82, 87, 89, 92, 93, 98, 102,
    107, 110, 112, 162, 163, 209, 217, 218,
    243, 245, 246, 247, 248, 250, 252, 264,
    265, 272, 273, 278, 280, 281, 298, 308,
    313, 314, 315, 318, 320, 326, 327, 332,
    341, 347, 348, 367, 371, 373, 413, 414,
    415, 453, 467, 469, 471, 475, 481, 482,
    483, 525, 620, 622, 633, 665, 683, 696,
    740, 743, 755, 758, 759, 764, 785, 800,
    803
cystine 162, 217, 218, 245, 247, 280, 447, 449,
    453, 469, 482
cystine stone formation 482
cysts 298, 348
cytoplasm 121
cytosine 76

d-alpha tocopherol (vitamin E) 407
d-penicillamine 299
DA. See dopamine
dairy products 368
Dalmane® (a benzodiazepine sedative) 193,
    426
dandruff 220, 471, 472, 744, 757, 758, 768
DBPC (di-tertbutyl para-cresol, BHT) 690
deactivators 771
DEAE (diethylaminoethanol) 495
Deaner® (dimethylaminoethanol p-
    acetamidobenzoate) 123, 124, 126, 134,
    135, 168, 170, 171, 175, 186, 193, 194,
    198, 211, 228, 274, 320, 431, 435, 439,
    465, 468, 483, 484, 495, 613, 649, 737,
    749, 750, 797
Deanol®. See Deaner®
death hormone (DECO, decreasing oxygen
    consumption hormone) 74, 98, 142
decarboxylase 130, 131, 646
DECO. See death hormone
dehydroascorbic acid (DHA, oxidized vitamin
    C) 417, 491, 790
dehydroepiandrosterone (DHEA) 286, 524
dehydrogenase 764
deoxyribonucleic acid (DNA) 76, 791, 802
deposits 121, 122, 215, 285, 307, 308, 324,
    364, 411, 466, 478, 750, 796
depressants 188, 251, 285, 289
DES (diethylstilbesterol) 54, 533, 704, 705
detergents 218, 254, 478, 495
DHA (dehydroascorbic acid, oxidized vitamin
    C) 417, 418
di-radical 376
dianhydrosorbitol 660
Diapid® (ADH, vasopressin) 128, 164, 168,
    173, 174, 190, 204, 229, 276, 277, 281,
    288, 320, 439, 465, 469, 483, 484, 613,
    763
diazoxide (Hyperstat®) 221
diethylaminoethanol (DEAE) 123, 495
diethylstilbesterol (DES) 54
dihydroergocornine 707. See also Hydergine®
dihydroergocristine 707. See Hydergine®
dihydroergocryptine 501, 707. See also
    Hydergine®
dihydroergotoxine 501, 640, 669, 701, 707.
    See also Hydergine®
dihydrotestosterone 139, 213, 219
dihydroxy vitamin D 152
dihydroxyphenylalanine (L-DOPA) 130

dilauryl thiodipropionate 465, 476, 483, 612
dill 334
dimethyl sulfoxide (DMSO) 237, 347, 662, 673, 686, 760, 791
dimethylaminoethanol. (DMAE.) *See* Deaner®
dimethylaminoethyl p-chlorophenoxyacetate. *See* Deaner®
dimethylbenzanthracene (DMBA, 7-12-dimethylbenz-a-anthracene) 33, 700
dinitrochlorobenzene 218
dinitrochlorophenol 218
diphenylhydantoin (Dilantin®) 168, 257, 258, 277, 643
disodium EDTA. *See* EDTA
disulfide 95, 790
disulfide bonds 95, 246, 467, 482, 789, 790
dl-alpha tocopherol (vitamin E) 407, 470, 692
dl-alpha tocopherol acetate (vitamin E) 31, 407, 465, 468, 611, 619
DMAE (dimethylaminoethanol). *See* Deaner®
DMAE bitartrate 484
DMBA (dimethylbenzanthracene, 7-12-dimethylbenz-a-anthracene) 144, 145, 333, 339, 700
DMSO (dimethyl sulfoxide) 214, 215, 237, 238, 298, 347, 348, 349, 477, 599, 663, 740, 759, 760, 791
DNA (deoxyribonucleic acid) 18, 21, 24, 68, 71, 75, 76, 88, 91, 92, 98, 101, 102, 103, 104, 106, 137, 138, 139, 144, 145, 146, 147, 148, 149, 150, 153, 206, 209, 213, 232, 241, 244, 250, 263, 264, 265, 269, 285, 286, 297, 331, 332, 402, 404, 422, 429, 472, 476, 479, 505, 506, 514, 515, 534, 550, 551, 645, 707, 709, 710, 744, 753, 770, 785, 786, 789, 791, 793, 795, 798, 802
docosahexanoic acid 111, 413
dolomite 249, 435, 436, 488, 489
DOPA (L-DOPA, dihydroxyphenylalanine) 127, 130, 197, 481, 641, 652, 661, 662, 698, 758
dopamine (DA) 127, 128, 129, 130, 132, 133, 134, 135, 136, 184, 185, 186, 197, 202, 236, 307, 414, 431, 474, 475, 479, 481, 487, 493, 505, 642, 643, 650, 653, 656, 662, 675, 701, 741, 788, 791, 796, 797, 798
dopaminergic stimulants 133, 136, 192, 197, 229, 236, 481
dressings 218, 379, 382
dry vitamin E 492
dyes 217, 420, 520, 621

E deficiency 78
EDTA 96, 97, 263. *See also* disodium EDTA
EGF. *See* epidermal growth factor
eggs 24, 53, 92, 102, 112, 117, 127, 138, 140, 142, 147, 148, 217, 243, 272, 292, 367, 371, 382, 482, 702, 759
EGTA 97
eicosapentaenoate 314
eicosapentaenoic acid 314
elastin 103
electrolytes 204
electrons 88, 95, 107, 118, 162, 227, 309, 310, 311, 312, 402, 406, 520, 527, 640, 644, 709, 799, 801, 804
elements 45, 88, 96, 245, 471, 495, 517
elevated serum cholesterol is an indicator of elevated free radical activity 367
emulsifiers 218
emulsion 352
endorphins 224, 236, 293, 343, 354, 478, 791, 792
enkephalins 186, 224, 293, 414, 792
enterotoxins 354
enzyme inducer 478, 479
enzymes 72, 76, 78, 87, 88, 89, 96, 99, 101, 103, 104, 106, 108, 119, 139, 140, 142, 144, 146, 162, 169, 170, 184, 186, 187, 206, 213, 227, 237, 244, 252, 265, 269, 270, 271, 273, 279, 280, 282, 289, 294, 297, 304, 313, 314, 315, 334, 337, 382, 384, 403, 409, 414, 451, 452, 470, 471, 422, 473, 475, 478, 479, 481, 494, 496, 502, 515, 516, 520, 617, 653, 665, 687, 696, 748, 752, 764, 769, 777, 787, 792, 793, 797, 799, 801, 803, 805
epidermal growth factor (EGF) 138, 165, 210, 211, 644, 646, 647, 658, 694
epoxides 264, 279, 341, 366, 770, 792, 797
epoxy 165, 279, 792
ergot 501, 640, 648, 664, 667, 676, 699, 733
ergot compounds 519, 520, 640
erythromycin 350
esters 92, 97, 199, 200, 209, 214, 215, 264, 406, 407, 462, 474, 484, 491, 492, 692, 792, 801
Estrace® (female sex hormone) 201
estradiol (female sex hormone) 199, 200, 201
estradiol cypionate (female sex hormone) 213
estradiol dipropionate (female sex hormone) 197, 199, 200, 201, 214, 215
estrogens (female sex hormone) 54, 55, 196, 199, 200, 201, 213, 214, 217, 236, 343, 407, 478, 792
ethane 404, 667
ethanol. *See* alcohol
ether 644
ethoxyquin (Santoquin®, 6-ethoxy-1-2-dihydro-2-2-4-trimethylquinoline) 55, 107, 112, 113, 114, 404, 636
euphoriants 288
exhaust 265, 413, 585, 783
experimental formulations 513, 520, 619, 776
experimental nutrient mix 210
extracts 54, 129, 377, 565, 581, 613, 767

fat soluble antioxidant 402, 419
fat soluble vitamin C (AP, ascorbyl palmitate) 369, 389
fats 5, 24, 44, 55, 66, 68, 77, 78, 83, 88, 101, 106, 108, 118, 119, 134, 165, 200, 210, 214, 215, 218, 220, 222, 223, 229, 235, 237, 238, 239, 243, 244, 247, 250, 273, 279, 280, 282, 284, 285, 286, 288, 289, 290, 291, 297, 308, 311, 312, 313, 314, 319, 337, 340, 363, 365, 366, 368, 369, 370, 371, 372, 376, 377, 378, 379, 382, 386, 388, 402, 403, 404, 409, 411, 413, 422, 424, 425, 432, 470, 475, 476, 478, 479, 481, 484, 503, 505, 515, 571, 637,

638, 650, 671, 687, 688, 690, 696, 735, 736, 741, 758, 774, 776, 777, 778, 780, 785, 787, 789, 796, 800, 802, 804. *See also* lipids

fatty acids 77, 111, 118, 175, 217, 314, 474, 636, 642, 668, 692, 793

feathers 97

feces 177, 339, 366, 410, 422, 446, 453, 489

female sex hormones. *See* estrogen, estradiol

fenfluramine 287

ferritin 443

fibroblasts 88, 137, 138, 144, 146, 336, 792, 796

fillers 273, 305, 306, 347, 407, 462, 485, 492, 619, 620, 621

fish 126, 141, 170, 171, 263, 313, 708

flatus 489

flavins 297

flavonoids. *See* bioflavonoids

fluoride 371, 689

fluorocarbons 351, 352, 524, 686

fly ash 264

folate (folic acid) 743, 758

follicle stimulating hormone (FSH, a gonadotropin) 765

food additive antioxidant 112, 465, 613

food additives 97, 218, 264, 336, 462, 573, 802

food preservatives 163, 195, 332, 333, 375, 376, 378, 384, 389, 478, 499, 663, 683, 689, 690, 752

formaldehyde 242, 269, 475, 784

frankincense 377

free fatty acids 448, 450, 495, 695

free radical, damage from 100, 102, 103, 104, 110, 111, 112, 124, 142, 29, 221, 265, 297, 313, 314, 318, 320, 324, 338, 347, 406, 413, 417, 482, 518, 560, 642, 665, 696, 729, 740, 758, 759, 785

free radical disease 793

free radical initiator 242, 475, 804

free radical scavengers 101, 265, 273, 274, 280, 298, 348, 354, 406, 477, 525, 740, 752, 758, 771, 793

free radical scavengers may help epileptics 642

free radical theory of aging 100, 103, 110, 146, 378, 496, 636, 637, 638, 639, 650, 690, 700, 702, 751

free radicals 66, 68, 70, 83, 88, 92, 96, 100, 101, 102, 103, 104, 106, 107, 108, 110, 111, 112, 115, 116, 117, 118, 119, 121, 124, 133, 135, 142, 146, 153, 161, 162, 165, 170, 177, 209, 237, 238, 243, 244, 246, 250, 254, 260, 263, 264, 265, 270, 271, 272, 273, 274, 275, 276, 280, 296, 297, 298, 299, 300, 304, 308, 311, 312, 313, 314, 316, 318, 319, 320, 324, 326, 332, 338, 339, 340, 341, 347, 348, 351, 354, 367, 368, 371, 376, 382, 402, 403, 404, 406, 409, 424, 470, 473, 474, 475, 481, 483, 484, 495, 502, 511, 514, 516, 518, 519, 520, 521, 524, 527, 534, 557, 559, 560, 563, 635, 636, 637, 638, 642, 643, 645, 665, 668, 682, 683, 685, 686, 692, 696, 701, 702, 729, 740, 742, 748, 751, 752, 758, 759, 760, 762, 769, 770, 771, 773, 783, 784, 785, 786, 787, 788, 790, 792, 793, 795, 796, 797, 799, 800, 803

Free Radicals in Medicine and Biology 639

fresheners 254

fructose 373

fruit 19, 55, 102, 110, 121, 237, 368, 371, 373, 376, 382, 404, 506, 507, 554, 616, 666, 684, 703

fruit juices 244, 491

FSH (follicle stimulating hormone, a gonadotropin) 236, 343, 478, 765, 799

fuels 206, 227, 265, 324, 391, 479, 688, 800

fumaric acid 79, 227

fumes 413

GABA (gamma aminobutyric acid) 190, 202, 282, 755, 793, 796, 798

gamma-1-glutamyl-l-cysteinylglycine (reduced glutathione) 764

garbage 120

garlic 472

Gas-X® 436, 489

gasoline 264, 337, 391, 560, 690, 786

gelatin 305, 347, 382, 407, 485, 619, 620, 737, 790

Gerovital (GH-3, diethylaminoethanol p-aminobenzoate, procaine, no relation to GH, growth hormone) 123, 184, 495, 651, 798

GH. *See* growth hormone

GH releasers, you should get a jeweler's ring size set 765

GH-3. *see* Gerovital

glass 80, 244, 272, 287, 354, 377, 378, 386, 387, 442, 453, 488, 704, 747

globulins 53, 146, 297

glucocorticoid 638

glucokinase 71

gluconate 465, 468, 612

glucose 71, 227, 246, 315, 373, 409, 415, 416, 425, 442, 443, 447, 448, 450, 467, 520, 777

glucose oxidase 416, 443, 520, 785

glucose-6-phosphate dehydrogenase (6-GPD) 453

glutamate 793, 802

glutamic acid 764, 793

glutaraldehyde 269

glutathione gamma-1-glutamyl-l-cysteinylglycine) 102, 107, 248, 280, 680, 764

glutathione peroxidase 78, 88, 101, 104, 146, 242, 280, 315, 333, 471, 637, 666, 671, 685, 698, 704, 793

glutathione reductase 162, 248, 280, 304, 472, 764

glycerol mono-oleate 380

glycine (aminoacetic acid) 613, 764, 784, 785, 794, 796

glycoproteins 794, 796

glydikin 605

gonadotropins 765

grains 147, 383, 613, 705, 767

grapes 102, 373

grass 242

gravy 382

grease 391, 478
growth hormone (GH) 73, 86, 123, 127, 129,
136, 139, 141, 165, 172, 176, 190, 192,
194, 223, 229, 236, 285, 286, 288, 289,
290, 323, 339, 342, 343, 345, 370, 373,
471, 477, 478, 480, 481, 509, 633, 635,
640, 652, 661, 662, 663, 671, 672, 701,
704, 735, 736, 741, 742, 765, 766, 771,
772, 774, 794, 799
growth hormone releasers 192, 233, 236, 286,
290, 342, 477, 478, 483, 509, 515, 640,
661, 662, 741, 771, 774
growth-hormone-releaser scandal 509
growth stimulants 213, 345
guaiac 447, 449, 453
guanine 76

Hadacol® 274
hair 8, 76, 81, 139, 175, 197, 212, 213, 214,
215, 216, 217, 218, 219, 220, 221, 382,
420, 471, 472, 473, 476, 479, 482, 516,
574, 659, 660, 742, 744, 745, 757, 758,
759, 768
hair pigment 757, 758
hamburgers 382
hamburgers, hot dogs, and sausages,
peroxidation and 369
hash 243
haze 349
HCl 465, 469, 612, 651, 671
HDL. See high density lipoproteins
HDL/LDL ratios 312, 324, 365, 367, 450,
466, 780
Head and Shoulders® 220, 471, 758
health food 5, 55, 83, 87, 89, 92, 102, 127,
135, 164, 169, 171, 192, 193, 195, 208,
217, 238, 239, 240, 243, 244, 251, 259,
272, 298, 348, 389, 462, 663, 670, 748,
776
heavy metals 96, 99, 244, 264
helium 804
Hemastix® 447
hematoporphyrin 743
hemoglobin 146, 177, 275, 297, 314, 406, 447,
449, 452, 453, 518
hemoproteins 297
herbicides 424
herbs 377
heroin 277, 293, 621, 671, 714, 715
heroinlike compounds 293
herring 689
hesperidin 465, 469, 477, 483, 612, 743, 758.
See also bioflavonoids
hexokinase 246, 416, 443, 447, 448, 450, 467,
777, 785
high density lipoproteins (HDL) 224, 229,
312, 324, 325, 339, 363, 364, 448, 450,
680, 692, 702, 777, 778, 779, 780, 781,
782, 794
high nicotine and low carcinogen cigarette
563
histamines 204, 205, 218, 219, 244, 282, 304,
327, 347, 413, 426, 754, 795
histidine 205, 754
histones 795
homocysteine 313, 314, 474, 674, 676, 678
homocystine 313, 674, 678
honey 373, 503

hormones 70, 72, 73, 76, 86, 89, 103, 108,
128, 129, 131, 137, 138, 139, 140, 141,
142, 164, 165, 169, 172, 173, 176, 180,
188, 190, 191, 196, 197, 199, 200, 201,
202, 210, 211, 213, 214, 215, 220, 228,
236, 276, 279, 285, 286, 287, 288, 290,
292, 304, 318, 321, 323, 336, 339, 343,
469, 471, 478, 482, 483, 484, 494, 495,
509, 510, 524, 534, 632, 634, 635, 641,
642, 652, 653, 656, 659, 662, 671, 678,
704, 758, 762, 766, 771, 784, 786, 794,
795, 798, 799, 800, 801
horseradish 104
horseradish peroxidase 104
humectants 163, 210
hyaluronate 104
hyaluronic acid 297, 298
Hydergine® 111, 112, 119, 124, 127, 128,
133, 135, 162, 168, 175, 176, 177, 178,
179, 187, 188, 194, 200, 201, 228, 244,
257, 258, 265, 272, 273, 274, 275, 276,
281, 304, 314, 318, 319, 320, 339, 348,
350, 439, 469, 482, 483, 484, 492, 501,
502, 503, 519, 520, 524, 525, 613, 641,
648, 650, 651, 664, 667, 669, 673, 676,
677, 681, 685, 699, 701, 702, 707, 726,
731, 732, 733, 734, 740, 749, 750, 758,
760, 798
hydrocarbons 260, 404
hydrocortisone 797
hydrogen 88, 107, 243, 424, 425, 784, 803
hydrogen peroxide 101, 102, 103, 133, 135,
170, 260, 279, 297, 298, 304, 324, 376,
518, 520, 769, 787, 788, 794, 795, 799
hydrolases 106
hydroperoxides 118, 279. See also ROOH
hydroquinones 297
hydroxyl radicals 102, 103, 135, 238, 279,
298, 760, 795
hyperbaric oxygen 119, 516, 665, 696
Hyperstat® (diazoxide) 221
hypochlorite 260, 279, 518
hypophosphite 112

idoxuridine 573
IGE (immunoglobulin E) 303
imipramine 136, 184, 185
immune system stimulant 87, 305, 323, 339,
419, 421, 477, 481
immunoglobulins 303, 448
immunostimulants 730
indoles 334, 338
inducers 187, 334, 516, 634, 683
inhibitors 31, 98, 184, 186, 241, 314, 332,
347, 479, 638, 651, 671, 672, 676, 678,
683, 691, 699, 702, 770, 798, 799
inhibitory neurotransmitters 134, 202, 793,
794, 796, 802
initiators 250, 312, 338, 368
inositol 162, 193, 216, 217, 282, 298, 300,
373, 465, 469, 476, 477, 483, 612, 755,
760, 797
insulin 72, 165, 246, 315, 370, 372, 373, 442,
443, 467, 476, 482, 675, 688, 762, 795
interferon 57, 82, 83, 85, 88, 335, 336, 411,
742, 796
intermediates 96, 103
intravenous ascorbate (vitamin C) 410

402

ions 96, 152, 254, 299, 391, 516, 635, 710
iron 78, 107, 108, 237, 299, 300, 311, 312,
    319, 338, 347, 369, 382, 417, 494, 718,
    759, 786, 787
irritants 103, 187, 218, 488, 515, 758
isocarboxazid 798
isocitric acid 79
Isoprinosine® 168
isoquinoline alkaloids 278

Jell-O® 91, 96, 330, 375, 382, 384, 522
jelly 479, 491
juice 97, 272, 388, 409, 749, 750
junk foods 224, 398, 399, 601

ketones 96

1-ascorbic acid 3-sulfate 366
L-DOPA 102, 107, 127, 132, 133, 134, 135,
    165, 192, 197, 202, 229, 236, 237, 288,
    289, 341, 345, 414, 431, 432, 435, 465,
    468, 471, 474, 475, 479, 480, 481, 483,
    509, 613, 622, 640, 641, 644, 652, 656,
    661, 699, 741, 743, 749, 771, 796
1-penicillamine 299
1-prolyl 1-leucyl glycine amide 168, 180
lactic acid 227
lactose 411
laetrile 575, 599
lard 377, 379
latex 95, 790
laxatives 187
LDH 448, 451, 479
LDL. See low density lipoproteins
lead 37, 51, 70, 72, 75, 81, 96, 97, 119, 121,
    136, 178, 184, 186, 202, 214, 217, 237,
    241, 244, 252, 260, 261, 263, 272, 277,
    300, 307, 312, 314, 318, 324, 338, 342,
 · 370, 372, 412, 422, 453, 473, 568, 599,
    728, 762, 767
leaded gasoline 263
leather 91, 92, 95, 163, 210, 269
lecithin 53, 126, 134, 135, 168, 170, 171, 187,
    193, 198, 228, 274, 365, 435, 649
leftovers 369, 378, 382
lemon 388
lettuce 52, 375, 643
leukotrienes 304, 642, 673
Levamisole® 340, 634
LH. See luteinizing hormone
LHRH. See luteinizing hormone releasing
    hormone
Librium® (see benzodiazapine) 193, 282, 426,
    477, 754, 755
limestone 244, 249, 415, 435, 488
linkers 106, 209, 475, 783
linoleic acid hydroperoxide 634, 636, 664,
    667, 700
linoleic acid 111
lipid antioxidant 402, 637, 673, 679, 692
lipid coat 206, 479, 657
lipid peroxides 109, 316, 366, 770
lipid-coated viruses 334
lipid-containing viruses 681
lipids (fats or oils) 24, 53, 55, 77, 97, 102, 103,
    108, 111, 123, 124, 175, 206, 209, 220,
    265, 279, 282, 297, 315, 318, 319, 364,
    365, 372, 376, 377, 402, 403, 404, 409,

410, 411, 413, 422, 425, 426, 434, 438,
    442, 448, 450, 463, 466, 470, 475, 476,
    478, 636, 639, 653, 667, 668, 678, 687,
    689, 691, 6792, 698, 702, 704, 758, 776,
    785, 787, 789, 790, 793, 796, 799, 800,
    801. See also fats
lipofuscin 103, 112, 120, 121, 122, 123, 124,
    127, 128, 138, 139, 174, 175, 176, 187,
    211, 320, 484, 495, 639, 640, 644, 649,
    750, 796. See also age pigment, age spots
lipopigments 121, 796. See also lipofuscin,
    amyloid, ceroid, age pigment, age spots
lipoprotein pigments 639, 649
lipoproteins 229, 312, 324, 325, 327, 364, 425,
    679, 680, 687, 692, 695, 777
lipovitellin 53
liquor 274, 279, 754. See also alcohol
lithium 182
litmus paper 249, 489
livetin 53, 702
Loniten® (minoxidil) 221
low cholesterol diets 308, 324, 364
low cholesterol levels are due to our high
    intake of other antioxidants 339
low density lipoproteins (LDL) 312, 324, 325,
    327, 339, 364, 365, 425, 448, 450, 692,
    777, 778, 779, 780, 781, 782, 796
low sodium antacid 488
LSD 174, 426, 718
lubricants 83, 103, 104, 161, 187, 621
Lucidril® (centrophenoxine, meclofenoxate)
    123
luteinizing hormone (LH, a gonadotropin)
    236, 343, 478, 765, 799
luteinizing hormone releasing hormone
    (LHRH) 131, 197, 236, 343, 478, 765, 795
lymph 57, 82, 85, 410, 796

Maalox® 345, 435, 488, 768
magnesium 415, 488, 677
magnesium pemoline (Cylert®) 168, 171, 174
malic acid 79, 227
malonaldehyde 106, 121, 325, 470, 481, 682,
    689, 784, 797
manganese 78, 297, 338, 643, 803
mannitol 373
MAO (monamine oxidase) 131, 172, 184, 186,
    797, 798
MAO inhibitor (monamine oxidase inhibitor)
    184, 798
marijuana 174
martinis 248, 275
mayonnaise 218, 379, 503
meat tenderizer 384
meats 24, 31, 127, 184, 192, 195, 202, 205,
    237, 251, 261, 288, 291, 312, 313, 314,
    337, 368, 369, 371, 377, 378, 382, 384,
    389, 474, 477, 509, 662, 688, 689, 705
meclofenoxate (centrophenoxine, Lucidril®)
    123
megavitamins 305, 443, 485, 729, 768
melanin 124, 175, 341, 750, 758, 770, 771
Mellaril® 283
membrane stabilizers 216, 217, 298, 300, 470,
    473, 477, 483, 760, 769, 797
membrane-binding factors 55
membrane-bound enzymes 642
menthol 255

403

meperidine 621
mercaptoethanol 86, 87
mercaptoethylamine 112
mercury 263, 653
mercury selenide 263
mesylates 501, 640, 701, 707
metabolites 144, 479, 563, 668
metals 76, 96, 205, 262, 264, 299, 391, 491, 788
methadone 621
methionine 218, 313, 314, 443, 471, 474, 702
methylcholanthrene 336
methylparabens 382
Metrazol® 168
milk 24, 135, 179, 184, 192, 251, 288, 312, 368, 371, 387, 411, 442, 471, 477, 643, 662, 802
milk of magnesia 415
minerals 78, 82, 86, 88, 89, 93, 99, 102, 104, 107, 175, 241, 245, 250, 252, 260, 268, 273, 291, 314, 315, 332, 367, 368, 371, 392, 393, 398, 399, 401, 431, 494, 510, 623, 726, 740, 756, 785
minoxidil (Loniten®) 221, 659
mixed-function oxidase enzymes 259, 334, 337, 797
moisturizers 53, 163, 208, 210, 741
monamine oxidase (MAO) 184, 414, 797, 798
monamine oxidase inhibitors (MAO inhibitors) 172, 495, 798
monamines 131, 184, 651
mono-tertiary-butylhydroquinone (TBHQ, 2-tertiarybutylhydroquinone) 379, 381
morphine 47, 293, 621, 643, 714, 725, 800
morphinelike hormones 293
mouthwash 371, 689
MSV (Moloney sarcoma virus) 87
mucin 53
mucous 131, 198, 205, 275, 419, 420
mushrooms 97, 650, 733
mutagens 24, 88, 106, 145, 241, 243, 265, 285, 308, 312, 326, 338, 339, 340, 366, 386, 404, 410, 475, 573, 783, 784, 797, 798
myelin 474
myrrh 377

Na-PCA (sodium salt of 2-pyrrolidone-5-carboxylic acid) 53, 163, 210, 620, 622, 647, 658, 741
NAD (nicotinamide adenine dinucleotide) 79, 665, 696
NADP (nicotinamide adenine dinucleotide phosphate) 424
NADPH (reduced nicotinamide adenine dinucleotide phosphate) 162, 280, 424, 425, 665
Naloxone® 354, 639
Naltrexone® 293
narcotics 575, 621, 713, 715
natural antioxidants 162, 367, 371, 424, 484, 639, 666, 690, 703
natural vitamin C 52, 54, 55
natural vitamins 52, 53, 55, 490
NDGA (nordihydroquaiaretic acid) 381, 404
NE. See norepinephrine
nerve growth factor (NGF) 128, 138, 176, 211, 276, 482, 502, 641, 648, 700, 798

neurochemicals 40, 128, 168, 169, 180, 639, 648, 798
neurohormones 290
neuromuscular messenger 228
neurotransmitters 126, 127, 128, 129, 131, 132, 134, 135, 153, 157, 169, 170, 171, 179, 184, 185, 186, 190, 192, 193, 197, 198, 228, 236, 274, 278, 287, 291, 295, 297, 409, 414, 431, 474, 479, 481, 498, 510, 650, 652, 741, 783, 788, 791, 793, 796, 797, 798, 799, 801, 803
NGF. See nerve growth factor
niacin (vitamin B-3) 24, 162, 193, 204, 205, 218, 243, 244, 245, 246, 247, 249, 279, 280, 281, 282, 283, 327, 347, 365, 424, 425, 426, 434, 435, 436, 462, 463, 465, 466, 469, 470, 483, 487, 488, 612, 643, 665, 688, 695, 696, 742, 754, 755, 758, 777, 798
niacin, reduction of paraquat toxicity in rats 665, 696
niacinamide (another form of vitamin B-3) 193, 245, 282, 426, 463, 469, 755
nicorette 256, 664
nicotinamide (niacinamide) 193, 227
nicotinamide adenine dinucleotide (NAD) 424, 665, 696
nicotinamide adenine dinucleotide phosphate (NADP) 424
nicotine 240, 241, 243, 244, 247, 249, 250, 254, 255, 256, 257, 258, 269, 275, 413, 424, 425, 563, 663, 664, 665, 803
nicotine/tar 255
nicotinic acid (niacin) 243, 327, 347, 424, 425, 434, 463, 469, 487, 488, 663, 685, 695, 700, 798
nitrates 31, 244, 261, 383, 384, 410, 798
nitric acid 413
nitrites 31, 244, 261, 336, 383, 384, 410, 798
nitrogen 89, 243, 403, 418, 443, 451, 491, 609, 610
nitrogen oxides (NOX) 147, 244, 246, 250, 257, 332, 349, 413, 516
nitrosamines 31, 244, 261, 336, 384, 410, 798
nonsteroid 196
Nootropyl® (piracetam) 168
noradrenaline (norepinephrine, NE) 734, 735, 799
nordihydroguaiaretic acid (NDGA) 381
norepinephrine (NE, noradrenaline) 126, 127, 128, 129, 130, 132, 136, 171, 172, 174, 176, 182, 184, 185, 186, 197, 202, 236, 251, 278, 287, 288, 289, 291, 295, 414, 479, 498, 641, 649, 734, 745, 788, 797, 798, 799, 802
NOX. See nitrogen oxides
nucleases 206
nucleoproteins 219, 795
nucleotides 550
nutrient mixes 464, 467, 619, 620, 742, 743, 750, 756, 760
nuts 383, 716

o-dianisidine 520
oils 24, 55, 77 88, 163, 165, 200, 209, 210, 232, 264, 279, 280, 319, 337, 347, 368, 369, 371, 375, 376, 378, 379, 381, 382, 386, 387, 388, 391, 402, 403, 407, 462,

492, 619, 627, 637, 639, 673, 690, 702, 705, 758, 787, 796. *See also* lipids
onions 254
opiates 293, 354, 669, 672, 686, 714, 715
opium 714
oranges 408
Orbit (a chewing gum) 498, 507
oregano 377
organic peroxides 24, 70, 107, 108, 116, 279, 280, 313, 319, 338, 368, 371, 378, 425, 515, 636, 740, 758, 783. *See also* ROOH; ROOR
ornithine 87, 89, 162, 192, 229, 298, 308, 315, 320, 332, 345, 443, 477, 483, 509, 640, 646, 661, 763, 771, 774
Orobronze® (canthaxanthin) 97
Ortho-Novum® (birth control pills) 201
orthotoluidine 416, 443, 785
ovalbumin 53
ovomucoid 53
oxalate 415, 447, 449, 453
oxaloacetic acid 79
oxalosuccinic acid 79
oxidants 102, 177, 259, 304, 376, 378, 386, 417, 422, 425, 473, 474, 475, 482, 518, 634, 636, 664, 667, 700, 785, 794, 796
oxidase 131, 651
oxidation 24, 66, 68, 88, 95, 101, 107, 110, 111, 118, 170, 175, 227, 242, 247, 250, 271, 299, 304, 308, 312, 338, 367, 376, 378, 381, 386, 391, 402, 403, 414, 418, 421, 472, 492, 636, 688, 689, 692, 786, 789, 797, 799
oxidized cholesterol 216, 312, 338
oxidized glutathione 248, 304, 764
oxidizers 250, 799
oxygen 55, 102, 104, 106, 107, 112, 119, 124, 135, 136, 146, 176, 177, 187, 227, 228, 243, 244, 250, 254, 257, 260, 265, 275, 285, 299, 300, 314, 318, 325, 350, 351, 354, 376, 378, 386, 391, 402, 403, 405, 406, 413, 417, 422, 452, 453, 470, 476, 482, 491, 502, 505, 524, 637, 638, 643, 668, 686, 771, 784, 785, 786, 787, 792, 795, 796, 799, 800, 802, 804
Oxygen Free Radicals and Tissue Damage 673
oxytocin 131, 469, 484, 642
ozone 31, 147, 248, 250, 260, 261, 332, 404, 422, 473, 516, 518, 636, 667, 668, 692, 698, 700, 790, 793, 799

p-acetamidobenzoate 484
p-acetamidobenzoate salt 123
p-aminobenzoic acid 97, 209, 217, 465, 473, 612
p-chlorophenoxyacetate 640, 649
PABA (p-aminobenzoic acid, para aminobenzoic acid) 55, 77, 78, 92, 93, 97, 162, 165, 209, 217, 245, 246, 248, 250, 252, 261, 263, 264, 298, 300, 422, 435, 465, 469, 473, 474, 483, 495, 612, 667, 698, 743, 756, 758, 797
PAH (polynuclear aromatic hydrocarbon, polycyclic aromatic hydrocarbon) 144, 146, 264, 279, 336, 337, 338, 339, 341, 364, 479, 797, 800

PAH epoxide (polynuclear aromatic hydrocarbon epoxide, polycyclic aromatic hydrocarbon epoxide) 279
painkillers 49, 335, 414
paints 165, 261, 299, 391, 747, 786
pancreatic enzymes 290
pantothenate (vitamin B-5) 55, 165, 210, 228, 245, 246, 291, 742, 755, 758
pantothenic acid (vitamin B-5) 31, 170, 187, 227, 246, 247, 430, 436, 492, 647, 657, 662, 686, 700
pantothenyl alcohol 479
papain 87, 89, 99, 163, 237, 384. *See also* proteolytic enzymes
papaya 87, 99, 163, 237, 384
para aminobenzoic acid (PABA, p-aminobenzoic acid) 217
Paraquat® 242, 243, 424, 665, 696
Parlodel® (bromocriptine) 133, 136, 139, 190, 197, 200, 201, 202, 229, 237, 288, 339, 465, 471, 613, 766
PBI. *See* protein bound iodine
PCA (2-pyrrolidone-5-carboxylic acid, pyrrolidone carboxylic acid). *See* Na-PCA
PCP 426
peanuts 383, 570
penicillamine 299
penicillin 350, 554, 761, 771
pentane 404, 692
pepper 52, 218
peptide 78, 180, 527, 624, 708, 800
peracetic acid 279, 340, 783
peristaltic stimulant 187
peroxidases 103, 106, 142, 515, 518, 520, 668, 692, 698, 799
peroxide value (pv) 378, 381
peroxides 24, 88, 104, 108, 115, 118, 285, 368, 376, 378, 386, 388, 403, 404, 470, 471, 476, 793, 799, 800, 802
peroxidized arachidonic acid 639
peroxidized fats 88, 106, 107, 108, 112, 121, 174, 285, 308, 325, 332, 367, 368, 376, 385, 386, 481, 784, 793, 800
peroxidized fats, reduction of PGI_2 production, 318
peroxyacetylnitrile 147, 515
peroxyl radicals 279
pertussis vaccine 357
pesticides 349
petroleum 102, 391, 560
PGH_2 109
PGI_2 70, 102, 103, 108, 279, 285, 311, 312, 316, 320, 366, 404, 799, 801
pH paper 489
phaseolamin 294, 671
Phenelzine® 798
phenobarbitol 643
phenolics 102, 107, 118, 689
phenols 702
phenothiazines 134, 283, 334, 585, 680, 702
phenylalanine 127, 130, 136, 172, 182, 184, 185, 186, 195, 202, 251, 252, 278, 287, 288, 289, 290, 291, 295, 341, 342, 374, 481, 483, 509, 619, 620, 701, 736, 745, 746, 752, 799
phenylbutazone (Butazolidin®) 769
phenylpropanolamine 171, 251, 287, 289, 295, 497, 498, 799

phosphates 53, 76, 227, 371, 406, 676, 679, 689, 698, 764, 786, 789
phosphatidyl choline 126, 170, 187, 228
phosphatidyl inositol 216
phosphodiesterase inhibitor 683
phospholipids 448, 450, 478, 776
phosphorus 478, 776
Phylan 100® (phenylalanine) 619
physiological saline 238, 348
pigments 81, 97, 103, 112, 120, 121, 122, 123, 174, 175, 208, 212, 341, 420, 451, 639, 640, 648, 649, 692, 710, 750, 758, 770, 784, 788, 796
pineapple 87, 99, 163, 237, 384, 801
pituitary hormone 190, 484, 765
placebo effects 47, 762
placebos 47, 49, 249, 302, 405, 411, 514, 642, 647, 649, 725, 762, 791, 800
plaques 81, 82, 83, 107, 108, 129, 190, 241, 307, 308, 312, 314, 315, 316, 317, 318, 319, 320, 326, 366, 368, 373, 408, 474, 483, 674, 677, 785, 786, 796, 800
plasma 96, 97, 327, 403, 410, 634, 652, 662, 667, 680, 681, 683, 685, 687, 695, 800
plastics 81, 91, 92, 102, 206, 378, 387, 390, 391, 499, 551, 560
plutonium 253, 263, 384
poisons 52, 54, 102, 120, 244, 271, 337, 354, 375, 376, 383, 413, 479, 570, 631, 797
pollen 54, 253
pollutants 104, 144, 147, 247, 259, 260, 261, 263, 264, 265, 266, 332, 340, 408, 516
polonium 244, 264
polyamines 345, 640, 661, 662
polycyclic aromatic hydrocarbons (PAH) 337, 800
polynuclear aromatic hydrocarbons (PAH) 241, 243, 256, 264, 278, 324, 337, 364, 413, 479, 682, 792, 800
polyoxyethylene 219
polypeptides 76, 82, 131, 138, 180, 469, 766, 784, 785, 791, 792, 794, 796, 800
polysaccharide 297
polysorbate 219
polysorbate 60 (Tween-60®) 218, 219, 659
polysorbate 80 (Tween-80®) 218, 219, 220
polysorbates 220
polyunsaturated fats 104, 110, 111, 304, 308, 312, 338, 363, 366, 367, 368, 371, 471, 800, 802. See also lipids
polyunsaturated fatty acids (see lipids) 111, 175, 314, 637, 648, 686, 689, 690. See also lipids
polyunsaturated lipids 111, 642, 797
polyunsaturated oil 347, 492. See also lipids
pork, 368, 478
potassium 447, 448, 449, 777
potassium sorbate 382
potassium-40 264
potato chips 380, 478
potatoes 54, 102, 294
preservatives 52, 206, 371, 375, 376, 377, 382, 414, 551
preservatives may be preserving you 375
preservatives might just be preserving you 52
primary antioxidants 476, 800
PRL-8-53 180
pro-oxidant 140, 313, 370, 764, 790

pro-vitamin A. See beta carotene
procaine 184, 495, 651. See also GH-3, Gerovital®
progesterone (female sex hormone) 644
progestins (female sex hormones) 199, 236, 343, 478
prolactin 190, 202, 236, 339, 343, 471, 478, 634, 641, 662, 671, 680, 702, 766
promoters 345, 366, 477, 660
propionic acid 382
propranolol (Inderal®) 110, 328, 734, 735. See also beta blockers
propyl gallate 368, 369, 376, 379, 380, 381, 389
propylene glycol 380
propylparabens 382
prostacyclin (PGI₂) 70, 102, 103, 108, 109, 312, 320, 366, 404, 638, 642, 676, 678, 680, 683, 799, 801
prostacyclin synthetase 108, 109, 285
prostaglandins 314, 638, 642, 643, 680, 801
proteases 87, 801
protectants 264, 265, 404, 421, 502, 664, 670, 679, 694, 700
protective antioxidant 104, 764
protective antioxidant cholesterol 338
protective enzyme inducers 559
protective enzymes 147, 248, 378, 425, 515, 516, 520
protein bound iodine (PBI) 448, 452
protein-digesting enzymes 99
proteins 44, 73, 76, 78, 82, 87, 91, 92, 93, 95, 96, 98, 99, 101, 103, 104, 105, 121, 123, 146, 163, 174, 176, 180, 184, 209, 237, 242, 269, 291, 294, 297, 303, 312, 320, 336, 363, 364, 370, 377, 382, 384, 403, 471, 472, 474, 514, 702, 784, 785, 789, 790, 796, 798, 800, 801, 802
proteolytic enzymes 163, 216, 237, 384. See also bromelain, Ananase®, Papain
psychedelics 240, 426
psychochemicals 243, 426
PV (peroxide value) 381
pyridoxine (vitamin B-6) 643
pyridoxine HCl (vitamin B-6) 465, 469, 612
pyruvate 764
pyruvic acid 79, 227

quenchers 107, 110, 112, 422, 773, 802

rabbits 89, 145, 308, 312, 315, 320, 348, 474, 483, 674, 687, 760
radicals 103, 104, 118, 146, 279, 297, 298, 316, 348, 363, 470, 496, 638, 643, 748, 760, 795, 803
radioisotopes 705
radioprotectants 728, 729
radium 264, 705
radon 264, 705
rags 786, 787
rancid fats (lipids) 92, 101, 102, 285, 308, 332, 370, 386
rancid oil (lipids) 386
raw egg 217, 272
reaction-controlling enzymes 95
reagents 214, 349, 624
recreational drugs 256, 268, 269, 274, 275, 564

reduced glutathione (gamma-1-glutamyl-1-
cysteinylglycine, see glutathione) 304,
472, 481, 680, 764
releasers 218, 483
residues 123, 509, 662, 753
resins 165, 279, 792
respirable particles 264
retinoic acid. See vitamin A
retinoids 261, 265, 421, 647, 658, 667, 681,
694, 695, 699, 801. See also vitamin A
retinol 666, 684, 703. See also vitamin A
riboflavin (vitamin B-2) 465, 469, 612, 764
ribonucleic acid (RNA) 76, 168, 472, 802
ribose 76
Rimso-50® (50 percent DMSO in water) 298,
348
Ritalin® 168, 171, 172, 174, 180, 287
RNA (ribonucleic acid) 66, 76, 91, 92, 98, 101,
103, 106, 121, 168, 169, 170, 171, 277,
332, 422, 429, 430, 435, 450, 465, 466,
468, 472, 473, 477, 483, 613, 648, 698,
744, 785, 789, 802, 805
ROOH (organic hydroperoxide) 107
ROOR (organic peroxide) 107
rose bengal dye 518
rosemary 377
rubber 91, 92, 93, 95, 102, 163, 206, 243, 269,
316, 319, 387, 391, 560, 746, 790
rutin 409, 465, 469, 477, 483, 612, 676, 678,
698, 743, 758. See also bioflavonoids
rye 268
RyKrisp® 292

saccharin 374, 498, 499, 570, 595, 599
safflower oil 111, 175. See also
polyunsaturated oils and lipids
sage 377, 493
salad 218, 379, 382
salmon 137, 140, 141, 644, 657, 786
salts 5, 260, 292, 298, 345, 347, 348, 410, 466,
473, 475, 484, 647, 658, 756, 763, 769
Santoquin® (ethoxyquin, 6-ethoxy-1-2-
dihydro-2-2-4-trimethylquinoline) 112,
113, 116, 117, 636, 689
saturated fats (lipids) 44, 110, 111, 338, 363,
366, 371, 802
sausage 369, 478
scavengers 106, 238, 298, 347, 348, 483, 742,
760
scopolamine 170, 642, 647, 649
seafoods 314
second messenger 176
secondary antioxidants 476, 802
sedatives 133, 193, 258, 269, 575, 754
seeds 44, 54, 137, 403, 636, 689, 692
selenite (a form of selenium, see sodium
selenite) 634, 666, 671, 672, 681, 685,
699, 702, 704
selenium 78, 82, 86, 88, 89, 93, 99, 102, 104,
107, 110, 112, 133, 135, 144, 162, 163,
165, 175, 196, 241, 242, 245, 247, 250,
252, 263, 264, 273, 280, 298, 300, 308,
314, 315, 318, 320, 324, 332, 333, 338,
341, 347, 348, 367, 371, 406, 415, 421,
465, 468, 471, 462, 483, 559, 612, 633,
634, 663, 664, 666, 671, 672, 681, 682,
683, 685, 698, 699, 702, 703, 704, 737,
740, 743, 758, 768, 785, 800

selenium sulfide 220, 758
selenized yeast 666, 671, 685, 704
seleno amino acids 242, 333, 666, 671, 685,
704
selenocysteine 471
selenocystine 242, 333
selenomethionine 242, 333, 666, 671, 685,
702, 704
Selsun Blue® (selenium sulfide shampoo) 220,
472, 758
semi-synthetic diet 112
serotonin (5-HT, 5-hydroxytryptamine) 130,
131, 134, 135, 179, 184, 192, 291, 796,
797, 798, 802
serum alkaline phosphatase 451
serum amylase 451
serum bilirubin 451
serum glutamic oxaloacetic transaminase
(SGOT) 447, 448, 452, 479, 776, 777
serum glutamic pyruvic transaminase (SGPT)
447, 448, 452, 479, 776
sewage 356
SGOT. See serum glutamic oxaloacetic
transaminase
SGPT. See serum glutamic pyruvic
transaminase
SH (sulfhydryl group) 263, 293
shampoos 218, 219, 220, 472, 758
shellfish 97, 422
shortening 388
sidestream smoke 252
silicon 722, 723
silicone 436
silicone antifoam 489
silver 205
Simethicone® (see silicone antifoam) 436, 489
singlet oxygen 260, 261, 263, 279, 304, 422,
423, 456, 518, 667, 773, 802, 804
slow-reacting substances 673
smog 92, 96, 162, 242, 244, 248, 250, 253,
261, 265, 340, 364, 385, 402, 404, 475,
481, 515, 783, 784
smoke 91, 92, 96, 162, 202, 209, 239, 240,
241, 242, 244, 247, 248, 249, 250, 252,
253, 254, 257, 258, 261, 263, 265, 266,
279, 314, 337, 339, 340, 350, 364, 369,
378, 385, 392, 404, 406, 413, 475, 481,
482, 664, 665, 666, 667, 684, 703, 706,
783, 784, 800
snacks 371, 398, 691
snuff 241, 256
soap 765
SOD. See superoxide dismutase
soda 374
sodium ascorbate (vitamin C) 247, 261, 345,
369, 377, 415, 462, 475, 488
sodium benzoate 382
sodium bicarbonate (baking soda) 249, 415,
488
sodium bisulfite 495
sodium hydrogen urate 103, 430, 805
sodium salicylate 748, 749
sodium salt of 2-pyrrolidone-5-carboxylic acid
(Na-PCA) 53, 163, 210, 741
sodium selenite (a form of selenium, see
selenite) 242, 245, 333, 465, 468, 471,
472, 612, 702, 737, 743, 750, 758
soft water 96, 260, 315

soil 332
solanine 54
solvent 214, 215, 220, 348, 349, 624, 714, 791
somatotropin (GH, growth hormone) 480, 481
sorbic acid 382
sorbitol 373, 477
soy 305, 485, 619, 621
soybean oil (see polyunsaturated oil, lipid) 381
spaghetti 294
sperm 139, 142, 147, 197
spices 163, 375, 377, 378, 689
spinach 334
sputum 449
stabilizers 177, 502
stainless steel 80
starches 44, 52, 77, 291, 294, 305, 375, 451, 485, 619, 672
steak 314, 369
stearates 660
steroids 196, 197, 200, 367, 623, 659
stimulants 88, 129, 139, 162, 171, 172, 174, 188, 197, 223, 276, 286, 287, 289, 291, 292, 304, 315, 341, 384, 411, 483, 575, 641, 650, 736
stimulatory neurotransmitters 802
stimulus barriers 240, 243, 250, 269, 274, 803
strychnine 168
succinic acid 79, 227
succinyl CoA 79
sucrose 315, 372, 373, 476
sugars 47, 71, 76, 77, 216, 246, 291, 298, 315, 370, 371, 372, 373, 374, 409, 411, 416, 442, 446, 451, 467, 476, 482, 498, 503, 520, 571, 595, 675, 688, 689, 760
sulfa (sulfa drugs) 248, 469, 474, 714
sulfanilamide (sulfa drug) 714
sulfation 366
sulfhydryl 87, 95, 244, 263, 293, 701, 803
sulfhydryl compounds 414, 483, 664, 670, 679, 694, 700, 803, 804
sulfhydryl group 95, 803
sulfinpyrazone (Anturane®) 328, 679, 717, 769
sulfoxide free radical 348, 298
sulfoxides 348
sulfur 95, 98, 107, 242, 327, 333, 385, 471, 483, 494, 668, 677, 789, 790, 803
sulfur-containing amino acids 471
sulfur-hydrogen bonds 95
sunblocks 92, 263, 474, 743, 761
sunscreens 209
superoxide dismutase (SOD) 78, 101, 104, 105, 106, 111, 119, 142, 146, 147, 175, 279, 280, 297, 298, 470, 496, 516, 518, 520, 645, 673, 748, 799, 803
superoxide radical 638, 673, 748, 803
suppository 201
suppressants 88, 263, 308, 323, 338, 339, 377, 497, 498
suppressors 303, 366, 573, 762
surfactants 218, 219, 478, 776
sweat 232, 241, 264, 472
sweeteners 570
synergists 381, 414, 416, 475, 483
synthetic vitamins 52, 53, 55
synethetics 374, 377, 389, 490
syrup 621

T-3 448
T-4 448
Talwin® 349
tars 241, 252, 253, 254, 255, 261, 279, 336, 339, 341, 563, 564
TBHQ (tert-butyl hydroquinone, monotertiary butyl hydroquinone, 2-tertiary butylhydroquinone) 368, 369, 376, 379, 380, 381, 389
TDPA (thiodipropionic acid) 381
tea 178, 188, 276, 292, 304
tears 515
teeth 8, 149, 371, 615
Tenox® (BHT or BHA) 379, 380, 381
Tenox 6® (antioxidant mixture) 380
Tenox 7® (antioxidant mixture) 380
Tenox S-1® (antioxidant mixture) 380
Test-Estrin® (androgen-estrogen preparation) 201
testosterone (male sex hormones) 138, 139, 196, 197, 199, 201, 213, 214, 659, 660, 765, 774, 795
testosterone 5-alpha reductase 139, 213
testosterone cypionate (male sex hormone) 197, 199, 200, 201, 214, 215
testosterone-producing cells 139
testosterone propionate (male sex hormone) 214, 215
tetracycline 350
tetrahydropteridines 297. See also folate
thalidomide 567, 571, 579, 583, 585, 589, 590
theobromine 292
theophylline 188, 276, 292, 304
thiamine (vitamin B-1) 87, 465, 466, 469, 475, 612, 804
thiodipropionates 298, 483, 702
thiodipropionic acid (TDPA) 381, 465, 476, 483, 612, 802
thiols 87, 297, 804
Thorazine® 283
thorium 264, 705
thromboxane synthetase 109
thromboxanes 108, 109, 314, 638, 642, 680
thymine 76
thymosin 86, 89, 278, 303, 305, 336, 565, 566, 634, 682, 715
thyroid 73, 236, 288, 323, 343, 452, 478, 613, 767
thyroid hormone 73, 141, 142, 323, 767
thyroid stimulating hormone (TSH) 236, 323, 343, 448, 478, 799
thyrotropin 323
thyroxine (a thyroid hormone) 142
Tice strain (BCG, Chicago BCG) 343
tin 241
tissue-dissolving enzymes 121, 797
titanium 96
toast 121, 382
tobacco 144, 209, 239, 240, 241, 243, 250, 252, 253, 255, 256, 264, 266, 275, 279, 337, 339, 479, 487, 563, 564, 571, 664, 665, 667, 706, 800
tocopherols 381, 407, 462, 491, 637, 673, 690, 692, 700. See also vitamin E
tocopheryl acetate 406. See also vitamin E
tomatoes 422
tonics 274, 479
topical hormones 200, 219, 220

total cholesterol 325, 45
total fatty acids 448
total lipids 448, 450, 478
total serum cholesterol 367, 368, 424
toxins 334, 354, 383, 411, 631, 797
trace elements 338, 679
tranquilizers 269, 282, 426, 585, 803
transmitters 169, 198, 783
Tranylcypromine® 798
TRF 236, 323, 343, 478
TRH 678
triamino acid 102, 107
tricarboxylic acid cycle 789
triglycerides 279, 324, 325, 373, 424, 425,
    434, 448, 450, 484, 680, 687, 688, 695,
    696, 751, 776, 777, 778, 804
trimethylamine 164
tripeptide 168, 180, 764
triplet oxygen 770, 771, 787, 804
trypsin 87, 89
tryptophan 131, 135, 179, 191, 192, 194, 289,
    291, 465, 468, 483, 509, 613, 622, 802
TSH. See thyroid stimulating hormone
tuna 263, 503
turkey 240
turnips 334
Tween® 660. See also polysorbate
tyrosine 102, 107, 127, 130, 172, 182, 184,
    186, 202, 291, 341, 342, 481, 509, 651

unpaired electrons 83, 102, 106, 107, 118,
    265, 297, 376, 403, 793, 804
unsaturated fats (lipids) 96, 103, 116, 121,
    279, 740, 742, 799
uranium 266, 705
urates 170, 430, 447, 448, 449, 466, 468, 473,
    769, 770. See also uric acid
urea 451
uric acid 103, 169, 170, 324, 415, 430, 435,
    447, 448, 449, 450, 466, 468, 473, 487,
    769, 776, 805
urine 128, 129, 173, 190, 204, 244, 246, 247,
    249, 256, 313, 315, 390, 391, 409, 416,
    446, 447, 449, 450, 451, 453, 464, 467,
    472, 487, 489, 621, 675, 688, 689, 762,
    763
usquebaugh 268

vaccines 308, 340, 730
Valium® 193, 282, 426, 477, 754, 755
Valium®-like nutrients 282
vanilla 377
vapors 377, 562
varnish 298
vasoconstrictors 425
vasodilators 425, 659
vasopressin (ADH, antidiuretic hormone,
    Diapid®) 128, 129, 164, 168, 173, 174,
    190, 194, 204, 228, 229, 276, 277, 288,
    320, 439, 465, 469, 483, 484, 509, 613,
    642, 647, 649, 670, 677, 701, 745, 762,
    763, 795, 799
vegetables 110, 334, 366, 368, 371, 376, 377,
    378, 379, 381, 666, 684, 703
velvet beans. See L-DOPA
very low density lipoproteins (VLDL) 327,
    424, 425, 463, 778
vinegar 270, 388

vinyl 300, 560
Viskane® 328
vitamin A 82, 87, 97, 112, 151, 165, 210, 245,
    247, 261, 264, 280, 298, 305, 313, 419,
    420, 421, 422, 465, 468, 470, 476, 483,
    485, 492, 540, 612, 633, 664, 665, 666,
    667, 680, 681, 684, 694, 695, 698, 699,
    703, 742, 746, 747, 756, 758, 762, 801,
    802
vitamin A acetate 492
vitamin A palmitate 492
vitamin B-1 (B-1 thiamine) 87, 92, 243, 245,
    272, 274, 280, 341, 415, 465, 469, 475,
    483, 612, 665, 696, 803, 804
vitamin B-2 (B-2, riboflavin) 245, 246, 248,
    280, 297, 304, 390, 464, 465, 469, 472,
    483, 612, 742, 758, 763, 764
vitamin B-3 (B-3, niacin, niacinamide,
    nicotinamide) 193, 218, 243, 245, 279,
    280, 282, 347, 365, 424, 434, 463, 465,
    467, 477, 483, 487, 612, 672, 696, 742,
    758, 798
vitamin B-5 (B-5, calcium pantothenate,
    pantothenate, pantothenic acid) 24, 31,
    51, 54, 165, 170, 187, 204, 210, 227, 228,
    245, 247, 274, 280, 291, 414, 430, 465,
    469, 479, 612, 742, 758, 789
vitamin B-6 (B-6, pyridoxine) 134, 205, 245,
    247, 280, 291, 299, 300, 312, 313, 314,
    431, 432, 465, 469, 474, 475, 483, 532,
    612, 632, 742, 754, 758
vitamin B-12 (cyanocobalamin) 78, 168, 170,
    277, 280, 465, 468, 473, 477, 483, 612,
    648, 758
vitamin C (C, ascorbate, ascorbic acid, sodium
    ascorbate, calcium ascorbate, mineral
    ascorbates) 14, 30, 31, 52, 53, 54, 55, 78,
    82, 88, 89, 92, 96, 111, 133, 135, 172,
    217, 243, 244, 245, 247, 249, 261, 263,
    272, 278, 280, 293, 298, 300, 304, 313,
    314, 315, 326, 327, 331, 334, 335, 336,
    341, 345, 347, 358, 360, 365, 381, 382,
    384, 390, 391, 393, 398, 399, 408, 409,
    410, 411, 412, 413, 414, 415, 416, 417,
    418, 429, 430, 431, 435, 436, 442, 443,
    446, 447, 453, 459, 462, 464, 465, 467,
    469, 470, 474, 475, 476, 477, 480, 482,
    483, 487, 488, 491, 531, 532, 536, 566,
    569, 599, 602, 611, 612, 620, 621, 634,
    663, 665, 673, 674, 675, 676, 679, 681,
    686, 687, 691, 693, 694, 696, 699, 701,
    727, 735, 740, 742, 743, 746, 749, 756,
    758, 762, 790, 795, 798
vitamin C content of your urine test 390
vitamin C pumps 111, 413, 639, 740
vitamin E (E, see alpha tocopherol, d-alpha
    tocopherol, dl-alpha tocopherol,
    tocopherols, and their acetates and other
    esters) 28, 31, 54, 55, 78, 82, 86, 101,
    106, 108, 110, 112, 114, 115, 116, 122,
    245, 263, 265, 280, 299, 327, 328, 347,
    371, 377, 393, 402, 403, 404, 405, 406,
    407, 410, 414, 465, 470, 471, 483, 491,
    518, 532, 611, 634, 636, 637, 638, 639,
    668, 673, 674, 676, 678, 679, 682, 691,
    692, 698, 699, 700, 727, 743, 747, 748,
    749, 750, 757, 758, 762, 768, 788, 794,
    797, 799

vitamin E acetate 86, 111, 112, 404, 405, 406, 407, 462, 468, 491
vitamin E esters 407, 462, 491, 492
vitamin E oil 347
vitamin E succinate 491
VLDL (very low density lipoprotein) 327, 424, 425, 448, 463, 688, 696, 777, 778, 780

warmed-over flavor 377, 689
wastes 120, 121, 211, 639
water-soluble antioxidant 247
water-soluble vitamins 369, 390, 464
wheat 55, 403, 407
whiskey 267, 268
whole-wheat bread 54
WI-38 137, 138
wine 97, 268, 272, 608

xanthine oxidase 103, 170, 769, 770, 805

xylitol 373, 498, 499
xylulose 416

yeast 242, 305, 333, 472, 473, 485, 619, 666, 671, 685, 701, 703, 704, 737
yogurt 164
yolk 702

zeaxanthin 53
zinc 78, 82, 86, 87, 89, 93, 102, 104, 110, 111, 112, 133, 135, 162, 163, 165, 175, 196, 241, 247, 250, 252, 264, 273, 280, 297, 298, 300, 308, 314, 315, 318, 320, 324, 332, 338, 345, 347, 348, 367, 371, 419, 420, 421, 465, 468, 470, 471, 483, 612, 643, 668, 698, 699, 740, 749, 756, 785, 800, 803
zinc gluconate 245
zinc pyrithione 220, 758
Zyloprim® 769

Index To Names:
Persons, Organizations, And Places

Abbott 168
Abkhasia villagers 615
ACS (American Chemical Society) 349, 667, 689
Adams 633, 644, 660, 709
Adelman 71, 72, 430, 632, 646, 697, 699
AEC (see Atomic Energy Commission)
AEI, Automated Equipment Inc. 625
Africa 570, 677
Ajinomoto Company, Inc. 622, 647, 658
Alabama 104, 146
Albers 706
Alchian, Arnen A. 718
Alcor Society for Solid State Hypothermia 720
Aldridge 644, 660
Alfin-Slater, Dr. 364, 680, 687
Alice in Wonderland 8, 23, 493
Allison 534
Almquist 639
Alpaire, Inc. 624, 666, 669
Altura 677
Alvares 681
Alzheimer's disease 129
AMA (see American Medical Association)
AMA Council on Drugs (see American Medical Association)
Amar, Inc. 446
Ambrose 676, 678, 698
American Aging Association (AGE) 535, 552, 621, 638
American Heart Association 329, 363, 366
American Chemical Society 349, 667, 689
American Oil Chemists Society (AOCS) 627
American Medical Association (AMA) 438, 588; Council On Drugs 582, 586
Ames, Bruce 339, 390, 446
Aminco® 640
Anastasi 638, 676, 678, 691, 699
Anderson 633, 648, 681, 693, 699, 709, 711, 718
Angeletti 641
Anisman 651
AOM (Active Oxygen Method) 378
Anthony Dowell 509, 653
Apollo 653
arctic 420
Aristotle 531
Armstrong, Dr. 104
Aslan, Dr. Ana 184, 495
Asmundson 644
Atlas ICI 218
Atomic Energy Commission (AEC) 560
Austin 669
Axelrod 650

Bacchi 643
Bacchus 653
Bach 673
Bacon, Francis 239, 437
Bada 721
Bahr 653
Bailey 674, 678, 692
Baldessarini 657
Baltimore Longitudinal Study Of Aging (BLSA) 223, 229, 661
Bamji, M.S. 764
Bangladesh 705
Banic 694
Banning 705
Barbul 633, 662, 671, 685, 700
Barnes, Dr. Broda 322, 323, 678, 679, 721, 767
Barrett 709
Barrington 656
Bartus 641
Baryshnikov, Mikhail 93, 509, 653
BASF Wyandotte 623
Basle 648, 681, 702
Bassett, Dr. 148, 150, 152, 645, 646
Basu 667, 681, 695
BATF (Bureau of Alcohol, Tobacco, and Firearms) 563, 564
Batta 706
Battig 665
Baum, Frank 554
Bazan, Dr. Nicholas 642
Beck, Dr. 140, 644
Becker, Dr. 150, 151, 152, 645, 646
Beckmann 708
Beeson 631
Bekey 711
Beller 671
Bellows 635
Benassi, Victor A. 46, 631
Bendat 711
Bender 540, 637, 647, 701
Benditt, Dr. Earl 307, 534, 674, 677
Bengal 518
Benolken 642, 648
Benowicz 532
Berde 640
Bergstrom 676, 678
Berkow 538
Bernard, Claude 91
Berntson 664
Berrios 642, 650, 662, 701
Beutler, E. 764
Bharadwaj, Dr. 140, 644
Biggert 702
Birmingham, Alabama, 104, 106

Bjelke 633, 664, 667, 680, 695
Bjorksten, Johan 98, 99, 115, 242, 332, 635, 674, 675, 677, 693
BLSA *See* Baltimore Longitudinal Study Of Aging
Blue Ridge Mountains Of Virginia 260–261
BNND (Bureau of Narcotics and Dangerous Drugs) 715
Boardman 653
Bodanszky 642
Bologna 653
Borek 629, 645
Borgeat 673
Borison 649, 651, 670, 672, 701
Bortz 679, 687
Bose 709
Bourne, Dr. G.H. 123, 412, 640, 649, 694
Bova, Ben 535
Bowie, David (rock musician) 653
Boyd 641, 652, 661, 662, 698
Bracco 639, 690
Brain Information Service 640, 652
Brandeis, Louis 717
Branen 653, 687, 689
Braughler 638
Braun 681
Bray 717
Brecher 653, 716
Bresler, Dr. David 326
Breslow 693
Briggs 696
Bristol-Myers Company 151
Britton 632, 697
Brizzee, Dr. Kenneth R. 122
Brody, H. 122, 639, 648
Bronowski 708
Bronson Pharmaceuticals 620
Brookings Institution 718, 720
Brozen, Dr. Yale 578
Bryan 631
Bucher 717
Buckley 695, 702
Bueding, Dr. Ernest 685
Buell 711
Bullworker® 233
Bureau of Alcohol, Tobacco, And Firearms (BATF) 563, 564
Bureau of Narcotics and Dangerous Drugs 715
Burgus 534, 641
Burkitt's Lymphoma 206, 308, 333
Burnet 534, 633, 682
Burroughs-Wellcome 769
Bussgang 711
Butler, Robert 557
Bylinsky 648, 653

Cadoret 669
Calabresi, Dr. Guido 569
California 104, 147, 173, 179, 224, 298, 348, 403, 449, 573, 640, 652, 657, 672, 709, 711, 756, 777
Calissano 648
Camanni 662
Cameron, Ewan 335, 411, 531, 633, 663, 681, 682, 693, 694
Campbell 633, 683
Canada 97, 98, 211, 256, 329, 332, 340, 357, 358, 405, 422, 596, 620, 623, 624, 635

Caproni AJ-21 527
Carrel, Alexis 30, 67, 81, 543
Carroll, Lewis 8, 23, 493
Carter 653
Cathcart, Dr. Robert F. 412
Catt 633, 662
Caucasus 65, 148
CEP (Council on Economic Priorities) 561
Cessna 185, 527
Chan 637, 668, 683
Chandrashekar 711
Chapman 661
Charman 663, 695, 700
Chemetics 702
Chemical Dynamics® Corp 622
Chicago BCG 343
Chieffi 635
Chio, Dr. 121
Chope 693
Chvapil 668, 698
Ciba-Geigy® 168, 171, 328, 673
Cicero 70
Cicone 683
Clark, Kenneth 653
Clark, Ronald W. 504
Clarke, Arthur C. 208
Cleveland, Ohio 104, 147, 561
Cline, Dr. Martin J. 21, 506
Cohen 646, 667
Coker 638, 680
Collier 403
Comfort 636, 647
Commodore® computer 675, 688
Comtel Imaging Systems® 527
Condorcet, Antoine Nicholas Marquis de 614
Cone, Dr. Clarence 152, 518, 646
Congress 39, 41, 398, 400, 508, 558, 562, 563, 564, 567, 569, 570, 571, 577, 578, 590, 594, 595, 596, 714
Consumer Product Safety Commission (CPSC) 561
Consumers Union® 563, 595, 715, 716
Cort 637, 673, 690, 692, 700
Cott 643
Cotzias, Dr. George C. 134, 479, 641, 699
Council On Economic Priorities (CEP) 561
Cox 631, 708
CPSC (see Consumer Product Safety Commission)
Cranston 716
Crick, Francis 505, 534, 550, 632
Criley, Dr. J. Michael 352
Cristofalo 646, 699
Crout, J. Richard 587
Crowell 678, 721
Cumming 709
Cutler, Dr. Richard 20, 106, 629, 645, 647

Darwin, Charles 189, 718
David McKay Co. 629, 721
Davidson 534
Davignon 683, 686
da Vinci, Leonardo 367, 487, 493, 505, 653, 675
Davis 403
Dawkins, Richard 19, 630, 718
Dean, Kris, 731, 732, 733
Dean, Sandy 444

Debono 631, 643, 656
Deitrich 670
Deitz 667
Del Maestro 639
Delaney 705
Delaney amendment 570, 571, 704, 705
Demartino 656
Dement 652
Demopoulos, Dr. Harry 100, 119, 135, 273,
    275, 299, 318, 319, 338, 348, 354, 367,
    406, 519, 638, 667, 668, 681, 683
Demsetz, Dr. Harold 716
Denckla, Dr. W. Donner 73, 98, 141, 142,
    632, 644
Department Of Energy (DOE) 560
Department Of Health, Education, and
    Welfare (DHEW) 357, 393, 398, 501, 686,
    706
Department Of Health And Human Services
    357
Descartes 167
Detroit, Michigan 104, 146, 561
Deusen 659
Devo (rock group) 718
Deyl 635
Di Luzio 668
Diaz 669
Dicke 524
Dietrich 643
Dillard 692
Disney, Walt 708
Division Of Cancer And Prevention, National
    Cancer Institute 563
Dixon 630
Djerassi 656
DOE (see Department of Energy)
Dohme Research Laboratories 538
Doll 695, 702
Donatello 653
Donne, John 41
Donsbach, Dr. Kurt 763
Doors, The (rock group) 653
Dow Chemical Co. 256
Dowell, Anthony, 509, 653
Down's syndrome 20
Doyle, Margot 565
Drachman 641, 647, 649
Du Mez 715
DuPont Corporation 561, 562, 631
Dube 659
Dubos, Rene J. 424
Dumm 647, 657, 662, 686
Dunhill Scale 286
Dunlop, Sir Derrick 572
Dykstra 641, 648, 652, 657

Eastman Chemical Products, Inc. 379, 622
Eastman Kodak 706
Echternacht 660
Ecuador 65, 615, 632, 721
Eddy 115, 636, 639
Egyptian 263, 268
Ehrlich ascites tumor 242, 333, 633, 682
Ehrman 711
Einstein, Albert 56, 402, 419, 504, 550, 551
Elden 659
Elliot 720
Elliott, Ebenezer 125

Ellis, Dr. John M. 299, 300, 302, 532, 643,
    697
Emmenegger 641, 650, 676
Enesco 648
England 329, 628, 648, 677, 679, 681, 702,
    717
Environmental Protection Agency (EPA) 252,
    259, 260, 264, 266, 561
Epson MX-80® 625, 724
Ermini, Dr. Marco 536
Eros 653, 656
Eskimos 44, 313, 314
Ettinger, R.C.W. 34, 720
Europe 123, 175, 177, 257, 275, 276, 322,
    328, 339, 572, 577, 596, 760, 766
Evans 702

Faber 675, 688
Fabricant 676
Faden 686
Falzone 647
Faraday, Michael 30
Farrant 720
Farrar 671
FASEB. see Federation Of American Societies
    For Experimental Biology
Fausto 646
FDA (Food And Drug Administration) 4, 5, 7,
    14, 40, 41, 86, 89, 98, 99, 124, 148, 150,
    152, 173, 174, 176, 180, 218, 219, 221,
    242, 255, 256, 257, 258, 261, 273, 274,
    275, 278, 281, 290, 294, 298, 305, 328,
    332, 336, 340, 343, 348, 349, 350, 352,
    368, 374, 376, 384, 392, 393, 394, 395,
    396, 397, 398, 399, 400, 416, 417, 422,
    438, 439, 469, 476, 479, 497, 501, 502,
    503, 514, 539, 555, 558, 564, 565, 566,
    567, 569, 570, 571, 572, 573, 574, 575,
    576, 577, 578, 581, 582, 583, 584, 587,
    588, 589, 590, 591, 592, 593, 594, 595,
    596, 599, 601, 602, 605, 607, 635, 677,
    690, 691, 704, 706, 707, 713, 714, 716,
    720, 730, 734, 744, 748, 760
federal 337, 400, 563, 574, 580, 591, 714
Federal Trade Commission (FTC) 41, 255,
    497
Federation of American Societies for
    Experimental Biology (FASEB) 634, 636,
    649, 651, 670, 674, 682, 687, 700, 701
Feigan, Dr. 410
Feinleib 679
Fender, Dr. Derek 522, 709
Fenoglio 629, 645
Fernstrom 534, 641, 649, 663
Ferris 649
Finch 641, 646, 649, 699
Finnie 711
Fisher 631, 674, 676, 678, 697
Flamm 638, 639, 683
Food And Drug Administration. See FDA
Forbes 776
Foreyt, John Paul 293, 672
Forman 632, 721
Fortune® 717
Foundation For Experimental Ageing
    Research 536
Framingham study 324, 679, 687
France 127, 177, 194, 272

Frankenstein 36
Franklin, Benjamin 14, 75, 608
Franklyn 681, 701
Freas, Kelly 747
French Guiana 240, 664
Freudenthal 682
Fridovich 637
Friedman, David 129, 533, 715, 717
Friedman, Milton, 533, 558, 577, 716
Friedman, Rose 716
Froeb, Dr. Herman F. 252
FTC (see Federal Trade Commission)
Fund For Integrative Biomedical Research
    (FIBER) 536

Galapagos 616
Galileo 572
Galton 678, 721
Gamow, George 550
Gardner 473, 701
Gebhard 656, 721
Gee 634, 636, 664, 667, 700
Geist 657
Gelenberg 651
Genazzani 656
General Foods 632, 689
General Mills 399
General Motors 27
Genetech 662
Georgieff 636, 682
Germany 296, 336, 337, 550, 585
Gibbs, Dr. James G., Jr. 287, 290, 672
Gilliland 718
Gillin 642, 647, 649
Gilman, A., 327, 688, 695–696, 777
Ginter 679, 687, 694, 701
Giroux 671
Gitler 702
Glogar 686
Glomset 675, 677
Goetzl 633, 694
Goldstein, Dr. Allan L. 89, 336, 634, 640, 663,
    667, 668, 680, 682, 687, 689, 692, 698, 700
Goldstick 674
Gompertz, Benjamin 9
Gompertz Law 9, 70, 794
Goodman, L.S. 327, 474, 537, 650, 656, 687,
    688, 695–696, 719, 764, 777
Gordon 679, 687
Gori, Dr. Gio B. 563, 706
Gould, Leonard A. 712
Goyan, Jere E. 593, 594, 691, 716
Graham, J.W. 711
Grant, Richard, 717
Grant, M. 656
Great Smoky Mountains 261
Greece 653
Greeder 633, 682
Greengard 650
Greenland 314
Gregory 632
Griffin, Merv, 516, 537, 736
Gross 661, 662, 671
Growdon 652
Gruberg, Edward 474, 674, 676, 678, 687
Guillemin 534, 641
Gunther 666, 671, 685, 704
Gutman 668, 683

Hagen, Lynn 625
Halliday, Dr. 138
Hambrugh 656
Hamby 679
Hamilton 659
Hamlet 95, 96
Hanawalt 534
Hanna 673
Hansen 672
Happle 660
Harang, Dr. Hunter 305, 306, 485
Harman, Dr. Denham 100, 103, 108, 110,
    115, 122, 535, 636, 637, 638, 639, 645,
    648, 650, 668, 689, 690, 692, 700, 701,
    702, 751
Harris poll 720
Harrison Anti-Narcotics Act 713–714
Hart, Ronald W. 146, 645
Hawkins 656, 695, 698
Hawthorne (effect) 510, 537, 623, 658
Hayashi 689
Hayek, Friedrich A. 717
Hayflick, Dr. Leonard 137, 138, 152, 534,
    644, 646, 699
Haynes 534
Hayward 625
Hazum 643
Heath 286
Heathkit® 731
Heetderks 712
Heisenberg, Werner 504
Heitkamp 665, 696
Helm 487
Henn, Frank 675, 688
Herophilus 356
Hershey, Daniel 645
HEW. See Department of Health, Education,
    and Welfare
HHS. See Department of Health and Human
    Services
Hicks 631, 708
Hilton 685, 695
Hindmarch 648, 664, 667, 676, 699
Hirsch, Dr. Gerald P. 19, 630, 649
Hirshleifer, Jack 630, 721
Hochschild 673, 700
Hodge 689
Hodgkin's disease 730
Hoekstra 637
Hoffer, Eric 631
Hoffmann-La Roche 193, 305, 566, 622, 744
Hofmann, Dr. Albert 650–651, 718, 733
Hollaender 534
Holmes, Oliver Wendell, Sr. 143
Holmes, Sherlock 153, 531, 707
Honeywell 625, 666, 669
Honn 683
Hoover 537, 544
Hoover Institution, the 691
Huang 644
Hughes, Howard 294
Hume 674, 678, 693
Hunzas 65, 615

IBM 723
ICI 659
ICN 168
India 656

414

Indians 261, 268, 271, 272, 616, 653
Indostan 63, 64
Institute Of Electrical And Electronic
    Engineers 646, 711, 712, 717
Irish people 271, 405
IRS (Internal Revenue Service) 536
Israel 336
Italians 177
Italy 272, 677

Jacobs 686
Janker Clinic 336, 337
Japan 110, 252, 263, 351, 376
Japanese 180, 325
Jeanes 689
Jefferson Airplane (rock group) 344, 375
Jerne 634
Jetten 647, 658, 694
Johns Hopkins 566, 657, 685, 721
Johnson, 640, 644, 661
Johnson, Samuel 539
Johnson, V.E. 204, 282, 656
Jondrow 587
Jones, Marvin L. 616, 721

Kabara 639, 702
Kalaba, R. 711
Kalokerinos, Dr. A. 621, 686
Kantner, Paul, 344
Kappas 681
Karel 638, 690
Kashmir people 65, 615
Katzenelson, Jacob 712
Kavanau, J.L. 181
Kefauver Amendments 98, 578, 580, 581,
    588, 704, 705, 714
Keith 409, 632, 693, 702
Kellogg 399, 635
Kelner 712
Kennedy, John F. 398, 400
Kent, Saul 532
Kesavan, H.K. 711
Khandwala 634, 636, 664, 667, 700
Kielholz 721
Kiev 652
King, Billie Jean 629, 645, 653
Kinsey 656, 721, 765
Kirk 632, 635
Kirkwood, Thomas 19, 630
Kiss (rock group) 653
Kitamura 667, 673
Klayman 666, 671, 685, 704
Klein 697
Klenner 693
Kodak 494, 706
Koestler, Arthur 363
Kohn 644
Kolata, G. 719
Kolb 715
Kontos 638, 643
Koo 325, 679
Koppers Co., Inc. 690
Kormendy 540, 637, 647, 701
Kornbrust 691
Korsakoff's psychosis 220, 221, 273, 276, 669
Kovanen 680, 687
Kraft Foods 503
Krebs (citric acid) cycle 79, 187, 227, 475, 479

Kristensen 679
Kugler 532
Kyros Vitamin Bill 400, 401

Laden 632, 647, 659
Lakein, Alan 13, 553
Lal, Kannar 656
Lancaster, Don 553
Landau, Dr. R.L. 565, 566, 569, 573, 580, 716
Lane 620
LaPlace, Pierre Simon 302
Larner 689
Larocca 653
Lasagna, Dr. Louis 565, 566
Lasalle 720
Lasker 108
Latshaw 782
Lauda 671
Laughlin 674, 676, 678, 697
Lave, L.B. 720
Lavins, L.S. 646
Lawrence, T.E. 37, 224
Leaf, Dr. Alexander 42, 554, 556
Leake 662, 673, 686
Leavitt 641, 647, 649
Ledingham 638
Lee, Y.W. 708, 711
Legros 642, 647, 649, 670, 677, 701
Lehninger 632
Lentz 668
Levenson 684
Levi-Montalcini 641, 648
Levine 672, 689
Levy, D.D. 646
Lewes, George Henry 504
Lewin, Sherry 693, 699
Leydig cells 138, 221
Lichstein 679
Lieber 669
Lieberman 667
Lions 616
Lipson, E.D. 712
Litton 492
Loliger 639, 690
Loompanics Unlimited 631, 718
Los Angeles (LA) 36, 104, 146, 224, 261, 454,
    515, 527, 537, 561, 620, 640, 652, 666,
    671, 672, 675, 685, 688, 704, 721, 724
Lowery, Alfred H. 706
Lowrey 252, 665, 667
Luce, Gay Gaer 644
Lundberg 377, 636, 689
Lundgren, Dr. 640, 644, 777
Lysenko 572

Maass, J.A. 646
Macfarlane 651
Mack Publishing Co. 537, 541, 544
Maeda 678
Mahley, Dr. Robert W. 687, 695–696, 777
Mackinodan, Dr. Takashi 89
Malitz 656
Maniatis, Tom 76
Mann, Dr. D.M.A. 121, 532, 639, 649
Manne 718
Marek's disease 208
Marmarelis, P.Z. 711, 712
Marryat, Frederic 268

Mars 704
Marshal, Elliot 720
Marx, Jean L. 433, 634, 683
Marx brothers, 433
Massachusetts Institute Of Technology (MIT) 126, 138, 164, 170, 251, 474, 511, 512, 709, 711, 728, 751, 768
Massey 630
Mathews-Roth, Micheline M. 744
Mattick 636, 689, 692
Maugh, 664, 680, 695, 690
Maugham, Somerset 15
Mavis 691
Maxim, M. 646
Mayo Clinic 325, 335
Mazess 632, 721
McCord, Dr. Joe M. 297–298, 638, 673
McCoy 631
McCully, Dr. Kilmer 313–314, 674, 676, 678
McDaniels, Allen 720
McDermott 631
McGinness 666, 671, 685, 703
McGoohan, Patrick 718
McKinnell 708
McLearn 670
Mead Johnson 201
Medawar, P.B. 266, 331–332, 559
Medical Hotline 535, 538, 706
Medicare 556
Medlars (National Library of Medicine computer literature search service) 540, 543, 544, 545, 546, 547, 712, 729
Medline (National Library of Medicine computer literature search service) 543, 544
Mehlman 667, 681
Mehta 679
Meier-Ruge 641, 650, 676
Meites, Joseph 196, 634, 641, 662, 671
Mellini 648
Melville, R. 656
Merck Sharp & Dohme 538, 623, 697
Merimee 62, 672, 701
Mesopotamian 268
Metchnikoff, Elie 81, 84, 125, 129, 137, 212, 554
Methuselah 500, 614
Mexico 596, 753
Michelangelo 653
Michigan 104, 145, 561
Mickel 639
Micronetic Laboratories 449
Micropro 723
Mideast 705
Miettinen 695
Milgram, Stanley 719
Miller, Dr. Sanford 571, 690, 718
Milner 633, 682
Miquel 640, 644, 692
Misha 93
Miss Cee 745, 746
Miss Jones 740, 757, 758, 759, 760, 761
MIT. *See* Massachusetts Institute Of Technology
Mitchell 661
Mittermeier 664
Modan, B. 666, 684, 703
Mojave Desert 391

Moloney murine sarcoma virus 421
Moncada, S. 108, 312, 404
Monsanto 113, 509, 636, 689
Montagna 660
Montaigne 385
Montgomery Ward 262, 329, 624, 625, 666, 669
Morehouse, Dr. Lawrence 224–225, 446, 532, 661, 662, 671
Morley 672
Morrison, Jim (The Doors, rock group) 653
Mount Everest 506
Mudd 674, 678
Mukai 682, 689
Mulas, A. 656
Muller 635, 663, 704
Mumma, Dr. Ralph 366
Myers 666, 669, 671, 685, 703
Myers, R.D. 641, 648, 657
Mytilina Brevispina 637

Naka, Ken-Ichi 711, 712
Nanda 639, 648
Nandy, Dr. Kalidas 123, 640, 649, 701
NAS. *See* National Academy Of Science)
NASA (National Aeronautics And Space Administration) 527, 709, 747, 753
Nathanson 650
National Academy of Science (NAS) 644, 709
National Cancer Institute (NCI) 242, 332, 558, 559, 560, 564
National Institute Of Aging (NIA) 42, 551, 555, 557, 558, 559, 560, 661
National Institute Of Mental Health (NIMH) 715
National Institute Of Occupational Safety and Health (NICSH) 561
National Institutes Of Health (NIH) 559, 560, 568, 661, 719
National Library Of Medicine (NLM) 393, 527, 543
National Research Council (NRC) 398, 416, 691, 693
National Security Agency (NSA) 509
Nauss, Dr. 421
Navarro, J.M. 711
Nepalese 653
Nestoros 669
New Jersey 104, 146, 515, 561, 668, 670, 683, 697
New York University (NYU) 299, 348, 354
Newark, New Jersey 104, 146, 515, 516, 561
Newton 526
NIA. *See* National Institute Of Aging
Nicholas, Antoine, Marquis de Condoret 614
Nicholson 632
Nicolas 642
Nicolle, Charles, 490
Nightingale 674, 687
NIH (National Institutes Of Health) 559, 568, 661
Nijinsky, Vaslav 653
NIMH. *See* National Institute of Mental Health
NIOSH. *See* National Institute of Occupational Safety and Health
Nockels, Dr. Cheryl F. 86, 634, 636, 682, 700
Noffsinger 636, 639

Normanskii interferometer 527
Northstar® computer 723
Novi 680, 764
Nugent, Ted 653
Nureyev, Rudolf 509, 515, 653
NYU. *See* New York University

Occam, William of 45
Occam's razor 45
Occupational Safety And Health
    Administration (OSHA) 266, 561, 562
Odens, Dr. Clifford 430, 648, 698
Oeriu 701
Ohio 104, 147, 533, 561
Oi, Dr. Walter 567, 719
Okrent, David 705
Oliveros 642, 649, 670, 677, 701
Oman, G.S. 720
O'Neill 708
O'Neill, Gerard K. 708
Ono 645
Ordy, J. Mark 12, 639, 648
Orwell, George 593
Osborne-1® computer 724
OSHA. *See* Occupational Safety and Health
    Administration
Oz 392, 554, 576, 630

Pan 369
Parker 647, 676, 694
Parkinson's disease 133, 134, 229, 414, 431,
    432, 474, 475, 766
Parratt 638
Passwater, Richard 532, 663, 674, 678, 681,
    687
Pastan 534, 650
Patterson 417
Pauling, Linus, 334, 335, 408, 411, 415, 416,
    418, 464, 531, 536, 633, 634, 656, 663,
    681, 682, 691, 693, 694, 695, 698, 699
Pavlidis 644, 660
Pawluk 645, 646
Pearson, Durk 35, 97, 177, 212, 214, 219,
    229, 230, 231, 232, 267, 271, 304, 367,
    429, 430, 473, 505, 510, 516, 527, 532,
    534, 535, 537, 562, 612, 613, 629, 640,
    641, 650, 653, 654, 658, 663, 664, 670,
    688, 696, 709, 724, 729, 733, 768, 770,
    771, 772, 773, 774, 775, 776, 777, 778,
    782
Pecile 635, 663, 704
Peele 657
Pelletier and Keith study 409, 632, 693
Pelton 700
Peltzman, Dr. Sam 533, 567–568, 578–589,
    594, 691, 704, 706, 716
Peng 631, 709
Pengelley 644
Pennsylvania 104, 146, 268, 561, 638, 673
Perry, M.A. 709
Pert, Candace 293
Peters 670
Peto 695, 702
Petrakis 325, 679
Pfeiffer 641, 643, 650, 699
Pfizer, Inc. 623
Phillips, 657
Philips, Michael 553

Picasso 15
Pietronigro 638, 683
Pike 633, 663
Pilla 645, 646
Pinckney 687, 697
Pinder, Mike 32
Pinocchio 501
Pittsburgh, Pa. 104, 146, 561
Playboy 751
Plotkin 664
Poincaré, Henri 3
Polynesians 99
Pomeroy 656, 721, 765
Pompey 656
Poser, Dr. R. 135
Posner, Richard A. 718
Povlishock 643
Powell 637
President's Commission On Aging 42, 554,
    556
Presley 532
Priestley, Joseph 75
Prinz 652, 661
Prometheus 148
Proxmire Vitamin Bill 400–401
Pryor, William A. 115, 534, 636, 637, 668,
    690
Ptashne, Mark 76
Pure Planet Products 620

Quaife, Arthur 720

Rabelais 284
Radden 633, 683
Rader, Dr. William 672
Ralli 647, 657, 662, 686
Ralston Purina Co. 398
Ranney 636
Ratcliff 554
Rawls 649
Rayleigh, John W.S. 505
Raymond, Stephen 474, 674, 676, 678, 687
Reade 633, 683
Reichel 639, 692
Reichlin 633, 657
Rekers 694, 699
Remington's Pharmaceutical Sciences 537,
    541, 544, 628
Repace, James L. 252, 665, 667, 706
Research Foundation 343
Rettura 684
Rheinwald 644
Rhoads 325
Richardson 648, 681, 702
Richter, Jean Paul 675
Rieley 667
Rigg, Diana 653
Riker 123, 126, 135, 168, 171, 193, 194, 228,
    274, 320, 465, 468, 484, 613, 749
Riley, Vernon 634, 652, 683
Rinfret 720
Rizzino 689
Robbins 659, 674, 676, 678, 699
Roberts 646, 699
Roberts, G.T. 711
Robertson 473, 701
Robinson 629, 644
Roche 407, 462, 611

Rochefoucauld, La 454
Rodale, J.I. 52–53
Rodale, Robert 53
Roehm 636, 668, 692
Roentgen 694, 699
Romania 184
Romano 663
Rorer 237, 422, 623
Rosenfeld, Albert 531
Rosenfeld, Beatrice 302, 304, 756
Rosenthal, Dr. S.R. 343, 685
Ross 675, 677
Ross, Irwin 717
Roth 632
Rotruck 698
Rouser, Dr. George 334, 657
Rubin 670
Rubinstein, Arthur 15
Rubinstein, Helena, 15
Ruspini, E. 711
Russell, Bertrand, 17
Russell, Eric Frank 718
Russia 65, 572

Sachar 652
Sacher 629, 645
Sacks, Oliver W. 133, 650
Sahara Desert 163, 210
Sahley 664
Samis 647
Samorajski 669
Samson 669
Samuelson, Dr. Bengt 304
San Bernardino, Cal. 732
San Francisco, Cal. 104, 147, 348, 515, 533,
    561, 669
Sandoz 111, 124, 127, 128, 133, 136, 139,
    162, 164, 168, 173, 175, 179, 187, 188,
    190, 194, 197, 202, 204, 228, 229, 237,
    257, 272, 273, 275, 276, 281, 288, 304,
    318, 319, 320, 348, 350, 465, 469, 471,
    482, 484, 501, 502, 613, 640, 651, 681,
    702, 707, 766, 798
Sato 689
Saunders Co. 631, 656, 697, 721
Saxe, John Godfrey 63, 64
Schaal Oven Test 380
Schacter, Stanley 249
Schaffner M.R. 711
Scheef, Wolfgang 337
Schellenberg 673
Schetzen, M. 711
Schiefelbein 646
Schild 648
Schmidt, Dr. A. 567
Schneider 640, 701
Schneiderman 674
Schopenhauer, Arthur 259
Schrauzer 663, 666, 671, 682, 685, 698, 703
Schubert 649, 700
Schuckit 670
Schwartz, Dr. Arthur 524, 645, 700
Schwarzenegger, Arnold 226
Schweikert 659
Schwing, Richard C. 27, 630, 706
Scott Tips, Esq. 537, 757
Scripps Institute 721
Seabury Press 653

Sears and Roebuck 624
Seiden, L.S. 641, 648, 652, 657
Seifter 684
Seil 642, 646
Seligman, Martin E.P. 181, 638, 651, 683
Setlow, R.B, 146, 645
Settel 649
Shakespeare 95
Shamberger, Dr. Ray 242, 332, 636, 663, 664,
    682, 683, 690, 693, 698
Shansky 672, 696
Sharrett 679
Shaw, George Bernard 15, 532, 535, 614, 670
Shaw, Sandy 177, 232, 233, 234, 235, 267,
    284, 429, 442, 443, 455, 510, 527, 532,
    535, 537, 612, 613, 629, 650, 651, 655,
    658, 670, 688, 696, 708, 724, 726, 727,
    728, 729, 730, 731, 732, 733, 734, 735,
    736, 738, 739, 764, 770, 771, 774, 775,
    777, 777, 781
Shekelle 665, 684, 703
Sherbourne Press 687
Sherrard 674, 676, 678, 697
Sherwin 637, 690
Shieh, L.S. 711
Shulgin, Alexander 275, 733
Shute, Dr. Wilfred E. 108, 532, 674, 678, 692
Shute Clinic 405
Shiebke 686
Siiteri 656
Simic 638, 690
Simon 708
Simon and Schuster 532, 661, 662, 671
Sincock 637
Sitaram 640, 642, 647, 649, 664
Skoff 683
Slater, Dr. 363, 680, 687
Slavs 285
Slick, Grace, (Jefferson Starship rock group)
    52, 375, 653
Sloan 671, 721, 774
Smith, Dr. Stephen 150, 304, 647, 672, 676,
    694, 697, 720, 737, 737, 740, 741, 742,
    743, 744, 745
Smithells 695, 697
Snipes 657, 681, 701, 702
Social Security 40, 42, 556
Sokoloff 675, 676, 678, 693
Sorensen, R.C. 657
Song 670
Soviet Union 509, 615
Spallholz 634, 666, 671, 672, 681, 685, 699,
    703
Spector 639
Spittle 675, 676, 679, 694
Spitzer 632, 647, 659
Spock, Mr. 392
Sporn 664, 667, 681, 682, 695, 699, 702
Sprince, Dr. Herbert 93, 243, 272, 475, 647,
    663, 664, 668, 670, 676, 677, 679, 694,
    700
Springer Publ. Co. 444, 656, 697
Stanley, Paul (Kiss rock group) 653, 249, 719
Stapleton 534
Stare, Dr. Frederick J. 497, 566
Stastny 646
Stein 641, 469

Stein and Day 657, 659, 721
Steiner 638, 676, 678, 691, 699
Sternlieb, Dr. 325
Stone, Dr. Irwin, 293, 418, 532, 682
Stossel 668
Strauss, Erwin S. 751
Strehler, Bernard L. 65, 115, 461, 629, 646
Streissguth 669
Sumatran 616
Sundaram 692
Sunde 637
Surinam 240, 664
Swanson, Robert A. 662
Swern 636
Swets, John A. 712
Swidler, Gerald 531, 670
Switzerland 112, 134, 256, 479, 536, 651, 700, 708
Syrian 616
Szent-Gyorgyi, Albert 331, 429

Takashima 660
Takeda Inc. 622
Talalay, Dr. Paul 685
Tanzer 635, 658, 670
Taplinger 657
Tappel, Dr. A.L. 121, 403, 404, 636, 637, 668, 673, 678, 679, 691, 692, 698
Tarrant, Dr. 638
Taylor, Dr. E.L. 322
Televideo® 723
Telser, Lester G. 597–580
Temin, Peter 714, 716
Tennov, Dorothy 657, 721
Tera Pharmaceuticals® 298, 348
Thijssen 656
Thomas, Dylan 34
Thomas, E.V. 712
Thompson, 421, 637, 679, 687, 690
Thompson, Sir George 161
Thomson 161
Tibetan 653
Tice Strain 343
Tissuemat® 527
Tietze 657
Toda 660
Toffler 708
Tolmasoff 645
Toto 630
Toussaint, Casserine 77
Treasury Department 255, 275, 563
Tsen 403
Turlapaty 677
Twain, Mark 441
Tyndall, John 120, 370

UCB 168
Underwriters' Laboratories® (UL) 717
Ungar 685, 693
Unimate Puma 527
United States Department of Agriculture (USDA) 308
United States Pharmacopoeia (USP) 420

Vajk 708
Valentino, Rudolf 653
Valley of Ten Thousand Smokes 261

VanDeusen, E.L. 657
Vane 108, 404, 676, 678
Van Rijn, Nicholas 718
Varian Co. 521, 527
Vernon 634, 652, 683
Verrochio 653
Verzar 534, 635, 659, 675
Veterans Administration 557
Vietnam 398
Vilcabamba, Ecuador 65, 615, 632, 721
Viret 639, 690
Virgil 317
Vitamin Research Products 620
Vochitu 701
Volterra 712
Von Mises, Ludwig 15, 718

Wadsworth 631
Walford 634, 672
Wardell 565
Washington, George 268
Watergate 398
Watson, James 44, 232, 505, 550, 633
Wattenburg 681, 683
Wei 643
Weil, Dr. Andrew 47, 631, 733
Weingartner 642, 647, 649
Weir 671, 721, 774
Weiss, Dr. J. M. 182
Weissman 669
Weitzman 668
Weksler 636
West, Mae 652, 653
Wheeler, Dr. Jack 3, 629, 642, 648, 721, 733, 756
Whelan 651, 682
Whipple, Chris 706
White, Dr. James R. 252
Whitehead, Alfred North 153
Wholesale Nutrition Club 390, 621
Wiener, Norbert 511, 522, 709, 711
Wiener analysis, 511, 512, 516, 521, 522, 524, 527, 709
Wiksell 639
Williams Dr. Roger J. 51, 430, 479, 696, 700, 712
Williams, W.J. 712
Wilson, E. Bright 45, 533, 630, 631, 659, 718
Windholtz 538
Winfree 644
Wulff 647
Wurtman, Dr. Richard J. 281, 535, 641, 649, 663
Wyden 553
Wyngaarden 631

Yakush, A. 711
Yalow, Rosalyn 290
Yanofsky 534
Yates, Dr. P.O. 121, 631, 639, 649, 711

Zeiss Axiomat 527
Zeitlin 638
Zierler 676, 679, 698
Ziman 630
Zola, Emile 392

INDEX TO NAMES:
PERSONS, ORGANIZATIONS, AND PLACES

ROMAN NUMERAL PAGE NUMBER SECTION

Adams, K. J. xxxvii
Adelman, Richard C. xxxii
American Heart Association xxxv

Bacall, Aaron xxxiv
Britton, Gary W. xxxii
Brody, H. xxxiii
Brozen, Yale xxxvi

Calbiochem xxxii
Cort, W. M. xxxv
Cranston, Alan xix
Crick, Francis v
Curie, Marie vii

Dean, Sandy xxxv
Demopoulos, Harry B. xix, xxxiv
Donsbach, Kurt xxxiv
Dow Jones and Company xxxiv
Dykstra, Linda A. xxxiii

Eastman xxxv

FDA xxiv
Fels Research Institute xxxiii
Fishscent Music xxxii
Frank, Sanders T. xxxiv
Franklin, Benjamin xxi
Friedman, Milton xxxvi

Gemrod Music xxxii
General Motors xxxi
Gilliland, Alexis xxxiv
Gregory, Roberta xxxvi
Gryglewski, R. J. xxxiii
Gutman xix

Harman, Denham v, xxxiii
Harris, Sidney xxxi, xxxii, xxxiv, xxxv
Hart xxxiii
Houle, Sue xxxi
Hylkema, Randall xxxvii

Japanese xvi
Johnson, Samuel xxvi

Kaufmann, William xxxi, xxxii
Kuschner, Marvin xviii

Landau, Richard xxxvi
Litton xxxiii

Loompanics Unlimited xxxiv
Los Angeles xxv

Maniatis, Tom xxxii
Mann xxxiii
Massachusetts Institute of Technology (MIT)
  xxxiii
Medicare xviii, xix
Medlars xxxvi
Mehlman, M. A. xix
MIT xxi
Monsanto xxxiii

National Institute of Health xviii
New Jersey xix
New York University xxxiv

Ordy, J. Mark xxxiii

Parkinson's disease xxiv
Pearson, Joe xxxii
Pearson, Durk xiii, xxi, xxv, xxxiv, xxxvi, xxxvii
Peltzman, Sam xxxvi
Playboy xxxiv
Ptashne, Mark xxxii

Remington's Pharmaceutical Sciences xxxvi
Robinson, Arthur B. xxxi
Roitt, Ivan xxxiii

Schwartz, Arthur xxxiii
Schweiker, Richard xix
Seiden Lewis S. xxxiii
Semmelweis xvii
Setlow xxxiii
Shaw, Sandy xiii, xxi, xxv, xxxiv, xxxvi, xxxvii
Shea, Ed V. xxxiv
Strehler, Bernard vii

Telser, Lester G. xxxvi
Thomas, Dylan xxxii
Tietze, Christoper xxxiv
Todd, Leonard xxxv
Toussaint, Casserine xxxii

Washington xxxvi
Watson, James v
Worthington Diagnostics xxxvii

Yates xxxiii

SAFETY INDEXES TO:
The Life Extension Companion and Life Extension, a Practical Scientific Approach

The Life Extension Companion

SAFETY INDEX TO:
WARNINGS, CAUTIONS, DANGERS, HAZARDS, AND PRECAUTIONS

IMPORTANT NOTICE:

Do not use any information from our *Life Extension Companion* or our *Life Extension, A Practical Scientific Approach* without first checking the Safety Indexes for both books for the supplement, drug, or action that you plan to take. Also check the Safety Indexes for any illness that you might have and for any drugs that you are now using, since this may influence the safety of your intended actions. It is important that you heed these warnings.

Live Long and Prosper,
Durk Pearson & Sandy Shaw

A

Hazard	A: Excess vitamin A, 8, 87
CAUTION	A: Overdose symptoms of vitamin A, 8, 51, 87
Danger	A: hypervitaminosis (overdose) A, 58
Hazard	Alcohol intoxication, 16
CAUTION	All Cautions, check index for, 299
CAUTION	All Cautions, discussion of index of, xvi
WARNING	All Warnings, check index for, 299
WARNING	All Warnings, discussion of index of, xvi
WARNING	All Warnings, follow appropriate, xiv
WARNING	All Warnings, watch for, xvii
CAUTION	All Cautions, watch for, xvii
WARNING	All substances: See warnings before using substances, 299
WARNING	Antidepressants, monamine oxidase inhibitor type: Don't use phenylalanine or tyrosine with MAO inhibitors, 7, 28, 34, 48, 111, 140
CAUTION	Arginine and ornithine: effect on herpes infection, 53
CAUTION	Asthma: No propranolol in asthma, 103

B

WARNING	B-6: Don't take B-6 in Parkinsonism, 9, 26
WARNING	BHT: Clinical tests required in BHT use, 156
WARNING	BHT: Do not use BHT with liver disease, 156
Hazard	BHT and driving or operating other dangerous equipment: Operating a car on BHT, 157
WARNING	BHT should not be used with sedatives (downers), 156
Precaution	Before using products, 299
Danger	Birth control pills, 158
CAUTION	Blood pressure, high: Tyrosine and phenylalanine and high blood pressure, 7, 28, 33, 48, 111, 140

C

CAUTION	C: Take vitamin C with cysteine to help prevent cystine stones, 9, 13, 24, 27, 53, 78, 81, 82, 99
Hazard	Capsules: Vitamin E in oil filled capsules, xiii, 189
Hazard	Char, combustion: Polynuclear aromatic hydrocarbons, 172

421

WARNING Clinical tests required in BHT use, 156
Danger Clotting: Deep vein clotting, 159
WARNING Cysteine: Diabetics should not use cysteine, 81
CAUTION Cysteine: Take vitamin C with cysteine to help prevent cystine stones, 9, 13, 24, 27, 53, 78, 81, 82, 99
Danger Cystine stones, 82

D

CAUTION D-Penicillamine should be administered by physician, 98
Danger DMSO: FDA says DMSO use may be, 126
Hazard DMSO: Industrial solvent grade DMSO, 65
Danger Deep vein clotting, 159
CAUTION Diabetics: No propranolol for diabetics, 103
WARNING Diabetics should not use cysteine, 82
CAUTION Diapid® is vasopressin: Do not use vasopressin if you have angina, 39, 146
WARNING Don't take B-6 in Parkinsonism, 9, 26
WARNING Don't use if tryptophan excites, 25, 27, 36, 110, 118, 143
WARNING Don't use phenylalanine or tyrosine with MAO inhibitors, 7, 28, 33, 48, 111, 140
WARNING Downers: BHT should not be used with sedatives (downers), 156
Hazard Driving or operating other dangerous equipment: Operating a car on BHT, 157
WARNING Do not use BHT with liver disease, 156
CAUTION Do not use vasopressin if you have angina, 40, 146

E

Hazard E in oil filled capsules, xiii, 189
Hazard Ergot alkoloids with vasocontrictor properties, 209
Hazard Excess vitamin A, 8, 87

F

Danger FDA says DMSO use may be, 126
Hazard Fat, burned: Polynuclear aromatic hydrocarbons, 172
Danger Food without antioxidants, 202
Danger Free radicals, 92, 175, 196, 322, 326, 332
Hazard Free radicals, 25

G

Danger Government safety regulations: Ping pong balls, 168
Hazard Government safety regulations: Accelerated high-dose test, 168, 169, 170

H

Hazard Health food store products, 66
WARNING High blood pressure: Tyrosine and phenylalanine and high blood pressure, 7, 28, 34, 48, 111, 140
WARNING High blood pressure from phenylalanine, tyrosine, and MAO inhibitors, 34
WARNING Hypertension: Tyrosine and phenylalanine and high blood pressure, 7, 28, 34, 48, 111, 140
Danger Hypervitaminosis (overdose) A, 58

J

Hazard Jet lag, 113

K

CAUTION L-Dopa cautions, 300
Precaution L-Dopa, 303
WARNING L-penicillamine is dangerous, 98
WARNING Lecithin probably rancid, 119, 142
WARNING Lecithin warning, 147
WARNING Liver disease: Do not use BHT with liver disease, 156

M

WARNING MAO inhibitors: Don't use phenylalanine or tyrosine with MAO inhibitors, 7, 28, 34, 48, 111, 140
WARNING Monamine oxidase inhibitors: Don't use phenylalanine or tyrosine with MAO inhibitors, 7, 28, 34, 48, 111, 140
Danger Myth of natural versus synthetic substance, xii

N

Danger Night environment, 121
CAUTION Non-scientific applications, xiv

CAUTION   Non-scientific health care, xiii
Hazard   Noradrenaline is norepinephrine: Low levels of norepinephrine, 6
Hazard   Norepinephrine: Low levels of norepinephrine, 6
Hazard   Nucleic acid analog, 151
Hazard   NE is norepinephrine: Low levels of norepinephrine, 6
CAUTION   No propranolol for diabetics, 103
CAUTION   No propranolol in asthma, 103

O

Hazard   Oil filled capsules: Vitamin E in oil filled capsules, xiii, 189
CAUTION   Ornithine and arginine: effect on herpes infection, 53
CAUTION   Overdose symptoms of vitamine A, 8, 51, 87
Hazard   Overwork: Long grueling hours of work, 17
Danger   Oxygen, water, 171

P

WARNING   PABA counteracts sulfa, 27
Danger   PAH carcinogens, 172
WARNING   Parkinsonism: Don't take B-6 in Parkinsonism, 9, 26–27
Hazard   Peroxidized lipids: Vitamin E in oil filled capsules, xiii, 189
WARNING   Phenylalanine: Don't use phenylalanine or tyrosine with MAO inhibitors, 7, 28, 34, 48, 111, 140
CAUTION   Phenylalanine and tyrosine and high blood pressure, 7, 28, 33, 48, 111, 140
Danger   Pollutants, 94
Hazard   Polynuclear aromatic hydrocarbons, 172
Danger   Power: risks of coal or water vs. nuclear, 172
Precaution   Products: Before using products, 299
Hazard   Products: Health food store products, 66
CAUTION   Products: Read before using suppliers' products, 299

R

Hazard   Rancid oil: Vitamin E in oil filled capsules, xiii, 189
Danger   Rancid oil: Vitamin E in oil filled capsules, xiii, 189
CAUTION   Read before using suppliers' products, 299

S

WARNING   Sedatives: BHT should not be used with sedatives (downers), 157
WARNING   See warnings before using substances, 299
Precaution   Side effects, 33
Hazard   Stress, 26
Danger   Sulfoxide free radical, 128
WARNING   Sulfa drugs: PABA counteracts sulfa, 27
CAUTION   Suppliers' products: Read before using suppliers' products, 299

T

CAUTION   Take vitamin C with cysteine to help prevent cystine stones, 9, 13, 24, 27, 53–54, 78, 81, 99–100
Hazard   Tars, combustion: Polynuclea aromatic hydrocarbons, 172
WARNING   Tryptophan: Don't use if tryptophan excites, 25, 27–28, 36, 110, 118, 143
WARNING   Tyrosine: Don't use phenylalanine or tyrosine with MAO inhibitors, 7, 28, 34, 48, 111, 140
CAUTION   Tyrosine and phenylalanine and high blood pressure, 7, 28, 34, 48, 111, 140

V

CAUTION   Vasopressin: Do not use vasopressin if you have angina, 40, 146
Hazard   Vitamin A: Excess vitamin A, 8, 87
Danger   Vitamin A: hypervitaminosis (overdose) A, 58
CAUTION   Vitamin A: Overdose symptoms of vitamin A, 8, 51, 87
WARNING   Vitamin B-6: Don't take B-6 in Parkinsonism, 9, 26
CAUTION   Vitamin C: Take vitamin C with cysteine to help prevent cystine stones, 9, 13, 24, 27, 53–54, 78, 81, 99–100
Hazard   Vitamin E in oil filled capsules, xiii, 189

W

WARNING   Warnings, check index for, 299
WARNING   Warnings, discussion of index of, xvi
WARNING   Warnings, follow appropriate, xiv
Danger   Water, oxygen, 171

SAFETY INDEX TO:
WARNINGS, CAUTIONS, DANGERS, HAZARDS, AND PRECAUTIONS

IMPORTANT NOTICE:

Do not use any information from our *Life Extension Companion* or our *Life Extension, A Practical Scientific Approach* without first checking the Safety Indexes for both books for the supplement, drug, or action that you plan to take. Also check the Safety Indexes for any illness that you might have and for any drugs that you are now using, since this may influence the safety of your intended actions. It is important that you heed these warnings.

Live Long and Prosper,
Durk Pearson & Sandy Shaw

DISCLAIMERS:
Principles for reasonable use of the book:
IMPORTANT—READ BEFORE USE OF ANY INFORMATION FROM THE BOOK!, xiii–xxiv, 246, 281, 485
Suppliers' products: read before use, 618

A

Precaution	A vitamin, proper dosage importance, 93
CAUTION	A vitamin: high dosages can foster development of some cancers, 87; overdose symptoms, 420–21, 756
Danger	Acetaldehyde, 270
WARNING	Acetylcholine precursors (choline, lecithin, Deaner®): do not take in depressive phase of manic-depressive psychosis, 187
CAUTION	Acidic vitamins: un-neutralized megadoses can have harmful effects, such as gastric acidity, hemorrhoids, ulcers, xxiv, 244, 246–47, 249, 281, 415, 426, 436, 462, 488–89, 755–56; use caution if ulcers develop, xxiv, 426
WARNING	Add only one new supplement at a time, 432
Danger	Aflatoxin, 383, 384
Hazard	Aging, smoking, and the birth control pill all increase requirements for B-6 and C, deficiency may cause abnormal blood clots, 202
Hazard	Alcohol, tobacco, 564
Hazard	Alcohol, 267, 274
CAUTION	Alcohol: BHT and tranquilizers enhance effects of, do not use together, 206, 282, 751–52; with antihistamines can depress nervous system, 282; phenothiazines are additive with, 283
WARNING	Alcohol: and barbiturate interaction, often deadly when used together, 193, 206–207, 571; and drug interactions, 281–283; do not drink during pregnancy and FAS (Fetal Alcohol Syndrome) risk, 277; BHT with alcohol interferes with rate of liver alcohol clearance, do not use together, 751–52
CAUTION	Allergic reactions to vitamin tablet fillers and binders, 305–06, 462, 485
CAUTION	Allergic reactions: to RNA injections, 170
CAUTION	Alpha tocopherol: vitamin E in vegetable oil containing capsules might be rancid, 407, 462, 492

CAUTION | Anemia: might be cause of several disorders, see physician, 165, 168, 207
WARNING | Angina pectoris: vasopressin (Diapid®) use may cause pain, do not use, 174, 204–05, 229
CAUTION | Antibiotics: use care in self-treatment with, 350
CAUTION | Antihistamines: with alcohol depress nervous system, 282
CAUTION | Antioxidants: as only part of cancer treatment, surgery and radiation necessary, 351
WARNING | Antioxidants taken during radiation therapy (including large doses of antioxidant nutrients) can interfere with radiation therapy, Sandy's case history should not serve as model, 728, 730
CAUTION | Arginine and other growth hormone (GH) releasers: coarsening of skin, joint diameter increase, larynx growth, voice pitch lowering due to larynx growth; all can be caused by excess GH release, 236, 342, 477
CAUTION | Arginine: may increase schizophrenia symptoms, 640, 661–62
Precaution | Ascorbic acid, high doses and hemorrhoids, 755
CAUTION | Atherosclerosis: may develop with B-6 deficiency and high-protein diet, 291, 313
WARNING | Atherosclerotic disorders: physician's treatment necessary, 316

B

CAUTION | B-1, C, cysteine: use of, 281
CAUTION | B-1 vitamin with C, cysteine combination, and diabetes mellitus, 246, 373, 467, 482; megadoses and blood sugar test results, 415–16, 442–43, 520; dosages and neutralization of, 246, 435, 462; possible scurvy symptoms if suddenly discontinued, 416, 470
CAUTION | B-2: antioxidant supplements needed with high doses to prevent photosensitization, 764
CAUTION | B-5. See Calcium pantothenate.
WARNING | B-6 supplements should not be used with L-Dopa in treatment of Parkinson's disease, xxiv, 134, 431–32, 474–75
Danger | Bacteria, virus, cancer cells, 83, 85
Hazard | Barbiturates, 571
WARNING | Barbiturates: alcohol interaction, 193; withdrawal and physician care necessary, 193–94; BHT with barbiturates and/or alcohol interfers with rate of liver barbiturate and/or alcohol clearance, do not use together, 206, 751–52
CAUTION | Barbiturates: interaction with BHT, do not use together, 206
CAUTION | BHT: enhances effects of alcohol and barbiturates, do not use together, 206; experimental use for herpes virus, 753
WARNING | BHT: with alcohol interferes with rate of liver alcohol clearance, do not use together, 751–52
CAUTION | Binders: allergic ractions to vitamin tablet fillers and binders, 305–06, 462, 485
Hazard | Birth control pills: aging, smoking, and the pill all increase requirements for B-6 and C, deficiency may cause abnormal blood clots, 202
Danger | Birth control pills: dangers of use are widely exaggerated, 202
CAUTION | Blood pressure changes: vasopressin when naturally released in severe injuries or with large intravenous doses, 484; vitamin E and heart disease patients, 328, 406; phenylalanine and tyrosine, 172, 185–86, 251
Danger | Blood pressure: increases with phenylpropanolamine, 289
CAUTION | Blood sugar tests: C vitamin megadose effects on, 415–16, 443, 520
Hazard | Blood transfusions, 524
WARNING | Brain damage: and physician's treatment, 316
CAUTION | Bromocriptine: doses over 30 milligrams can have adverse effects on schizophrenics, 640
WARNING | Bromocriptine: postmenopausal women may restart menstrual cycle with use, 136, 139, 197, 471
Danger | Bureau of Narcotics and Dangerous Drugs is dangerous to everyone, 715

C

CAUTION | C, B-1, cysteine: use of, 281
CAUTION | C vitamin: with B-1, cysteine combination, and diabetes mellitus, 246, 373, 467, 482; megadoses and blood sugar test results, 415–16, 442–43, 520; dosages and neutralization of, 246, 435, 462; possible scurvy symptoms when suddenly discontinued, 416, 470
WARNING | C vitamin: in cancer treatment, surgery and radiation necessary, 341; children's need for, 358, 686
CAUTION | Calcium pantothenate (B-5): dosage caution, 187, 246, 390
CAUTION | Cancer treatment: antioxidants are only part of cancer treatment, surgery and radiation necessary, 341
WARNING | Cancer treatment: antioxidants taken during radiation therapy (including large doses of antioxidant nutrients) can interfere with radiation therapy, Sandy's case history should not serve as model, 728, 730
WARNING | Cancer treatment: Sandy's should not serve as model, 730
WARNING | Cancer: large antioxidant dosage experimental, 341, 728; excessive A vitamin dosage and, 87; need for professional care, xxiv, 341
CAUTION | Cancer: high doses of vitamin A and development of, 87
Danger | Carbon monoxide and nitrogen oxides, 244
Danger | Carcinogenic coal combustion products, 705
CAUTION | Case histories: how to properly use, not complete, self-diagnosis danger, individual choice of supplements, nonendorsement, physician must be consulted, 725–26
WARNING | Children: immunizations of sick or vitamin-deficient child and SIDS, 358, 360, 686; life extension nutrient program are for, xxiv, 431, 468, 611
WARNING | Choline should not be used with manic-depressive psychosis, 187
CAUTION | Choline: intestinal bacteria and fishy smell side effect, 164
Hazard | Cigarettes, 256
WARNING | Circulation: poor leg circulation needs professional treatment, 316
CAUTION | Circulation: cold extremities and thyroid function, 767
WARNING | Clinical lab tests: authors' life extension formula and, 611; experimental nutrient program and, xxiv, 166, 430, 442, 458, 462, 463, 467
CAUTION | Clinical laboratory tests: regularity and importance of, xiii–xxiv, 166, 430, 458, 462, 466
Precaution | Computer systems, buying of, 724
CAUTION | Cysteine, with vitamins B-1, C combination, and diabetes mellitus, 246, 373, 467, 482; megadoses and blood sugar test results, 415–16, 442–43, 520; dosages and neutralization of, 246, 435, 462; possible scurvy symptoms if suddenly discontinued, 416, 470
CAUTION | Cysteine, B-1, C: use of, 281
CAUTION | Cysteine: proper dosage, 93, 217, 247, 280, 469, 482; and diabetics, 246, 373, 467, 482

425

WARNING	Cysteine: can block the effects of insulin, 482
CAUTION	Cysteine: can cause cystine urinary bladder or kidney stone formation, 217, 247, 482
CAUTION	Cystine: bladder/kidney stone formation, 217, 247, 482

D

Danger	Danger: Keeping eyes open for, 14
Hazard	Delaney Amendment can be hazardous to your health, 570
CAUTION	Depression information: not offered as substitute for professional help, 182
CAUTION	Diabetes mellitus: cysteine blocking of insulin effects, 246, 373, 467, 482; physician's care important, 373, 467, 671; mistaken symptoms, 165, 168, 207, 212; use of B-1, C, and cysteine, 467
Danger	Diabetics: How to reduce chances of developing cardiovascular disease and blindness, 373; use of niacin, 425
WARNING	Diabetics: cysteine can block the effects of insulin, 482
Precaution	Dimethyl sulfoxide, antioxidant supplements required, 348–49, 760
Hazard	Dimethyl sulfoxide impurities, 349
Danger	Dinitrochlorobenzene or dinitrochlorophenol, 218
WARNING	Disclaimers: principles for reasonable use of book, 485
Hazard	Diseases, 595
Precaution	DMSO, antioxidant supplements required, 348–49, 760
Hazard	DMSO impurities, 349
Precaution	Dosages: how to reduce, 436, 470
Precaution	Drug interactions: purchase *Clinical Guide to Undesirable Drug Interactions and Interferences*, see page 444

E

CAUTION	E vitamin: in vegetable oil containing capsules and rancidity, 347, 407, 462, 492; read before taking, 406
WARNING	Exercise: do not attempt peak-output program without professional guidance, 225

F

WARNING	FDA regulation: *opt-out* warning, 591
WARNING	FDA regulation: "This drug has not been FDA approved," 592
Danger	FDA's "You can get all the nutrients you need with a knife and fork" claim, 392
CAUTION	Females: side effects if systemic testosterone is used to excess, 197
CAUTION	Fillers: allergic reactions to vitamin tablet fillers and binders, 305–06, 462, 485
Danger	Food preservatives: their elimination from many foods can lead to growth of carcinogen and ultratoxin producing microorganisms, 376
Hazard	Foods without additives can be a major health hazard, 383
Danger	Free radical chain initiators, 368
Danger	Free radicals, 271, 273, 280, 348

G

CAUTION	Glucose tolerance tests: vitamin C megadoses and test results, 415–416, 442–43, 520
Precaution	Gout susceptibility, and uric acid test to be taken before using RNA, 169–70, 430, 435, 466, 473
CAUTION	Gout: do not use RNA supplements, 169–70, 429–30, 435, 466, 473
Precaution	Government grants a two edged sword, 558
CAUTION	Growth hormone (GH) releasers: coarsening of skin, joint diameter increase, larynx growth, voice pitch lowering due to larynx growth; all can be caused by excess GH release, 236, 342, 477
Precaution	Growth hormone (GH) releasers: If you use GH releasers you should get a jeweler's ring size set to monitor finger joint diameter, 765
CAUTION	Growth hormone (GH): excess release and consequences, 236, 342–43, 477–78, 774; schizophrenics should not use GH releasers, 640, 661–62.

H

CAUTION	Hair loss: physical checkup to determine cause, 212
WARNING	Hangovers: do not use BHT with alcohol, 751–52
CAUTION	Heart disease: gradual increase in vitamin E dosage, 328; physician's treatment necessary, xxiv, 328; sodium restrictions, xxiv, 294
WARNING	Heart attacks: physician's care necessary, 316
WARNING	Heart disease: E vitamin dosage, 328; and peak output exercise program, 225; physician's treatment necessary, xxiv, 328; sodium restrictions, xxiv, 294
Danger	Herpes: FDA approved treatments, 479
CAUTION	High blood pressure patients: use of baking soda, 244, 249, 345, 415, 426, 436, 462, 488; and kidney disease, 191–92; phenylalanine use in 136, 172, 186, 251, 288–89, 736; sodium restrictions, xxiv, 293–94; sodium-free vitamins, 619; tyrosine use in, 186
WARNING	High blood pressure: do not take phenylalanine or tyrosine with MAO inhibitors, 172, 184, 186, 204; use tyrosine and especially phenylalanine with great caution and only under a physicians very close supervision with very frequent self measurement of blood pressure, 136
Danger	High-energy radiation, 100
CAUTION	High-fat diet: experimental, 368

CAUTION	High-protein diet: B-6 supplements needed to avoid atherosclerosis, 291, 313
Danger	Home, yours, far more dangerous than almost any workplace, 562
Hazard	Homocysteine, a metabolite of methionine, 313
Precaution	Hydergine®, 320
Precaution	Hydergine® side effects with large amount of caffeine or theophylline, 178, 188, 276
CAUTION	Hydergine®: contraindication for use with acute or chronic psychosis, 257
Danger	Hydroxyl free radicals, 101
CAUTION	Hyperbaric oxygen: use of, 119

I

WARNING	Immunizations: vitamin-deficient children vulnerable to SIDS, 358, 686; index to, 510
CAUTION	Immunizations: smallpox, may cause acceleration of growth of pre-existing tumor, 730
CAUTION	Insomnia: consult with physician for cause, 189
Precaution	Insulin requirement calculated by home computer program, 675, 689
WARNING	Insulin: cysteine can block the effects of insulin, 482

J

CAUTION	Joint diameter increase with excess GH (growth hormone) release, 236, 342, 477

K

CAUTION	Kidney disease: cysteine must be taken with vitamin C to prevent cystine stones, 217, 247, 482; and high blood pressure, 191–92; RNA supplements and, 169–70, 466; and sodium use, xxiv; damage to from high doses of thiol compounds, 87
WARNING	Kidney disease: do not take author's experimental life extension formula, 611; physician's treatment necessary, xxiv, 316
CAUTION	Kidneys: proper cysteine/vitamin C ratio is necessary to avoid development of cystine stones even in normal kidneys, 217, 247, 482

L

Precaution	L-Dopa, side effects, 192
Precaution	L-Dopa, excess dosage, 127, 134
CAUTION	L-Dopa: antioxidants needed with, 133, 202, 237, 481; may increase schizophrenic symptoms, 640, 661–62
WARNING	L-Dopa: in treatment of Parkinsonism, do not use B-6 supplements with, xxiv, 134, 431, 474; high doses may cause preexistent melanoma growth, 127, 341, 481
CAUTION	L-penicillamine: lethal nature of, 299
CAUTION	Laryngeal spasm: vigorous "snorting" of Diapid® may cause, 174
CAUTION	Larynx growth with excess GH (growth hormone) release, 236, 342, 477
Danger	Lead compound pigment painted buildings, 261
Hazard	Lead paint chips: eating, 261
Danger	Lead water pipes, 261
Hazard	Lead: in gasoline, hazard often exaggerated, 263
WARNING	Legs, poor circulation in and need for physician's treatment, 316
Danger	Liberty: government safety regulatory agency danger to liberty, 717
CAUTION	Librium®: will enhance alcohol effect, do not use together, 282
CAUTION	Life extension drugs: read before taking, 7
Precaution	Life extension formulas, how to start, 463
WARNING	Life extension nutrient program: do not use authors' dosage levels, 462–63; authors experimental formula must *not* be used by children, pregnant women, persons with kidney/liver damage, 611; clinical lab tests monitored by research-oriented physician necessary, xxiv, 166, 430, 442, 458, 462, 467; personal responsibility for, xxiii, 725–26
CAUTION	Life extension nutrient program: older people and altered drug tolerance, 430–31
WARNING	Liver damage: do not take authors' experimental life extension formula, 611
Precaution	Low-sodium diets and baking soda, 244, 247, 249, 345, 415, 426, 436, 462, 488

M

CAUTION	Male impotence: for cause, consult physician, 207
WARNING	Manic-depressive psychosis: do not take acetylcholine precursors in depressive phase, 187; professional psychiatric treatment necessary, 182
WARNING	MAO inhibitors: do not use when taking phenylalanine and/or tyrosine, 172, 184
WARNING	Melanoma, pigmented malignant, use nutritional restraint, and PKU-type diet, without L-Dopa, phenylalanine and tyrosine, 341–42, 481
WARNING	Melanoma, pre-existing: L-Dopa, phenylalanine, tyrosine should not be used, 127, 136, 481
WARNING	Menopausal women: bromocriptine (Parlodel®) may reinstitute menstrual cycle, 136, 139–40, 471
CAUTION	Menopause: with estrogenic stimulation, annual Pap smear necessary, 200
CAUTION	Metrazol®: danger of, 168
Danger	Microorganisms, 82
Danger	Molds and bacteria in foods can produce carcinogens and ultra-toxins, 382
WARNING	Monamine oxidase inhibitors: do not use when taking phenylalanine and/or tyrosine, 172, 184
Danger	Motorcycle helmet: not using, 574

N

Precaution	Niacin, gradual increase of dosage, 247, 249, 283, 426, 435
Precaution	Niacin acidity must be neutralized, 243, 247, 249, 426, 435–36, 487–88

427

CAUTION	Niacin: dosage should be gradually increased and taken with full stomach, acidity should be neutralized, 247, 249, 283, 426
Danger	Nitrosamine carcinogens: formation of, 410

O

CAUTION	Obesity: with heart disease or high blood pressure, consult physician, 294: sodium restriction, 294
Danger	Obesity, cancer, and cardiovascular disease, 249
WARNING	*opt-out* warning, 591
CAUTION	Oral anticoagulants: and alcohol interaction, do not use together, 283
CAUTION	Ornithine and other growth hormone (GH) releasers: coarsening of skin, joint diameter increase, larynx growth, voice pitch lowering due to larynx growth; all can be caused by excess GH release, 236, 342, 477
CAUTION	Ornithine: may increase schizophrenic symptoms, 640, 661–62
Danger	Oxidants, 425
Hazard	Oxidation products, 338

P

Precaution	PABA, discontinue use when taking sulfa drugs, 248, 469, 474
Precaution	PABA, neutralization of acidity, 435–36
Precaution	Papaya, raw, can cause sore mouth and lips, 99, 237
CAUTION	Papaya: do not eat raw with ulcer, 99, 237
Precaution	Para-aminobenzoic acid, discontinue use when taking sulfa drugs, 248, 469, 474
CAUTION	Paraquat-contaminated cannabis: mutagenic and fibrotic cross-linker health hazard, 242–43
Hazard	Paraquat: a free radical poison, on cannabis, 243
WARNING	Parkinson's disease: antioxidants should be taken with L-Dopa, 133; B-6 supplements should *not* be taken with L-Dopa, xxiv, 134, 431–32, 474–75
CAUTION	Parlodel® (bromocriptine): doses over 30 milligrams can have adverse effects on schizophrenics, 640
WARNING	Parlodel® (bromocriptine): postmenopausal women may restart menstrual cycle with use, 136, 139, 197, 471
WARNING	Parotid cancer treatment: Sandy's should not serve as model for similar cancers, 730
Precaution	Phenylalanine, high dosage side effects, 136, 185–86
WARNING	Phenylalanine and high blood pressure: do not take phenylalanine with MAO (monamaine oxidase) inhibitors, 172, 184, 186, 204; use phenylalanine with great caution and only under a physicians very close supervision with very frequent self measurement of blood pressure, 136
WARNING	Phenylalanine: do not take with PKU, 136, 252, 289, 341–42; do not use with MAO (monamine oxidase) inhibitors, 172, 184; do not use with pre-existing melanoma, 127, 136, 341–42, 481
CAUTION	Phenylalanine: elevation of blood pressure side effect, 136, 172, 185–86, 251; with high blood pressure extreme caution in dosage, very close supervision of physician, and very frequent self blood pressure measurement 136, 172, 185–86, 204, 251, 288–89, 736; chronic high dosage toxicity not studied, 252; 736; overdose symptoms, 172, 185–86
WARNING	Phenylketonuria (PKU): do not use phenylalanine, 136, 341–42, 481
CAUTION	Phenylpropanolamine: can cause high blood pressure, 289; NE (norepinephrine) depletion side effect, 498
CAUTION	Physicians: consultation needed for serious illness, xxiv, 168, 189, 321, 328, 341, 373, 440, 467, 671, 675, 689, 767; medical records and lab tests results sent to, xxiv, 430, 437, 611; consult to determine causes of sexual decline and hair loss, 207, 212
WARNING	Physicians: anecdotal reports no substitute for, 726; required for barbiturate withdrawal, 194; life extension experimental program MUST be monitored by 189, 321, 328, 341, 440, 467, 611; need for treatment in serious illness, xxiv, 168, 189, 316, 321, 328, 341, 373, 440, 467, 671, 675, 689, 767
Precaution	Pineapple, raw, can cause sore mouth and lips, 99, 237
CAUTION	Pineapple: do not eat raw with ulcer, 99, 237
Hazard	Polyunsaturated fat, 265
Danger	Polyunsaturated fats: substituting for saturated fats can be dangerous, 363
WARNING	Pregnancy: drinking of alcohol during and FAS risk, 277; do *NOT* follow life extension experimental program if pregnant, xxiv, 431, 468, 611
DISCLAIMER	Principles for reasonable use of the book, READ BEFORE USE OF ANY INFORMATION FROM THE BOOK!, xxiii-xxiv, 246, 281, 485
Precaution	Procaine as a mild MAO inhibitor and monamines, 184
DISCLAIMER	Products, suppliers', read before use, 618
CAUTION	Products: nutritional, purchase of, advertised in magazines, 495
Precaution	Protein-rich diet requires B-6 suppplements, 291, 313
WARNING	Psychosis: professional treatment necessary, 182. (See also Manic-depressive psychosis.)
CAUTION	Psychosis: Hydergine®contraindication for use, 257
CAUTION	Purchase of nutritional products: advertised in magazines, 495

R

Hazard	Radiation released by coal-burning power plants is more hazardous than that released by nuclear power plants, 264, 705
WARNING	Radiation therapy and the thymus gland: protection for in radiation therapy, 342, 728
CAUTION	Radiation therapy cancer treatment: antioxidants (including large doses of antioxidant nutrients) can interfere with radiation therapy, Sandy's case history should not serve as model, 728, 730
Danger	Radioactive heavy metals, 264
Hazard	Rancid fats and oils: eating, 378, 386
Danger	Random damage, 67
WARNING	Regulation, FDA: "This drug has not been FDA approved," 592

WARNING	Regulation, FDA: *opt-out* warning, 591
CAUTION	RNA supplements: due to danger of gout, take serum uric acid test first, 169–70, 430, 435, 466, 473
CAUTION	RNA: allergic reactions to RNA injections, 170

S

Hazard	Sandy's cancer case history, do not use as a model, 370
CAUTION	Schizophrenia: symptoms may worsen with GH releasers such as arginine, ornithine, Parlodel® (bromocriptine), 640, 661–62
CAUTION	Selenium: proper dosage and symptoms of toxicity, 93, 472
Danger	Self-diagnosis, 296
CAUTION	Self-diagnosis: danger, 168, 189, 302, 725
CAUTION	Self-experimentation: be very careful, physician supervision necessary, 725
Hazard	Side effects of nutrients, 246, 281
Danger	Singlet oxygen, 260, 423
CAUTION	Skin: coarsening of with excess GH (growth hormone) release, 236, 342, 477
CAUTION	Sleeplessness: consult physician for causes, 189
CAUTION	Smokers: with diabetes, and physician's treatment, 246; with ulcers, and acidic vitamins, 258; with high blood pressure and acidic vitamins, 244; nutrient supplements dosage procedure, 246, 258
Hazard	Smoking, 239, 242
Hazard	Smoking, drinking, and other lifestyle hazards: keep records of, 459
CAUTION	Sodium containing preparations: and heart disease, high blood pressure, and kidney disease, xxiv, 294
Precaution	Starting out with a life extension formula, 463
CAUTION	Stroke: physician must review nutrient use, 321
CAUTION	Strychnine: danger of, 168
Hazard	Sugar: eating large quantities, 370, 371, 595
Precaution	Sulfa drugs, discontinue use of PABA (para-aminobenzoic acid) when taking sulfa drugs, 248, 469, 474
Hazard	Sulfoxide free radical, 298
WARNING	Supplement: add only one new one at a time, 432
DISCLAIMER	Suppliers' products, read before use, 618

T

CAUTION	Tablets: allergic reactions to vitamin tablet fillers and binders, 305–06, 462, 485
CAUTION	Thiol compounds: and kidney damage, 87
WARNING	"This drug has not been FDA approved," 592
WARNING	Thymus gland: protection for in radiation therapy, 342, 728
CAUTION	Thyroid function: and cold extremities, 767
Hazard	Tobacco smoke: involuntary exposure to may cause cancer, 253
Precaution	Tranquilizers and interaction with alcohol, do not use together, 282
Precaution	Tryptophan, side effects, 135, 179–80
CAUTION	Tumors, pre-existing: possible increase in rate of growth from smallpox vaccinations, 730
WARNING	Tyrosine and high blood pressure: do not take tyrosine with MAO inhibitors, 172, 184, 186, 204; use tyrosine with caution and only under a physicians close supervision with very frequent self measurement of blood pressure, 136
WARNING	Tyrosine: do not use with MAO inhibitors, 172, 184, 186; do not use with pre-existing melanoma, 127, 341–42, 481
CAUTION	Tyrosine: gradual increase in dosage, 186

U

CAUTION	Ulcers: megadose of niacin and neutralization, 426, 487; raw papaya and pineapple caution, 99, 237; smokers with, and acidic vitamins, especially niacin and ascorbic acid, 258
CAUTION	Urinary bladder: proper cysteine/vitamin C vitamin ratio to avoid development of cystine stones, 217, 247, 482

V

CAUTION	Valium®: will enhance alcohol effect, do not use together, 282
Hazard	Varying the dose of prescription drugs, 435
Precaution	Vasopressin, 321
CAUTION	Vasopressin (Diapid®): angina pectoris patients may experience pain, do not use, 174, 204, 229, 469
Danger	Vegetable oils, 379
Precaution	Vitamin tablet fillers and binders can cause allergic reactions, 305, 462, 485
Precaution	Vitamin A, proper dosage importance, 93
CAUTION	Vitamin B-1, C, cysteine: use of, 281
CAUTION	Vitamin B-1, with C, cysteine combination, and diabetus mellitus, 246, 373, 467, 482; megadoses and blood sugar test results, 415–16, 442–43, 520; dosages and neutralization of, 246, 435, 462; possible scurvy symptoms if suddenly discontinued, 416, 470
CAUTION	Vitamin B-5. See Calcium pantothenate.
WARNING	Vitamin B-6 supplements should not be used with L-Dopa in treatment of Parkinson's disease, xxiv, 134, 431–32, 474–75
CAUTION	Vitamin C, with B-1, cysteine combination, and diabetes mellitus, 246, 373, 467, 482; megadoses and blood sugar test results, 415–16, 442–43, 520; dosages and neutralization of, 246, 435, 462; possible scurvy symptoms if suddenly discontinued, 416, 470
CAUTION	Vitamin C, B-1, cysteine: use of, 281

WARNING   Vitamin C: in cancer treatment, surgery and radiation necessary, 341; children's need for, 358, 686
CAUTION   Vitamin tablet fillers and binders: allergic reactions, 305–306, 462, 485, 619
CAUTION   Vitamin tablets: allergic reactions to vitamin tablet fillers and binders, 305–06, 462, 485
CAUTION   Voice pitch lowering due to larynx growth with excess GH release, 236, 342, 477

                                        W

DANGER   Water, 706
Hazard   Withdrawal from alcohol, 277

                                        X

Hazard   X-rays, 793